The Life and Work of Judith S. Kestenberg

In this volume, Janka Kormos offers a comprehensive historical and theoretical analysis of the life and work of Judith S. Kestenberg, exploring her pioneering contributions to the somatic foundations of psychic development.

The volume traces Kestenberg's journey as a Polish-Jewish émigré in New York's psychoanalytic circles, illuminating her psychodynamic theory of movement and method of movement analysis within postwar American mental health sciences. Kormos presents Kestenberg as a nonconformist, an innovative and eclectic thinker who gravitated towards the unknown and unspoken, highlighting the somatic precursors of psychic development and the kinaesthetic imprints of transgenerational trauma. Through Kestenberg's work, the book explores questions of disciplinary positioning, transdisciplinarity and the evolving relationship between the arts and psychological practice throughout the 20th century. It also contributes to our understanding of postwar American psychological sciences, within which the study of bodily movement became increasingly central.

QR codes throughout the volume offer readers exclusive access to archival material compiled by Kormos. Previously unavailable to the public, these documents reveal intimate details of Kestenberg's life and work and will be invaluable to graduate students and researchers in psychoanalytic studies, body-oriented psychotherapy, dance/movement therapy and the history of psychology. *The Life and Work of Judith S. Kestenberg* is a vital resource for scholars in the history of psychological sciences, psychoanalysts, arts and dance therapy practitioners, and trainees seeking insight into somatic approaches to trauma and the integration of embodied practices within therapeutic frameworks.

Janka Kormos is a Marie Skłodowska-Curie Postdoctoral Fellow at the University of Cyprus, and a scholar of movement studies and embodied practices in the history of the psychological and medical sciences. Kormos led the creation of the Kestenberg Papers, a stand-alone archival collection housed in the Manuscript Division of the Library of Congress.

"This fascinating book is the result of rigorous, long-term research into the work of a largely forgotten innovator in the fields of psychoanalysis, child development, movement and trauma studies. It presents not only a long-awaited intellectual biography of Judith Kestenberg, but also places her work into a historical and scientific context that helps the reader to both understand and evaluate it. Kestenberg's psychoanalytic account of movement development and somatisation will be of great value to anyone interested in the role of the body in psychoanalysis, but also to psychologists, somatic therapists, historians, women's-history and gender studies scholars. Kormos' work also provides essential links between two parts of Kestenberg's work that are rarely viewed as a continuum: her studies of body movement and her pioneering work with child survivors of the Holocaust. A truly interdisciplinary, enjoyable and accessible read."

Ana Tomčić, *PhD, is a Postdoctoral Researcher in History at the Department of Psychoanalysis and Psychosocial Studies at the University of Essex (UK), where she is involved in the research of early free and low-cost psychoanalytic clinics in the UK and Central Europe*

"This wonderful book offers a rigorous examination of Judith Kestenberg's intellectual legacy, tracing her trajectory from Tarnów to Vienna to New York. It synthesises her diverse professional pursuits to highlight central themes of embodiment, social justice, and communal responsibility. By situating Kestenberg's work within shifting sociopolitical, cultural, and religious frameworks, Kormos clarifies her engagement with and contributions to broader psychoanalytic traditions, further contextualising her among other often-marginalised foremothers, including Hug-Hellmuth, Spielrein, Deutsch, Benedek, and Mahler. This volume is an essential resource for scholars of psychoanalysis, psychiatry, dance/movement therapy, Jewish women's history, and comparative genocide studies."

Klara Naszkowska, *PhD, is an Adjunct Professor of Gender, Sexuality, and Women's Studies at Montclair State University (New Jersey, USA), Founding Director of the International Association for Spielrein Studies, and editor of the 2025 Gradiva award-winning volume,* Early Women Psychoanalysts: History, Biography, and Contemporary Relevance (Routledge)

"This book offers a rigorous, in-depth intellectual biography of a pioneering twentieth-century psychoanalyst. Through her research into child development, body movement and child survivors of the Holocaust, Judith Kestenberg developed a body of knowledge whose relevance and richness have yet to be fully recognised. An essential reading for anyone interested in the field."

Fátima Caropreso, *PhD, is a Full Professor in the Department of Psychology at the Federal University of Juiz de Fora (Brazil) and Visiting Fellow in the Department of Psychosocial and Psychoanalytic Studies at the University of Essex (UK)*

"Janka Kormos's intellectual biography of Judith Kestenberg is an enjoyable and engaging read for anyone interested in the lesser-known life and oeuvre of this Polish-Jewish psychoanalyst émigré to the United States. Between the 1940s and the 1970s, Kestenberg forged a distinctive career in the male-dominated worlds of American psychiatry and psychoanalysis. The author skillfully shows how Kestenberg's original contributions - her somatic approach to psychoanalysis, her developmental movement therapy, and her research into the psychosocial effects of the Holocaust - were interwoven and shaped by her experience and perspective, with the body at their centre. The book will be especially relevant to psychotherapists with a somatic orientation, as well as to readers interested in the history of psychoanalysis in this period. In tracing Kestenberg's life and work, it also opens onto a wide range of issues that remain pressing in contemporary psychology and psychotherapy."

Agnes Szokolszky, *PhD, is a Docent at the University of Szeged (Hungary) and a researcher in the history of psychology, embodiment, and ecological approaches*

"Janka Kormos's book presents Judith Kestenberg's life and work with remarkable breadth and sensitivity, examining her contributions through personal, professional, social, cultural, and critical lenses. The result is a richly layered scholarly portrait balancing curiosity with critical rigour, capturing the scope and originality of Kestenberg's career. This volume is a significant contribution to the field and a fitting tribute to the exceptional richness of Kestenberg's oeuvre."

Katalin Vermes, *PhD, is an Associate Professor of Philosophy at Eszterházy Károly Catholic University (Hungary), Course Leader of the Movement and Dance Therapy Postgraduate Training at Eötvös Loránd University (Hungary), and a researcher in the phenomenology of the body*

The Life and Work of Judith S. Kestenberg

The Body on Trial

Janka Kormos

Routledge
Taylor & Francis Group
LONDON AND NEW YORK

Designed cover image: Designed by Janka Kormos. Images courtesy of Child Development Research, comprising K. Mark Sossin's private collection.

First published 2027
by Routledge
4 Park Square, Milton Park, Abingdon, Oxon OX14 4RN

and by Routledge
605 Third Avenue, New York, NY 10158

Routledge is an imprint of the Taylor & Francis Group, an informa business

British Library Cataloguing-in-Publication Data
A catalogue record for this book is available from the British Library

ISBN: 978-1-032-90823-6 (hbk)
ISBN: 978-1-032-90198-5 (pbk)
ISBN: 978-1-003-55995-5 (ebk)

DOI: 10.4324/9781003559955

Typeset in Times New Roman
by Taylor & Francis Books

To my beloved grandparents:
Zsuzsanna Mindszenty and Károly Tulipán

Contents

Illustrations

Figures

Table

Data Availability Statement

A large portion of the data that support the findings of the research was derived from the following resources available in the medical, psychoanalytic, and institutional archives in the public domain: Kestenberg's training documents can be accessed from the University of Vienna Archive, the Freud Museum London, and the A. A. Brill Library and Archive of the New York Psychoanalytic Society. Professional connections and correspondence were found in Paul Schilder's papers in the Brooklyn College Library; the papers of Anna Freud, Berta Bornstein, Edith Jacobson, and Marianne Kris in the Manuscript Division of the Library of Congress; Margaret Mahler's papers in the Beinecke Rare Books and Manuscript Library at Yale University; and the Martha Davis and Irmgard Bartenieff collections in the Michelle Smith Performing Arts Library of the Clarice Smith Performing Arts Center at the University of Maryland. Information on her clinical appointments was obtained from the Oskar Diethelm Library of the DeWitt Wallace Institute of Psychiatry at Weill Cornell Medicine, the Archives of Mount Sinai Hospital, and the Archives of the New York Academy of Medicine. Newly discovered material that the book draws upon can be consulted in the Kestenberg Papers, Manuscript Division, Library of Congress, Washington, DC, United States. Data supporting the findings of this study are primarily available in the book and its supplementary material in the online curated archive accessible via a QR code provided in the Introduction of this book. Additional data from unpublished oral history interviews are available from the corresponding author upon reasonable request.

Disclaimer

In case of any disruptions of the QR codes, readers can access the curated archive via this link as well: https://drive.google.com/drive/folders/1ApJddr_KGr9jbUGknsXEba_NCfPvCKNJ?usp=drive_link

Acknowledgements

An earlier version of this manuscript was submitted as a doctoral dissertation at the University of Pécs, Hungary. As a first-generation scholar, I want to emphasise that neither this book nor my dissertation is a personal accomplishment; both are collective achievements. Neither would have been possible without a state education system, and without the devoted teachers, mentors, colleagues, family, and friends who offered guidance, opened doors, and sustained me with encouragement – support that not only allowed me to take paths that diverged from the family background but also inspired me to carve out space for myself and my thoughts in the world. This is an enormous privilege, one that is not available to most. For me, this book is proof that collective support and mutual aid really can break social barriers. Along the way, I was carried by many forms of generosity – from accommodation to intellectual space, inspiration, and freely shared knowledge – and I take it as my responsibility to pass on the access and support I've been given.

While working on this book, I was helped, supported, and encouraged by many people. My academic advisor, Katalin Szili, offered me guidance and support throughout the process. I am grateful to Melanie Johnson French for her continuous encouragement and for sharing her expertise in the Kestenberg Movement Profile. This project is greatly indebted to the Hungarian Fulbright Foundation, whose grant enabled the extensive archival study in the USA that became the backbone of this book. I'm deeply grateful to Susan Loman, K. Mark Sossin, Silvia Birklein, and Martha Davis for their generosity in sharing their knowledge, expertise, memories, and networks, without which this book could not have been completed. Special acknowledgement is due to Janet Kestenberg Amighi, who kindly hosted me at her home for days as I searched through boxes of her mother's life's work. I also thank my generous hosts – Klara Naszkowska, Ann-Aliki Antoniou, Ines and Thom Hilde, and Arnold Lopez – who opened their homes to me while I was on my research visits in the USA. I'm grateful to Joshua Levy at the Library of Congress for welcoming the Kestenberg Papers into the collection of the Manuscript Division. I'm thankful to Liesbeth Manders and Sherry Goodill for connecting me with experts and for supporting me with grant applications, and Miriam Gassner for her assistance in translating German letters. Heartfelt thanks go to Klara Naszkowska for the inspiring discussions about our shared interest in Kestenberg and to Hedda Lausberg for sharing her personal library on movement behaviour research with me.

I also appreciate the editors and peer reviewers at *Imagó Budapest, Lélekelemzés, Replika, Journal for the History of the Behavioural Sciences,* and *Psychoanalysis and History* who helped me refine my ideas and publish my work. I am thankful to the Hungarian Association for Movement and Dance Therapy and the European Society for the History of the Human Sciences for supporting the development of my ideas during their conferences. I am indebted to the History of Science Society for their scholarship, which enabled me to participate in their summer school programme and receive expert advice on research in the history of science. Special thanks to Gerardo Con Diaz for sharing his professional network and facilitating the presentation of my work at the University of California, Davis. Heartfelt appreciation goes to my teachers and fellow PhD candidates in the Theoretical Psychoanalysis Doctoral Program – especially Kiss Kata Dóra – for their guidance throughout the years.

Finally, my deepest gratitude goes to my family and friends, whose ceaseless support sustained me in completing this book. My mother, Zsuzsanna Tulipán, with her sharp intellect and insatiable thirst for knowledge, inspired my love of learning from the very beginning. László Százados, through his devotion and hard work, showed me what dedication to one's craft looks like. My father, Ferenc Kormos, with his innovative spirit, gave me the confidence to think independently. I am also immensely grateful to Bean, who has been a source of inspiration and my firmest support during this work. I'm also thankful to Anna Kormos, Elena Botts, Júlia Hadi, András Juhász, Olívia Reschoffsky, Marc Andrews, and Mariana Waligora for their friendship, care, and encouragement throughout the years. Last, I want to thank my grandparents, Mindszenty Zsuzsanna and Károly Tulipán, to whom I dedicate this book. They lived long and memorable lives, and they passed away before I could place this book in their hands. They raised seven children and worked tirelessly, laying the foundations that later made it possible for me to pursue my interests. My grandmother's unconditional love, kindness, wisdom, and perseverance continue to inspire me every day. My grandfather, who spent his life as a manual labourer, believed in me, and this fills me with pride. Without them, none of this would have been possible. As they did not speak English, I write this to them in Hungarian: *Köszönök mindent drága Nagyi és Nagypapa!*

Introduction

On 23 February 1971, at the 565th meeting of the New York Psychoanalytic Society, Judith S. Kestenberg presented, for the first time, her psychodynamic theory of movement, "Development of the Young Child as Expressed Through Bodily Movement I." At the symposium, Margaret Mahler (1971, p. 1) remarked that "Dr Kestenberg's research has placed psychoanalytic observation in a truly new key." She predicted that her "alphabet and grammar will be learned" and that "her interpretations of the kind of body language [...] will become a source for enriched understanding of psychoanalytic theory and practice" (p. 15). Mahler's forecast proved overly optimistic. Kestenberg's psychodynamic vocabulary of movement and her developmental assessment method remained largely unreflected within psychoanalysis. In the 1970s, Kestenberg shifted her focus to a new research direction. Collaborating with her husband, Milton Kestenberg, and several mental health professionals, she led one of the largest international research projects on the psychohistorical study of the Nazi Holocaust. Kestenberg's work received a selective reception. Disciplinary alliances and ambitions within American psychological sciences contributed to the fragmentation of her legacy along the lines of her two principal projects. Her movement studies became influential in the emerging field of dance/movement therapy, whereas psychoanalysis acknowledged her Holocaust research.

The pages that follow present an intellectual biography of Judith Silberpfennig Kestenberg (1910–1999), a Polish-Jewish émigré psychiatrist who arrived in the United States a few years before the outbreak of the Second World War. Kestenberg's life reflects the specific challenges that Eastern European Jewish women psychoanalysts faced in the early twentieth century, including forced migration, loss of family and social connections, language barriers, and financial precarity. Her oeuvre also illustrates the intellectual potential of the inside-outsider position, which enabled her to attend to underexplored topics and bring fresh perspectives to the largely male-dominated fields of American psychiatry and psychoanalysis.

Kestenberg's work is most often encountered through her two seemingly disparate projects: her developmental movement studies and psychohistorical

DOI: 10.4324/9781003559955-1

research on the effects of the Nazi Holocaust. Rather than treating these as complete dislocations of interest, this book takes their apparent disjunction as a point of entry. It asks what personal and professional experiences shaped her enduring investment in bodily movement, and whether and how they were woven into her later psychohistorical studies. I foreground a somatic orientation as the interpretive lens for reading Kestenberg's work and argue that her attention to the body provides the connective tissue across her life-work. Kestenberg brought the body 'to trial' not only conceptually but also literally. For her, the body both testified and acted. It offered a path towards personal and collective development and an instrument to process the traumas of the twentieth century.

If the reader permits a brief personal note, I first encountered Kestenberg's work during my graduate training in dance/movement therapy. With a background in contemporary dance and the social sciences, and a long-standing interest in how movement research and choreographic exploration might contribute to psychosocial support, I was initially drawn to a set of questions. What does psychology want from dance? How does it imagine the moving body, and how does it conceptualise movement as evidence? As my training progressed, a more reflective question was added. What might dance and dancers seek from psychology? Learning about the Kestenberg Movement Profile left me intrigued and apprehensive. It offered a theoretically anchored account of movement development, but it also felt too confident in assigning meaning to movement for someone like me coming from postmodern traditions of dance. Kestenberg's aspiration to look for the mind in movement and the body in mind drew me in further. It resonated with my experiential understanding that movement and dance are modes of thinking. This book is shaped by this encounter.

Reading her work revealed further depth and specificity, as well as tensions and unresolved questions. As a psychiatrist and psychoanalyst, she sought to bridge a significant gap by crafting a language for the moving body in her field. Her psychodynamic theory of movement remains the only comprehensive, structured framework in psychoanalysis that places bodily movement at its centre. I sensed the endurance Kestenberg brought to this quest in the sheer attention and effort required to take in the density of her texts, as she tried to translate lived movement experience into written language. I have come to regard Kestenberg's theory as a uniquely detailed approach within the depth psychology of movement, offering concepts that may inform not only clinical contexts but also artistic practice, philosophical inquiry, and cultural analysis. At the same time, understanding the intellectual underpinnings and the socio-political conditions in which the method emerged is essential not only for recognising its limitations but also for identifying the cultural and political implications, and the potentially harmful dimensions, that accompany any system that claims interpretive authority over bodies. This book aims to stimulate further study of the specific clinical, cultural, and historical visions of the moving body, which may be especially relevant in the context of the growing attention paid to bodily processes in contemporary psychoanalytic practice and infant mental health.

The principal orientation of this book is historical, and history is applied at several registers.[1] First, history is used as a goal: uncovering the narrative of Kestenberg's life-work is the argument itself. The winding roads she took, from Poland to Vienna to New York, from a wealthy family background to forced emigration and financial hardship at the outbreak of the Second World War, from neurology to psychoanalysis to developmental movement studies, and from the murder of her parents to psychohistorical studies on the Nazi Holocaust, seemed to call for a connecting lens. I attempt this integration while honouring the dislocations, complexities, and imperfect circles one walks in a lifetime. Despite Kestenberg's contributions to psychoanalysis, developmental study, child guidance, dance/movement therapy, and psychohistory, no comprehensive research has traced the evolution of her concepts or examined the significance of the bodily dimension within her work. This book seeks to fill that gap by restoring Kestenberg's legacy to the historical memory of American psychological sciences.

My objective, however, is not only to place her contributions firmly in the historical record but also to draw on her work to deepen contemporary understanding of professional belonging, evidence hierarchies, and disciplinary boundaries in mid- to late-twentieth-century American psychological sciences. I approach these questions through two closely related concerns: what her career reveals about broader mid-century trends, and what it shows about the place of movement studies within the Cold War context of American psy-sciences. To do so, I use history as a tool to challenge the assumption that disciplinary memory reliably tracks the significance of a legacy or an idea. Through a reception study, I trace the processes, disciplinary ambitions, and conceptual and methodological alliances that contributed to the overall uneven reception of Kestenberg's work and the selective reception of her developmental movement studies. In this sense, the book offers a case study of how specific theories and theorists become overlooked by their own fields in their own time. This case study also shows how scientific objects and evidence are constructed, and how disciplines negotiate boundaries of legitimacy and demarcation in a given historical moment. In this same register, I also map links between Cold War psy-science discourses and the study of movement behaviour in the United States. Finally, the reception history also serves as a kind of laboratory for testing psychoanalysis's apparent concern with the bodily in psychic life.

This history-of-science perspective underscores the importance of studying psychological theories and methodologies within their socio-political contexts, illuminating how they reflect broader narratives of health and well-being and carry concomitant cultural and political implications. Kestenberg's work exemplifies the centrality of direct infant observation and developmental assessment to efforts to legitimise psychoanalysis within American psychiatry, and it also illustrates the shift towards community-based approaches and prophylactic psychiatry in the 1960s. Her formulations on the meaning of bodily movement and its significance for individual and societal well-being clarify the place of movement studies in Cold War psy-science discourses. Finally, her psychohistorical studies on the effects of the Nazi Holocaust reflect main currents in the growing Holocaust awareness of the 1980s, when personal narratives increasingly became tools of personal and political transformation. The book also makes a present-day intervention: it identifies resonances between Kestenberg's somatic ideas and contemporary theories of embodiment in infant mental health and psychological sciences, offering a guide to their conceptual lineages.

Several questions guided this study: what intellectual milieu did Kestenberg's theory of movement development and method of movement analysis emerge from, and what conceptual and historical influences shaped her thinking? What does a synoptic view of her life and work contribute to our understanding of the development of her ideas? How did shifts in theorising, methodology, and scientific orientation in mid-century American psy-sciences shape the reception of her movement studies? How did the close alliance between American dance/movement therapy and the Kestenberg Movement Profile emerge? How might a survey of her oeuvre contribute to our understanding of the twentieth-century history of American psychological sciences?

As my interest is primarily historical, my theoretical analysis draws upon Kestenberg's original publications. I also trace the afterlives of her ideas, showing that her concepts remain relevant in current research and clinical practice. However, I do not seek to evaluate their present-day accuracy, efficacy, or theoretical adequacy or to assess later revisions introduced by Kestenberg's followers. I take the sustained professional uptake across fields as an indicator that her concepts remain 'alive' and continue to address unresolved questions or fulfil needs that other frameworks do not fully meet. Readers interested in the ongoing developments of the Kestenberg Movement Profile and its broader adaptation are referred to the two volumes of *The Meaning of Movement* (Kestenberg Amighi et al., 1999, 2018).

This book is written for an interdisciplinary academic readership spanning the histories of the psy-sciences, psychoanalysis, infant mental health and development, dance/movement therapy, and trauma and Holocaust studies. It assumes a basic familiarity with foundational psychoanalytic concepts. At the same time, I aim to make the argument accessible across disciplines by introducing specialised terms and debates as they first arise, with additional information provided in the footnotes. Because Kestenberg's movement-based work encompasses theory, method, and empirical observation, I use a consistent set of terms throughout the book to distinguish between them. Developmental movement theory refers to her overarching model of how movement expresses and shapes psychological development; psychodynamic vocabulary of movement refers to the language she used to describe movement behaviour; infant observation studies refers to the longitudinal, direct observation research on which her formulations were built; and Movement Profile refers to her structured assessment procedure that translates coded movement observations into quantitative indicators, visualised as plotted graphs to support clinical and developmental interpretation. When I refer to her movement-related work as a whole, I use the term movement studies as shorthand for this constellation of concepts.

The content of this book is enriched by five oral history interviews with individuals who worked closely with Kestenberg or in the broader field of movement behaviour research: Janet Kestenberg Amighi (Kestenberg's daughter and close collaborator), Mark Sossin, Susan Loman, Silvia Birklein, and Martha Davis. These conversations make room for firsthand recollections and reflections from those who knew her and participated in the professional worlds this study reconstructs. In addition, the book draws extensively on never-before-seen documents I discovered during research visits to private collections held by Kestenberg's family members and former collaborators, namely Janet Kestenberg Amighi, Mark Sossin, Helene Bass-Wichelhaus, and Eva Fogelman. The first phase of this archival research was completed in 2022 under a PhD fellowship supported by the Hungarian Fulbright Foundation; a second phase followed over several months in 2025. As a result of this work, I assembled a stand-alone archival collection, the *Judith Kestenberg Papers*, now housed in the Manuscript Division of the Library of Congress (United States). The collection comprises more than 20,000 items spanning Kestenberg's life and work. It includes family correspondence from 1937–1940 documenting the tragic circumstances of her final exchanges with her parents before their deaths. It also contains Kestenberg's observational notes from her developmental movement studies; newsletters and administrative records from the Child Development Research; staff notes, parent journals, and proceedings from the Center for Parents and Children; original 8-mm film reels used to annotate movement; unpublished manuscripts; and artwork and poetry created by survivors of the Nazi Holocaust. It is my hope that the *Kestenberg Papers* will serve as a lasting resource for historians of the psy-sciences and medicine, mental health professionals, and students. I am especially pleased that Kestenberg's archive now sits within the Library of Congress's distinguished holdings alongside the papers of Sigmund and Anna Freud, Carl Rogers, Arnold Gesell, and many others. This book is accompanied by access to a curated online archive (accessible via QR codes located at the end of the Introduction), where readers can consult selected documents, some of which are now part of the *Kestenberg Papers*.

I wish to emphasise that this book represents the first comprehensive historical and theoretical study of Kestenberg's life and work. Given the breadth of her legacy, there remains a significant opportunity for further in-depth research. I encourage those interested in any aspect of her oeuvre to pursue this invitation, thereby contributing new perspectives to the scholarly record.

Structure of the Book

The book moves from biography and conceptual reconstruction to a reception history and disciplinary contextualisation, before taking an outlook on the contemporary afterlives of Kestenberg's concepts and concluding with an integrated reading of her oeuvre.

Chapter 1 reconstructs Judith Silberpfennig Kestenberg's life from her childhood in Poland to her final home in New York. It situates her upbringing, education, emigration, marriage, and professional formation, providing the biographical and institutional context for the detailed analyses that follow. The chapter draws on archival sources from medical, psychoanalytic, and university collections, as well as papers held in private collections.

Chapter 2 offers a theoretical analysis of Kestenberg's work, centring on her developmental movement studies that emerged between the 1940s and the mid-1970s. It situates her ideas within contemporaneous psychoanalytic discourses and traces the intellectual lineages, debates, and key figures that shaped her conceptual development, moving from psychoanalytic debates on female sexual development to psychoanalytic studies of movement to pioneering traditions of direct infant observation, before presenting Kestenberg's own formulations. Organised as a thematic chronology, the chapter follows the evolution of her core questions about bodily sensation, movement, personality development, and transgenerational trauma. The discussion moves from her early work on the libidinisation of internal organs to her first longitudinal infant observation studies (begun in 1953) and then traces the consolidation of her psychodynamic theory of movement across her key publications in the 1960s. The chapter then presents the culmination of these ideas in her movement-based developmental assessment framework, the Kestenberg Movement Profile, together with her principles of movement observation and notation. It also examines her application of movement theory in practice through child guidance and family support at her community project, the Center for Parents and Children. Finally, it introduces a later phase of conceptual expansion, as Kestenberg and her collaborators reworked earlier formulations from the late 1970s through the 1990s, placing greater emphasis on mutuality and object-relatedness and developing ideas concerning fetal movement patterns. The chapter concludes by introducing her psychohistorical Holocaust studies, highlighting their scope and orientation, her main trauma concepts, and the somatic emphasis that continued and extended her earlier concerns.

Chapter 3 compares the reception of Kestenberg's developmental movement studies across psychoanalysis, creative arts therapies, and movement behaviour research and contrasts this with the reception of her Holocaust studies in a concise format. It shows how her movement-focused work remained largely unreflected within psychoanalysis, while her Holocaust research gained greater recognition, and how her movement concepts found resonance in dance/movement therapy and, to a lesser extent, in movement behaviour research.

Chapter 4 examines theoretical alliances, disciplinary boundaries, and methodological shifts in postwar American psy-sciences to account for the selective reception traced in Chapter Three. It first offers a focused history of psychoanalysis and psychoanalytic psychiatry in the United States, with attention to shifts in theorising and methodology from the 1950s to the 1970s. It then turns to specific developments within American psychiatry in the mid-1960s before widening the frame to the broader socio-political context and the relationship between the trends of movement behaviour research and Cold War psy-science discourses.

Chapter 5 briefly traces the afterlives of Kestenberg's body–mind and transgenerational trauma concepts, showing how her ideas continue to circulate in research and clinical practice. By identifying tentative resonances between Kestenbergian formulations and contemporary approaches to embodiment in infant mental health and related fields, it positions aspects of her work as possible conceptual antecedents to these approaches.

Chapter 6 offers an integrated account of Kestenberg's life and work, tracing continuities and dislocations across her oeuvre and identifying recurring themes throughout her life. It focuses on the links between her personal circumstances and the professional choices that shaped the trajectory of her work.

The curated archive can be accessed by scanning the QR code, which directs the reader to the archive's main folder. Further information on the exact location of individual documents within the online archive is provided in the endnotes throughout the book.

Please refer to the reader's guide for instructions on using the online archive, which can be accessed by scanning this QR code:

Note

1 I am indebted to Professor Gerardo Con Diaz for the formulation of history operating at different registers, presented in his masterclass at the Interdisciplinary Summer School, organised by the History of Science Society, held at the Science History Institute, Philadelphia, USA, 1 July 2023.

References

Mahler, M.S. (1971). Discussion of Judith S. Kestenberg: Development of the young child expressed through bodily movement I. 565th Meeting Proceedings, New York Psychoanalytic Association and Society Meeting Notes, A. A. Brill Library, Archives and Special Collections.

Kestenberg-Amighi, J., Loman, S., Lewis, P., & Sossin, K.M. (Eds.). (1999). *The meaning of movement: Developmental and clinical perspectives of the Kestenberg Movement Profile.* Gordon & Breach.

Kestenberg-Amighi, J., Loman, S., & Sossin, K.M. (Eds.) (2018). *The meaning of movement: Embodied developmental, clinical and cultural perspectives of the Kestenberg Movement Profile* (2nd ed.). Routledge.

Chapter 1

Life Between Worlds

Roots and Early Influences

On 17 March 1910, Judyta Hadasa Silberpfennig (known to her friends and family as Ida or Iduś) was born in Krakow, as the third and youngest child of an Orthodox Jewish family. Her brother, Henry (1905–1961), was 5½, and her sister, Henda (later Helen Silving, 1906–1996), was 4 years older than her (Naszkowska, 2023). Judith was fond of her siblings. In her autobiographical essay she expressed that Henda remained a lifelong role model whom she admired for her intelligence and independence. She remembered her brother as an adventurous, fun-loving person from whom she inherited her sense of humour and laughter (Kestenberg, 1992).

Judith was born with cervical kyphosis (a forwards curvature of the neck often causing pain) and dorsal scoliosis (a sideways curve in the spine often associated with muscle strain and issues with breathing). This condition shaped her childhood, with daily rituals of lying strapped in a corrective brace. Judith recalled the physical discomfort this caused, as well as the comfort of her mother sitting with her and reading stories (Kestenberg, 1992, p. 151). Her posture remained a persistent concern throughout childhood, and she was enrolled in gymnastics classes alongside her brother. Judith recalled the pleasure of movement and physical freedom. Her fondness for gymnastics and physical movement endured throughout her life (Kestenberg, 1992).

Both her mother, Sara Salomea Silberpfennig (maiden name Bauminger, 1883/1884/1887–1941), and her father, Yeshayahu Silberpfennig (called Szaje, also Chaim, Jesaia Kaim, 1883/1884/1886–1941), came from wealthy Jewish families (Naszkowska, 2023). They made their home in Tarnów, a multicultural Galician town (now in Poland) with a large Jewish population (Naszkowska, 2023). The Silberpfenning family was affluent and well connected, living in one of Tarnów's most beautiful townhouses furnished with works of art (Silving, 1988, p. 36). They employed several household helpers and home tutors for their children (Kestenberg, 1992; Naszkowska, 2023). They also observed Jewish customs. Sara wore a half-wig, and the

DOI: 10.4324/9781003559955-2

family kept kosher and celebrated religious holidays. Sara appears in her daughters' recollections as a vibrant and deeply intellectual woman (Kestenberg, 1992; Silving, 1988). According to Henda, she spoke six languages, enjoyed Hebrew poetry, played the piano, and secretly attended courses at the University of Krakow, before women were permitted to enrol (Silving, 1988, p. 19). Later, she also audited political science courses at the University of Vienna while her son, Henry, studied there (Naszkowska, 2023). Sara "refused to be identified as a housewife" (Silving, 1988, p. 75). Judith also remembered her as an intellectually curious, psychologically gifted woman with an unending love for children. During the First World War, Sara visited an orphanage and took Judith with her, where they played with the children (Kestenberg, 1992, p. 157). Judith believed that her mother had dreamed of becoming a doctor, but, as women were not yet allowed to study medicine, she could never fulfil her intellectual ambitions. This may have strengthened her determination to support her children's further education (Kestenberg, 1992).

Judith's father, Szaje Silberpfennig, was an entrepreneur who accumulated great wealth through his investments. He owned a car and frequently took the family on lavish vacations (Naszkowska, 2023). He was a radiant, kind-hearted, and socially engaged person who was a prominent member of the Jewish community (Silving, 1988, p. 5). A committed socialist and generous philanthropist, he established an orphanage for toddlers in Tarnów after the First World War (Kestenberg, 1992, p. 157). Szaje was an authority figure to Judith, whom she greatly trusted, though she also recalled moments of disappointment. Owing to his business endeavours, Szaje was often absent from the family home, which took a toll on the family (Kestenberg, 1992, p. 160). Judith recalled that, perhaps strengthened by a young daughter's admiration for her father, she seemed to be the only one certain that he would return. During the First World War, Judith, her siblings, and her mother moved to Austria for several years. She recounted difficult memories of not knowing where her father was, sensing her mother's anxiety over their financial instability, experiences of xenophobia and anti-Semitism, and a pervasive sense of not belonging (Kestenberg, 1992, pp. 159–165).

In keeping with Orthodox Jewish customs, Judith was initially educated at home by private tutors. Her early studies focused on Hebrew reading and writing, as well as on Jewish religion and culture. As she later wrote, "The Bible was my elementary book, the source of my knowledge, what was allowed and what was not" (Kestenberg, 1992, p. 162; all quotations from this source are my own translation). She recalled her Hebrew teacher, Mr K., as an empowering educator who encouraged her to seek her own path to God and highlighted the cultural and social aspects of Judaism. Judith attended synagogue with enthusiasm, appreciating both the singing and the strong sense of community she found there (Kestenberg, 1992, p. 160). She was also fond of her Polish tutor, Miss Taubeles, who inspired her ongoing passion for learning. Judith was educated at home until the second grade of high school. After the war, when her family returned to Poland, Judith was enrolled in a private girls' gymnasium that offered a college-preparatory education. Naszkowska (2023, p. 201) noted that there were no public high schools for girls in Galicia at the time. In the interwar period, as anti-Semitism intensified in the Second Polish Republic, Judith recalled experiencing discrimination from a teacher at the school (Kestenberg, 1992, p. 165). During this period, the family's finances stabilised. Her father purchased a holiday home in Hinterbrühl, Austria, where the family spent many summers. In the early 1920s, however, a series of unfortunate investment decisions resulted in significant financial losses, ultimately forcing the sale of the holiday home (Kestenberg, 1992, p. 165).

From Poland to Vienna

In 1923, Judith's brother, Henry, graduated from high school and planned to study political science in Vienna. Sara and Henry relocated to Vienna, and, a year later, Henda and Judith joined them. Judith attended a private high school in Ottakring,[1] which was directed by Ludo Moritz Hartmann, a distinguished social democrat and historian and the father of Heinz Hartmann (1894–1970), who later became a prominent psychoanalyst. Here, Judith found new friendships and role models. She later attributed the origins of her world-view to these formative years, which reinforced her enduring commitment to socialist ideals and community welfare (Kestenberg, 1992, p. 165). Around this time, she experienced her first love with Walter, who introduced her to Freud's work, which she did not take to at first. As she explained, "My resistance to psychiatry and psychoanalysis was linked to my idea that a man must be flawless and heroic and not allowed to complain" (Kestenberg, 1992, p. 167).

Medical Training

Nevertheless, perhaps influenced by Walter, who also studied medicine, Judith enrolled at the University of Vienna Medical School in 1928. Her decision was also driven by concerns about her family's financial instability and by her desire to support them (Kestenberg, 1992). As a Polish citizen, she was initially required to pay higher tuition fees, which she could not afford. Determined to study, Judith boldly negotiated a tuition reduction. She first pursued a specialisation in neurology,[2] later changing to psychiatry to better meet practising requirements in Vienna (Transcript of Records, 1929–1933; Naszkowska, 2023, p. 202). As she neared the end of her studies, Vienna's political climate, once defined by strong Social Democratic leadership, had deteriorated and, by 1934, had given way to fascism. Judith once again found herself grappling with issues of belonging and mourned the loss of her "Red Vienna" (Kestenberg, 1992, p. 169).

She completed her final examinations in the summer of 1933 and graduated on 8 June 1934 (Transcript of Records, 1929–1933). In her final year, she published her first paper, based on work at the Neurological Institute under Professor Marburg, on pseudotabes[3] (Silberpfennig, 1933). Looking back, she recalled her specific interest in explaining patients' symptoms solely on the basis of the histological findings. She wanted to know whether alterations in the nervous systems could be inferred from changes in the patient's external behaviour (Kestenberg, 1992, p. 169). Judith went on to intern at the university's Neurology and Psychiatry Clinic (Nervenklinik). There, while working with patients with brain injuries, she returned to Freud's writings with renewed interest. "I started working in the psychiatric ward and slowly began to become acquainted with Freud for the second time. I soon saw the connection between body, brain, and psyche" (Kestenberg, 1992, p. 170). She worked with patients with aphasia who were confined to the psychiatric ward, which allowed her to continue pursuing her neurological interest within psychiatry.

It was at the Nervenklinik that she met Margaret Schoenberger (later Mahler, 1897–1985), who was a senior resident. Mahler taught Judith the Rorschach personality test, which they applied to assess people with brain injuries. They published their study in 1938, which, according to Judith, was the first psychoanalytically oriented paper for both of them (Silberpfennig & Mahler-Schoenberger, 1938; Kestenberg, 1992, p. 172). Between 1933 and 1941, Judith published a number of neurological studies, some under the name Ida Silberpfennig and others under Judith Silberpfennig (Silberpfennig, 1933, 1936a, 1936b, 1938, 1939, 1941a, 1941b; Silberpfennig & Urban, 1937a, 1937b; Silberpfennig & Mahler-Schoenberger, 1938; Silberpfennig & Birkmayer, 1938). These studies, examining the links between perception, cognition, and bodily movement, laid the foundation for her interest in the relationship between psychic functioning and bodily movement (Kestenberg, n.d.a, 1975a).

During this period, Max Schur[4] (1897–1969), who was involved with Judith's friend at the time, informed her that she exhibited symptoms of neurosis and recommended that she pursue treatment. Judith recalled: "That was too much for me. I did not want to be a patient" (Kestenberg, 1992, p. 170). Perhaps as a result of this encounter and her renewed interest in Freud, she applied to train at the Vienna Psychoanalytic Society in 1934. She was interviewed by the two Polish-speaking analysts, Ludwig Jekels (1887–1954) and Helene Deutsch (1884–1982) (Kestenberg, 1992, p. 170). She started her training analysis in February 1935 with Eduard Hitschmann (1871–1957), who saw her for 22 months until June 1937 (Hitschmann, 1941; WPV/01/228, 1937; WPV/01/230, 1937). In the autumn of 1936, she began her theoretical training and attended courses with Heinz Hartmann, Otto Isakover (1899–1972), Edward (1894–1959) and Greta Bibring (1899–1977), Paul Federn (1871–1950), and August Aichhorn (1878–1949) (Kestenberg, 1941). A note of 25 June 1937 from the Education Committee of the Viennese Psychoanalytic Society, reporting Hitschmann's evaluation, stated that, at the beginning of her training, Judith showed some 'syndromes' which were considered typical for that stage; thus, she was deemed fit to advance to practical training under supervision (WPV/01/230, 1937). As fascism spread across Europe, Judith's professional future became increasingly uncertain. In both Poland and Vienna, *numerus clausus* policies would have limited her ability to practise. As a Jewish woman, a socialist, and a psychoanalyst, she was in grave danger (Naszkowska, 2023, p. 204). Driven by necessity and her aspiration to collaborate with the psychoanalytic infant researcher Margaret Fries (1896–1987) in New York, she set out to emigrate to the United States (Naszkowska, 2023; Kestenberg, 1991).

From Vienna to New York

Judith's former neurology professor, Hans Hoff (1897–1969), facilitated her introduction to Paul Schilder (1886–1940), the director of the Child and Adult Psychiatry Department in Bellevue Hospital in New York, who invited her for a professional internship[5] (WPV/01/228, 1937). Hubert Urban (1904–1997), her former colleague at the *Nervenklinik*, helped her to secure an affidavit for her American visa application through a personal connection (Kestenberg, 1992). Initially, Judith could not afford the trip to New York, and her mother discouraged her from leaving. Her father sent her $100 from Poland, money intended as her dowry, which she used to purchase a ticket for the transatlantic journey (personal communication, Kestenberg Amighi, 13 November 2021). On the 30 June 1937, with heavy hearts, her mother and sister accompanied her to the train station (Kestenberg, 1975a, 1992; New York Psychoanalytic Society & Institute, 1937–1945). Judith recalled being scared and anxious upon arriving in New York (Kestenberg, 1992). She recalled that Schilder made deliberate efforts to facilitate her integration into the professional community. He invited her to clinical discussions and group therapy sessions even though she was not yet trained as an analyst (Kestenberg, 1992, p. 175).

Social and economic adversities defined the context in which Judith had to build her new home in New York. The lingering repercussions of the Great Depression throughout the 1930s, along with widespread anti-Semitism, intensified the challenges faced by newcomers (Hale, 1995; Aron & Starr, 2013, p. 112). Employment opportunities in state hospitals were equally limited, with institutions reducing both funding and staff. Under these conditions, it was particularly difficult for émigré professionals to secure positions, given the abundance of well-trained American psychiatrists competing for supplementary income (Hale, 1995). Judith was in a precarious financial situation during her internship. As a foreigner, she was not paid and received only food and board. Max Schur connected her with someone at the Council of Jewish Women, an organisation that provided help to immigrants at the time. She received a $20 monthly stipend from them to cover her commuting expenses. She became friends with two women from this organisation, who later sent her clients for analysis. They also helped her with publishing her papers in English (Kestenberg, 1992). Kestenberg (1992) recollected that "the first thing I noticed in the psychiatric ward at Bellevue Hospital was that my English, which I had learned from a Scot, was not sufficient to understand the colleagues and the patients" (p. 164), which caused her further hardships in grounding herself within the new professional community. Nevertheless, in 1938, she passed the State Board examination and became a licensed medical professional.

After the annexation of Austria in March 1938, Judith realised she would not be able to return to Europe (Kestenberg, 1992). Her family attempted to send her personal belongings and their china, but she could not afford the customs fee, and the shipment was returned (Janet Kestenberg Amighi, personal communication, 13 November 2021). Anxious for her mother and siblings in Vienna and her father in Poland, Judith poured her fears and hopes into letters between 1937 and 1940, desperately working to bring them to New York (Kestenberg, 1937–1940). Even her safety became uncertain when she had an issue with her US residence permit because of a missing document. The matter was resolved when her father arranged the necessary paperwork through a public notary in Poland (Kestenberg, 1937–1940). Amid the emotional strain of the escalating war, Judith began personal analysis in 1938 with the Viennese émigré Edith Buxbaum (1902–1982) (Naszkowska, 2023; Kestenberg, 1992).

Determined to rescue her siblings, Judith secured funds from the Emergency Committee on Relief and Immigration of the American Psychoanalytic Association to support her brother's journey (Naszkowska, 2023). Henry first travelled to Cuba and later settled in Florida (Kestenberg Amighi, personal communication, 13 November 2021). Her sister, Henda, fled Vienna on her own on 15 March 1939 and went to New York. Despite holding two doctorates, she first worked as a maid for a wealthy woman and subsequently as a teacher at a small school (Kestenberg, 1992, p. 179). Henda later went on to lead a pioneering life and became one of the earliest women to hold a professorship in criminal law in the United States (Paz, 2014; Gassner, 2024, 2026).

As the war broke out in 1939, Judith's mother, Sara, fled Vienna to Stanislav, which belonged to Soviet-occupied Poland. Judith kept in touch with her through letters and sent her clothing packages. However, tragedy struck, as Judith recalled:

> She received permission from the Russians to leave. I sent her a ticket immediately (with Kubie's help), but it was too late. She could not leave anymore. I do not know what happened in this little town of Stanislavow. (Kestenberg, 1992, p. 180)[6]

On 26 July 1941, Stanislav was taken by the Germans, and Sara was murdered in one of the three massacres that year (Naszkowska, 2023, p. 206).

Judith's father, Szaje, who remained in Poland, was imprisoned in Tarnów. After December 1941, their correspondence ceased (Kestenberg, 1992). He was deported to the Auschwitz extermination camp, where he was murdered. His death was recorded on 23 December 1941 by Stanislav Ryszter in a secret notebook (Naszkowska, 2023, p. 206).

It was only after the end of the war, in 1946, that Judith received the heartbreaking confirmation that both her parents had been killed in the Nazi Holocaust. This is when she realised the unbelievable truth that her mother would not speak to her again (Kestenberg, 1992, p. 182). Burdened by guilt, Judith fell into a deep depression and defended against the trauma by throwing herself into her work (Kestenberg, 1992). For the next 22 years, she refused to speak about the Nazi Holocaust, even within the family (Naszkowska, 2023, p. 207). She struggled to find a way to process the loss of her parents and the destruction of her home country and culture. She remembered that each new wave of disappointment made it harder for her to feel at home, especially after discovering the limited action taken by the Roosevelt administration to stop the mass murder of Jews in Europe (Kestenberg, 1992, p. 180). During these years, Judith quietly wrestled not only with the loss of her parents but also with the challenge of piecing together her identity in yet another unfamiliar land.

Marriage and Family

In 1942, about a year after losing contact with her parents, Judith met Milton Kestenberg[7] (1913–1991), who would become her lifelong companion, both professionally and personally. Milton, a Polish-Jewish lawyer, had arrived in the United States by chance and, like Judith, found himself unable to return to Europe after the outbreak of the war. They shared the reality of immigrant life, the loss of their home and loved ones in the Nazi Holocaust, and the struggle to build a new future in New York (Kestenberg, 1992). As Judith put it, "The war, our families in the war, became entangled with the need to live" (Kestenberg, 1992, p. 181).

Milton, determined to continue practising law in the United States, enrolled in university while working full-time. He worked as a real estate agent and managed properties across New York City, including the Apthorp Building on the Upper West Side of Manhattan, where Judith had her clinical office for several years (Kestenberg Amighi, personal communication, 13 November 2021).

Judith recalled that, after a series of losses and the collapse of idealised paternal figures, Milton restored in her a sense of trust and inspiration reminiscent of what she had once felt for her father: "The trust that I had in my father as a child was reawakened. […] I felt like a new person and wanted to have children right away" (Kestenberg, 1992, p. 181). In 1944, amidst their busy schedules, they got married during their lunch break and welcomed their first child, Janet, in 1946. In 1956, they adopted a second child, Howard (Kestenberg Amighi, personal communication, 13 November 2021). The Kestenberg family moved to Long Island, New York, in 1959. Their home soon became a hub for fundraising and community-development events (Kestenberg, 1992). In the decades that followed, Judith and her daughter, Janet, worked closely, ultimately for much of their lives, on developmental movement studies. Milton, psychologically minded and deeply admiring of Judith's work, became involved in her professional world, leading to their psychohistorical studies on the effects of the Nazi Holocaust.

The New York Psychoanalytic Community

With Eduard Hitschmann's enthusiastic recommendation, Judith enrolled at the New York Psychoanalytic Institute (NYPI) on 18 September 1937,[8] with Herman Nunberg (1884–1970) becoming her supervising analyst (Kestenberg, 1937, 1941, 1991, 1992; Hitschmann, 1941; WPV/01/228, 1937). During her training, she worked on three cases: one on ejaculation praecox, one on compulsion neurosis, and a final case on alcoholism. She completed her required hours of control analysis by 1940 and continued to work on all three cases independently (Kestenberg, 1941). In parallel, she pursued further clinical experience in child psychiatry. Between 1939 and 1940, she served as a psychiatric consultant for New York University Hospital's child psychiatry unit and for an orphanage for children of colour. Between 1939 and 1943, she served as an assistant child psychiatrist at the Payne Whitney Psychiatry Clinic (Kestenberg, n.d.c).[9] She was a clinician at Mount Sinai Hospital between 1941 and 1942, alongside René Spitz (1887–1974) (Kestenberg, 1992). Judith was dedicated to child guidance and community mental health. Between 1939 and 1945, she taught social workers of the Community Service Society, a major non-profit social welfare organisation in New York. She also took an active part in the New York Mayor's Committee Project for Day Nurseries between 1945 and 1946, a wartime movement to maintain day nurseries to support working mothers (Kestenberg, n.d.c).[10]

Judith joined the NYPI at a tumultuous time, when various battles over theoretical and methodological orthodoxy divided the psychoanalytic community (Kestenberg, 1992). The intellectual and cultural orientations of the American and European analysts were somewhat different. European émigrés were, in larger proportions, politically left-leaning and often gravitated towards topics in social work and psychosomatic medicine. Questions regarding theoretical orthodoxy versus eclecticism rippled through the American psychoanalytic community. Diversions from Freudian theory created severe ruptures, particularly within the New York Society (Hale, 1995, pp. 116–118).

However, Judith remembered that her first years at the NYPI were permeated by familiar feelings of reunion with former colleagues and friends from Vienna (Kestenberg, 1992). According to her recollections, Hartmann read and commented on her manuscripts with great care. However, she also reported that he labelled her neurotic because her perspective on the origins of the ego differed from his (Kestenberg, 1975a, 1992). Judith found generous support from colleagues who shared her interest in child analysis, namely Margaret Mahler, Berta Bornstein (1899–1971), Phyllis Greenacre (1894–1989), and Marianne Kris (1900–1980) (Kestenberg, 1975a). Bornstein referred patients to her to support her professionally. Judith and Greenacre first met at one of Nunberg's private seminars. Greenacre described Judith as a gifted and devoted student who was well trained in neurology and presented a rare combination of interests (Greenacre, 1975, p. xiii). To pursue training in child analysis, Judith joined Marianne Kris's seminars in the 1940s. As formal child analysis training was unavailable at that time, the seminars were held at Kris's home (Naszkowska, 2023; Kestenberg, 1992). Kris (1942) wrote an approving note on Judith's year-long training progress and she sponsored her membership of the Academy of Child Psychiatry (Kris, 1960). In 1948, Kestenberg also began personal analysis with Kris (Kestenberg, 1992; Kris, 1959). They remained in close correspondence until at least 1975. Judith sent several papers to Kris for comments and corrections. She also organised a celebration for Kris's birthday (Kris & Kestenberg, 1959–1975).

As mentioned previously, Mahler and Kestenberg worked together at the *Nervenklinik* in Vienna in the 1930s (Kestenberg, n.d.a; Kestenberg, 1992). They maintained a close friendship and followed each other's work with enthusiasm. They were both committed to child guidance and mental hygiene, sharing a particular interest in the relationship between movement and psychic development. However, their long friendship was not without conflicts – a letter correspondence between them from 1955 documents a period of tension. Kestenberg had offered critical comments on Mahler's work, which Mahler received negatively during a plenary discussion (Kestenberg, 1955b). In response, Kestenberg expressed surprise at Mahler's reaction and sent a letter to reassure Mahler that no harm was intended. Mahler wrote a reply on the back of the letter, but ultimately marked it as "file to no response necessary" (Mahler, n.d.). In her handwritten note, Mahler described her perception of Kestenberg as unpredictable, marked by "strong hostility mixed with guilt-driven bursts of goodwill and generosity" (Mahler, n.d.). Nevertheless, they appeared to resolve this conflict, as their correspondence continued in subsequent years. Kestenberg invited Mahler to family celebrations and also organised a party to mark the publication of the collection of essays honouring Mahler's work (Kestenberg, 1971). Mahler was one of the few people in the psychoanalytic community who deeply understood Kestenberg's psychodynamic theory of movement. It is evident from their correspondence that Kestenberg viewed her as a sort of translator and proponent of her ideas to the wider psychoanalytic community (Kestenberg, 1970, 1971). Some tensions also marked the New York community of child analysts. Kestenberg (1992) remembered that differences between Bornstein and Mahler led Bornstein to oppose Kestenberg becoming a training analyst on Mahler's recommendation.

In 1941, during a meeting at the psychiatric ward of the New York Hospital, Judith presented case studies of mothers she observed at a child guidance clinic, examining the relationship between maternal psychological issues and children's behavioural problems (Greenacre, 1975). In subsequent years, she published several papers on issues of child placement, separation from parents, and adoption (Kestenberg, n.d.a). In 1943, Kestenberg became an associate member of the New York Psychoanalytic Society and was elected a full member in 1945. Her first paper, "Early Reactions to Tensions," presented before the Society in 1945, already contained nascent ideas that later found expression in her formulations on vaginal sensations and the flow of muscle tension (New York Psychoanalytic Society & Institute, 1937–1945; Kestenberg, 1945). In 1952, Kestenberg sent Bornstein a proposal outlining a curriculum for a training centre in child analysis intended for trainees in psychiatry, neurology, and obstetrics (Kestenberg, 1952, 1992). Her proposal emphasised infant observation studies, with a particular focus on movement development. Bornstein received the idea with interest but also expressed that the plan was overly ambitious (Bornstein, 1952).

Building on these emergent interests, in 1953, Judith began her longitudinal infant observation study, following the development of three subjects over 24 years (Kestenberg, 1953–1978, 1975a). In 1954, she presented case studies from these observations at the Arden House Conference of the New York Psychoanalytic Society in a report titled "Preliminary Report on Three Infants" (Kestenberg & Friend, 1954; Kestenberg, 1965a, 1992). In the years that followed, her focus shifted to female sexual development. She shared her formulations on the subject in the mid-1950s, in her presentation "A Stage in the Development of Female Sexuality" and in her articles "Vicissitudes of Female Sexuality" and "On the Development of Maternal Feelings in Early Childhood" (Kestenberg, 1954, 1956a, 1956b, 1956c).

In pursuit of establishing her career as a psychoanalytic psychiatrist in the United States, Kestenberg held various clinical appointments. In 1956, she was appointed training analyst at the State University of New York (SUNY) and, with the recommendation of Sandor Lorand (1892–1987), she became a clinical professor of psychiatry in 1959 (Kestenberg, 1992). She lectured on the theory and technique of child analysis, child development, and psychopathology at the Department of Psychiatry at Downstate Medical Centre, Division of Psychoanalytic Education (Kestenberg, n.d.a;

State University of New York, 1964). Between 1956 and 1957, she was affiliated with the Vanderbilt Hospital Child Psychiatry Department's newborn nursery and well-baby clinic (Kestenberg, n.d.a). From 1960, Kestenberg taught general practitioners and paediatricians in the Psychiatry Department of the Long Island Jewish Hospital, where she also served as a paediatric research psychiatrist. She also lectured as part of the child analysis programme of the Washington Psychoanalytic Institute between 1963 and 1964 (Kestenberg, n.d.a).

Even though Kestenberg (1992, p. 182) stated that formal integration into the analytic circles was never her ambition, she actively presented at numerous conferences across the country throughout her career (Sossin, personal communication, 1 November 2022; Kestenberg, n.d.a). She was a member of several professional associations, namely the American Psychoanalytic Association's Committee for Psychoanalysis in Childhood and Adolescence, the New York Psychoanalytic Society, the Long Island Psychoanalytic Society, the Psychoanalytic Association of New York, the American Psychiatric Society, and the Association of American Academic Child Psychiatry (Kestenberg, n.d.a).

Developmental Movement Studies

A focused and enduring interest in somatic processes and bodily movement characterised Kestenberg's professional life. She recalled that her early studies of brain injury in the 1930s provided an opportunity to investigate the relationships between cognitive function, psychological experience, and bodily movement (Kestenberg, 1975a, 1992). As a psychiatry intern at the Bellevue, Kestenberg found the assessment methods in developmental psychiatry extremely limited and wondered whether assessment could be based solely on movement behaviour (Kestenberg, 1975a, 1992). She was also dedicated to child guidance and actively read developmental studies by Arnold Gesell (1880–1961) and Charlotte Bühler (1893–1974). She followed Anna Freud (1895–1982) and Dorothy Burlingham's (1891–1979) child guidance and psychoanalytic developmental research with enthusiasm. She visited the Hempstead Clinic in 1955 to deepen her understanding in Anna Freud's developmental approach (Kestenberg, 1955a).

These interests in movement and developmental research coalesced in her longitudinal infant observation study. Kestenberg recruited three mother–infant dyads from the Vassar Brothers Public Hospital's newborn nursery in Poughkeepsie (Kestenberg, n.d.a, 1953–1978). The families came from culturally diverse and economically marginalised backgrounds, and Kestenberg sought to establish a mutually beneficial relationship with them by offering gifts as a form of financial support. The children frequently sent letters to Kestenberg requesting specific items, such as winter boots and coats. Additionally, she facilitated referrals to medical specialists using her professional networks. While

Kestenberg's observations primarily focused on the children, they occasionally included interactions with parents and other family members. Notably, when scheduling research visits, she addressed correspondence directly to the children rather than the parents. As the children reached young adulthood, they maintained contact with Kestenberg through letters, updating her on their educational and professional pursuits (Kestenberg, 1953–1978).

During the early years of this study, in the 1950s, to record changes in the infants' movements, Kestenberg developed her method of muscle *Tension-Flow* inscription. To further advance her methods of documenting movement behaviour, she began studying Labanotation (a dance notation method) in 1957. Her first movement teacher was a German émigré dancer, Irmgard Bartenieff (1900–1981), who later became a pioneer of American dance/movement therapy. Later, Kestenberg continued her movement studies with London-based experts Marion North (1925–1992) and Warren Lamb (1923–2014) (Kestenberg, n.d.a).

In 1962, Kestenberg founded the Sands Point Movement Study Group, bringing together psychiatrists, dancers, and educators interested in movement behaviour. The group's founding members were Jay Berlowe, Hershey Marcus, Esther Robbins, and Martha Soodak (Kestenberg Amighi & Loman, 1990). The dancer Forrestine Pauley, the dance/movement therapist Penny Lewis and an early years educator, Arnhilt Buelte, joined the group later. Informal members of the group were Godfrey Cobliner (sociologist and collaborator of Rene Spitz), Warren Lamb, Marion North, and Irmgard Bartenieff (Kestenberg, n.d.d). They began meeting at Kestenberg's home on Fridays (Sossin, personal communication, 1 November 2022; Kestenberg Amighi, personal communication, 13 November 2021). Kestenberg recalled her first years of developmental movement studies:

> I was sort of a lone investigator, and I did not have anyone to talk to because you cannot talk to psychiatrists, apart from these [the members of the study group], about movement. When we first published a paper together on movement patterns, one of the people who read it called me the "Lady with the Rhythms." So, I was somewhat of a novelty then. (cited in Kestenberg Amighi & Loman, 1990, p. 18)

Marcus and Berlowe remembered their long conversations around the dining table at Kestenberg's home about how to document and analyse movement. They began experimenting with movement notations on paper and observing infants at local hospitals where they were affiliated (Kestenberg Amighi & Loman, 1990). Marcus noted that the group, primarily consisting of psychiatrists, lacked direct experience with movement exploration. He remembered the significant emotional impact embodiment sessions had on him in the beginning (cited in Kestenberg Amighi & Loman, 1990). The dancer,

Forrestine Pauley, facilitated their first movement classes, encouraging participants to embody the movement patterns they observed in infants, thereby deepening their understanding of the connection between psychic and somatic experiences. Kestenberg's daughter remembered the Group's early years as follows:

> I was an adolescent at the time and [...] [m]y reflection on the Group was that I was embarrassed to take my friends through the dining room because they (the Group) would be on the floor doing various strange movements. When they were not doing that, they were sitting at the table writing indecipherable little squiggles. (Kestenberg Amighi & Loman, 1990, p. 11)

Between 1962 and 1967, in collaboration with the study group, Kestenberg developed her psychodynamic vocabulary of movement and her movement-based developmental assessment method, the Kestenberg Movement Profile (Kestenberg Amighi et al., 2018, pp. 8–10; Kormos, 2021a). To test the validity of her developmental movement theory, she began applying her Movement Profile across various settings. She compared her movement data with developmental data recoded at the New York Child Development Centre (Kestenberg, 1975a). In 1965, Kestenberg visited Anna Freud at the Hempstead Clinic to conduct developmental assessments of children solely based on their movement behaviour. She compared her findings with the clinic's interpretations and identified substantial correspondence, supporting the view that bodily movement could serve as a reliable indicator of dynamic and developmental processes (Kestenberg, 1955a, 1965a, 1965b, 1975a; Kestenberg Amighi et al., 2018, p. 9). In a 1965 letter, Anna Freud (1965) also praised the developmental accuracy of Kestenberg's method. Emboldened by this encouragement, Kestenberg published her psychodynamic theory of movement in the *Psychoanalytic Quarterly* across three papers in the 1960s, entitled "The Role of Movement Patterns in Development" (1965a, 1965b, 1967).

Kestenberg conducted further validity tests by collecting infant observation data across several Israeli kibbutzim between 1968 and 1970 (Kestenberg, 1975a, 1975b). She took observational photographs and made films of children and their parents. She applied her movement notation technique and constructed movement profiles of about 150 children aged 4 months to 10 years, including twins and blind children (Kestenberg Amighi et al., 2018, p. 10; Kestenberg, 1968–1972). During these kibbutz studies, she developed her concepts about the motor aspects of the development of community spirit (Kestenberg, 1975a, 1992). On 19 July 1968, she presented a lecture entitled "Movement Profiles and Psychological Assessment" at Oranim College of Education, in which she described the *Movement Profile* as a diagnostic and developmental assessment framework useful for professionals concerned with personality (Kestenberg, 1968–1972).

Kestenberg synthesised her developmental movement theory, first publishing it in 1971 in the article "Development of the Young Child as Expressed Through Bodily Movement I" (Kestenberg et al., 1971). The most comprehensive version of the Movement Profile was presented in 1985 in the publication "The Role of Movement Patterns in Prevention and Diagnosis" (Kestenberg, 1985).

In 1970, Judith and Milton Kestenberg founded Child Development Research (CDR), a nonprofit, educational organisation that managed several projects such as the Center for Parents and Children between 1972 and 1989, the Sydney L. Green Prenatal Project, and later the Jerome Riker International Study of the Organised Persecution of Children (Child Development Research, n.d.b, n.d.c). Under the auspices of the CDR, further infant observation studies were conducted, prenatal and postnatal parental support was offered to families, and training on movement and psychic development was delivered to mental health professionals and parents alike (Kestenberg, 1975a). The aim of the work at the Center for Parents and Children was to prevent childhood trauma through early detection of emotional disturbance and potential pathogenic factors in the parent–child dynamic. Mental health professionals at the centre offered child guidance interventions through creative movement and play sessions (Kestenberg, 1972; Loman, 2016). Parents received training in developmental movement assessment and were encouraged to apply it to their own children to identify any developmental or psychological issues. The centre also served as a placement institution for dance therapists, psychiatrists, and clinical psychologists in training (Loman, 1980).

Holocaust Studies

In 1968, while treating a second-generation survivor, Kestenberg found that her long-buried feelings about the Nazi Holocaust resurfaced, which drew her attention to mechanisms of transgenerational trauma transmission. This moment marked the beginning of the second epoch of her career, which she devoted to exploring the psychological effects of the Nazi Holocaust. Seeking to understand existing clinical approaches, she distributed questionnaires to analysts worldwide regarding their treatment of second-generation survivors. The limited response she received underscored a serious gap in psychoanalytic knowledge and practice, prompting her to establish a group dedicated to the psychoanalytic study of the effect of the Nazi Holocaust on the second generation (Kestenberg, 1980). The group held its first meeting in December 1973 at Kestenberg's home. It was attended by 14 psychoanalysts, including Sandor Lorand (Kestenberg, 1974). In the course of their case discussions about survivors they had been treating, the analysts expanded the scope of their study to include child survivors of the Nazi Holocaust and war children. With this expansion, they aimed to address a broader range of severe psychological consequences resulting from mass dehumanisation in children (Jucovy, 1985). Judith and Milton Kestenberg devoted themselves to advocacy for an exceptionally disadvantaged group: child survivors of the Nazi Holocaust. Milton took on restitution cases of child survivors in indemnification trials. At the time, many German psychiatrists and much of public opinion maintained that children who could not recall specific details of their persecution were insulated from enduring psychological harm. As a result, their claims were frequently dismissed, and the suffering of child survivors went unrecognised. Judith Kestenberg developed a somatically oriented, psychoanalytically informed interview technique designed to elicit memories of early childhood experiences, which could potentially be used as evidence in restitution cases in court. Drawing on her somatic orientation, Judith also developed new embodied concepts on the mechanisms of transgenerational trauma transmission.

In 1981, the Kestenbergs launched the *Jerome Riker International Study of Organised Persecution of Children*, which became one of the largest international psychohistory projects on the transgenerational effects of the Nazi Holocaust (Kestenberg, 1972, 1992, n.d.a,; Naszkowska, 2023). Judith Kestenberg, together with collaborators K. Mark Sossin, Ira Brenner, Eva Fogelman, Helene Bass-Wichelhaus, and Robert M. Prince, conducted psychoanalytically oriented, narrative interviews with Nazi Holocaust survivors and with children of survivors, as well as with children of Nazi persecutors. They trained local interviewers worldwide and recorded interviews in several languages (Child Development Research, n. d.a). Judith Kestenberg received three awards for her Nazi Holocaust studies: the Holocaust Memorial Award from the New York Society of Clinical Psychologists on 14 May 1987, the Elise M. Hayman Award for Holocaust Research from the International Psychoanalytical Association on 28 July 1993, and the Eleanor Roosevelt Award from the American Jewish Congress Commission for Women's Equality on 14 June 1996 (Sossin, 1999, personal communication, 12 April 2024; Sossin et al., 1999; Holocaust Award, 1987, p. 28; International Psychoanalytical Association, 1992, p. 40).

On 16 January 1999, after a long illness, Judith S. Kestenberg died in Sands Point, New York (Sossin, 1999). Her publication record comprises seven books, 27 book chapters, and 129 articles[11] (Kestenberg, 1975b). She is remembered by her colleagues as an inspiring and generous mentor, a pioneer of psychoanalytic movement studies, and an industrious and determined theoretician, with unending sensitivity towards children (Sossin, 1999, personal communication, 1 November 2022; Loman, personal communication, 15 November 2022). Janet and Howard both think of her as an attentive and charismatic mother, a hardworking professional, and a socially engaged person with a strong Jewish identity (Kestenberg Amighi, personal communication, 13 November 2021; Naszkowska, 2023).

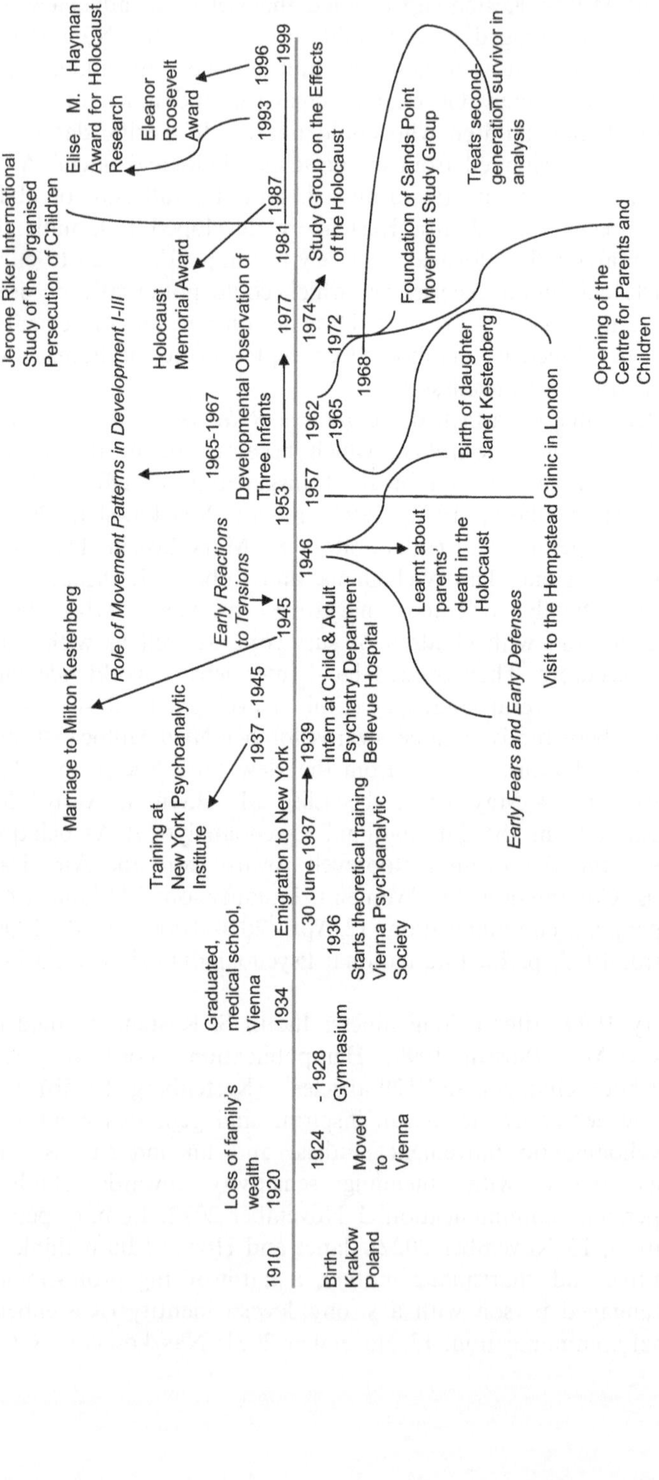

Figure 1.1 Timeline of significant events in the life of Judith S. Kestenberg.

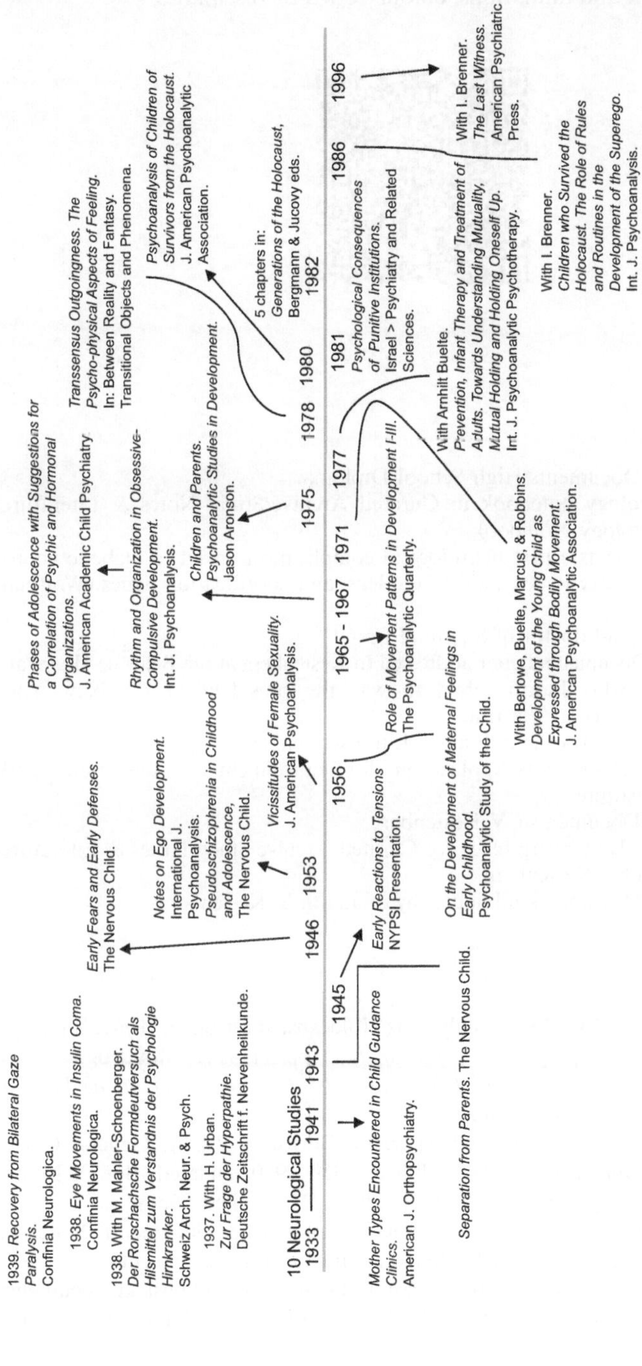

Figure 1.2 Timeline of Judith S. Kestenberg's most important publications.

Please scan the QR are code for a data visualisation of Judith S. Kestenberg's professional network and affiliations, colour-coded by disciplines.

Notes

1 Curated Archive/Documents/High School Diploma.
2 See Judith's neurology notebook in Curated Archive/Study Notes & Literature/Study Notes/Neurology Notebook.
3 Diabetic pseudotabes is a rare neurological complication linked to diabetic neuropathy. It causes sensory issues, pain in the legs, and coordination issues (Woltman & Wilder, 1929).
4 The family friend and doctor of Sigmund Freud.
5 Curated Archive/Documents/Letter addressed to Kestenberg at the Bellevue Hospital.
6 Lawrence Kubie who Judith refers to was the president of the New York Psychoanalytic Society at the time.
7 Curated Archive/Photos of Judith and Milton Kestenberg.
8 Curated Archive/Documents/Application for Enrollment to the New York Psychoanalytic Institute.
9 Curated Archive/Documents/CV Kestenberg.
10 On who and what Kestenberg read, see Curated Archive/Study Notes & Literature/Some Books of Judith Kestenberg.
11 Curated Archive/Documents/Bibliography of Judith S. Kestenberg.

References

Aron, L., & Starr, K. (2013). Psychoanalysis as Holocaust survivor. In *A psychotherapy for the people: Toward a progressive psychoanalysis* (pp. 111–127). Routledge.

Awards. (1992, Winter). *International Psychoanalysis: The Newsletter of the International Psychoanalytical Association*, 40.

Bornstein, B. (1952). *Letter to Kestenberg*, Berta Bornstein Papers, General Correspondence, 1933–1968, Kestenberg, Judith S. 1950–1960, undated, Box 2, Manuscript Division, Library of Congress, Washington, DC, United States.

Child Development Research. (n.d.a). 4R Policy [Unpublished document]. Materials discovered by the author in Janet Kestenberg Amighi's private collection.

Child Development Research. (n.d.b). Mission statement [Unpublished document]. Child Development Research, Box 34, Articles of incorporation, bylaws, and mission statement, Kestenberg papers (collection in process). Manuscript Division, Library of Congress, Washington, DC, United States. Materials discovered by the author in Janet Kestenberg Amighi's private collection.

Child Development Research. (n.d.c). An ounce of prevention CDR leaflet [Unpublished archival materials]. Child Development Research, Box 35, Brochures and Membership Forms, Kestenberg papers (collection in process). Manuscript Division, Library of Congress, Washington, DC, United States. Materials discovered by the author in Janet Kestenberg Amighi's private collection.

Freud, A. (1965, November 17). Letter to J. S. Kestenberg [Unpublished archival material]. Box 3, Kestenberg papers (collection in process). Manuscript Division, Library of Congress, Washington, DC, United States. Materials discovered by the author in Mark Sossin's private collection.

Gassner, M. (2024). Weiblich, jüdisch, vergessen? – Die Frauen des Wiener Kelsen-Kreises und ihr Beitrag zu Kelsens Rechts- und Demokratietheorie. In C. Jabloner & M. Gassner (Eds.), *Hans Kelsen und die österreichische Wissenschaftskultur.* (Schriftenreihe des Hans Kelsen-Instituts, Vol. 43, pp. 107–145). Manz. https://www.inlibra.com/10.5771/9783214262976.pdf

Gassner, M. (2026). Austrian jurists in US exile: Jurisprudence as a door opener to US law schools in the aftermath of World War II. *Journal of Austrian-American History,* 10(1–2), 174–194. doi:10.5325/jaustamerhist.10.1-2.0174

Greenacre, P. (1975). Foreword. In J.S. Kestenberg, *Children and parents: Psychoanalytic studies in development* (pp. xiii–xiv). Jason Aronson.

Hale, N.G. (1995). *The rise and crisis of psychoanalysis in the United States: Freud and the Americans, 1917–1985.* Oxford University Press.

Hitschmann, E. (1941, April 2). Letter to Dr Zilborg [Letter]. In *Training documents, Judith S. Kestenberg (1910–1999).* A. A. Brill Library, Archives and Special Collections, New York Psychoanalytic Association and Society, New York, NY, United States.

Holocaust Award. (1987, July 2). *New Jersey Jewish News,* 28.

Jucovy, M.E. (1985). Telling the Holocaust story: A link between the generations. *Psychoanalytic Inquiry,* 5(1), 31–49. doi:10.1080/07351698509533574.

Kestenberg Amighi, J., & Loman, S. (1990). The past of the Kestenberg Movement Profile: A panel discussion of Kestenberg, J. S., Buelte, A., Marcus, H., Berlowe, J., & Lamb, W. In S. Loman & P. Lewis (Eds.), *The Kestenberg Movement Profile: Its past, present applications, and future directions* (pp. 9–32). Retrieved from https://aura.antioch.edu/facbooks/25.

Kestenberg Amighi, J., Loman, S., & Sossin, K.M. (2018). Introduction. In J. Kestenberg Amighi, S. Loman, & M.K. Sossin (Eds.), *The meaning of movement, embodied developmental, clinical and cultural perspectives of the Kestenberg Movement Profile* (2nd ed., Kindle ed., pp. 3–12). Routledge.

Kestenberg, J.S. (n.d.a). CV [Unpublished curriculum vitae]. Documents of Judith S. Kestenberg (1937–1999). New York Psychoanalytic Association and Society A. A. Brill Library, Archives and Special Collections. New York, NY, United States.

Kestenberg, J.S. (n.d.b). CV [Unpublished curriculum vitae]. Box 1, Kestenberg Papers (collection in process). Manuscript Division, Library of Congress, Washington, DC, United States. Materials discovered by the author in Mark Sossin's private collection.

Kestenberg, J.S. (n.d.c). Notes, miscellaneous [Unpublished archival materials]. Box 6, Kestenberg papers (collection in process). Manuscript Division, Library of Congress, Washington, DC, United States. Materials discovered by the author in Mark Sossin's private collection.

Kestenberg, J.S. (n.d.d). Outline for a project for interdisciplinary center for child development. Materials discovered by the author in Mark Sossin's private collection.

Kestenberg, J.S. (1937). Application for enrollment. Documents of Judith S. Kestenberg (1937–1999). New York Psychoanalytic Association and Society A. A. Brill Library, Archives and Special Collections. New York, NY, United States.

Kestenberg, J.S. (1937–1940). Personal family letters [Unpublished manuscript]. Box 1, Kestenberg Papers, Manuscript Division, Library of Congress. Kestenberg Papers (collection in process). Library of Congress, Washington, DC, United States. Materials discovered by the author in Kestenberg Amighi's private collection.

Kestenberg, J.S. (1941). Application for endorsement of training completed. Documents of Judith S. Kestenberg (1937–1999). New York Psychoanalytic Association and Society A. A. Brill Library, Archives and Special Collections. New York, NY, United States.

Kestenberg, J.S. (1945). Early reactions to tensions. Presentation at the 283rd Meeting of the New York Psychoanalytic Society. Documents of Judith S. Kestenberg (1937–1999). New York Psychoanalytic Association and Society A. A. Brill Library, Archives and Special Collections. New York, NY, United States.

Kestenberg, J.S. (1952). Letter to Berta Bornstein. Berta Bornstein Papers, General Correspondence, 1933–1968, Kestenberg, Judith S., 1950–1960, undated, Box 2, Manuscript Division, Library of Congress, Washington, DC, United States.

Kestenberg, J.S. (1953–1978). Longitudinal study of infant observation [Unpublished archival materials]. Boxes 58–60, Kestenberg papers (collection in process). Manuscript Division, Library of Congress, Washington, DC, United States. Materials discovered by the author in Mark Sossin's private collection.

Kestenberg, J.S. (1954). A stage in the development of female sexuality. Presentation, Psychoanalytic Study Group, Seattle.

Kestenberg, J.S. (1955a). Letter to Anna Freud. Anna Freud Papers: Correspondence, 1902–1983, Box 54, Kestenberg, Judith, 1955–1969. Manuscript Division, Library of Congress, Washington, DC, United States.

Kestenberg, J.S. (1955b, February 22). Letter to Mahler. Margaret Mahler Correspondences. Margaret S. Mahler papers (MS 1138), Series IX. Box 184. Folder 2530. Beinecke Rare Book and Manuscript Library. Yale University, New Haven, United States.

Kestenberg, J.S. (1956a, March 16). On the development of maternal feelings in early childhood: Observations and reflections [Presentation]. Meeting of the New York Psychoanalytic Society, Documents of Judith S. Kestenberg (1937–1999). New York Psychoanalytic Association and Society A. A. Brill Library, Archives and Special Collections. New York, NY, United States.

Kestenberg, J.S. (1956b). On the development of maternal feelings in early childhood: Observations and reflections. *The Psychoanalytic Study of the Child*, 11, 257–291. doi:10.1080/00797308.1956.11822936.

Kestenberg, J.S. (1956c). Vicissitudes of female sexuality. *Journal of the American Psychoanalytic Association*, 4(3), 453–476. doi:10.1177/000306515600400303.

Kestenberg, J.S. (1965a). The role of movement patterns in development, I: Rhythms of movement. *Psychoanalytic Quarterly*, 24(1), 1–36. doi:10.1080/21674086.1965.11926334.

Kestenberg, J.S. (1965b). The role of movement patterns in development, II: Flow of tension and effort. *Psychoanalytic Quarterly*, 24(4), 517–563. doi:10.1080/21674086.1965.11926363.

Kestenberg, J.S. (1967). The role of movement patterns in development, III: Control of shape. *Psychoanalytic Quarterly*, 26(3), 356–409. doi:10.1080/21674086.1967.11926431.

Kestenberg, J.S. (1968–1972). Kibbutzim studies, Israel. Boxes 50–54. Kestenberg papers (collection in process). Manuscript Division, Library of Congress, Washington, DC, United States. Materials discovered by the author in Mark Sossin's private collection.

Kestenberg, J.S. (1970, 22 December). Letter to Mahler. Margaret Mahler Correspondences, Kestenberg, J.S. (1969–1975, n.d.). Margaret S. Mahler papers (MS 1138), Series I, Box 11, Folder 272. Beinecke Rare Book and Manuscript Library, Yale University, New Haven, CT, United States.

Kestenberg, J.S. (1971, April 14, 16). Letter to Mahler. Margaret Mahler Correspondences. Margaret S. Mahler papers (MS 1138), Series IX. Box 184. Folder 2530. Beinecke Rare Book and Manuscript Library. Yale University, New Haven, United States.

Kestenberg, J.S. (1972, September 7). Letter to Mahler. Margaret Mahler Correspondences, Kestenberg, J. S. (1969–1975, n.d.). Margaret S. Mahler papers (MS 1138), Series I, Box 11, Folder 272. Beinecke Rare Book and Manuscript Library, Yale University, New Haven, United States.

Kestenberg, J.S. (1974, July 14). Letter to Marianne Kris. Ernst Kris and Marianne Kris Papers, Correspondences, Box 36, Kestenberg, Judith S., 1959–1975, Manuscript Division, Library of Congress, Washington, DC, United States.

Kestenberg, J.S. (1975a). Preface. In *Children and parents: Psychoanalytic studies in development* (pp. xv–xxvii). Jason Aronson.

Kestenberg, J.S. (1975b). *Children and parents: Psychoanalytic studies in development.* Jason Aronson.

Kestenberg, J.S. (1980). Psychoanalyses of children of survivors from the Holocaust: Case presentations and assessment. *Journal of the American Psychoanalytic Association*, 28(4), 775–804. doi:10.1177/000306518002800402

Kestenberg, J.S. (1985). The role of movement patterns in diagnosis and prevention. In D.A. Shaskan & W.I. Roller (Eds.), *Paul Schilder: Mind explorer* (pp. 97–161). Human Sciences Press.

Kestenberg, J.S. (1991). Dr Judith S. Kestenberg talks to Kristina Stanton. *Free Associations*, 2(2), 157–174.

Kestenberg, J.S. (1992). Kindheit und Wissenschaft. Eine biographische Skizze. In L. M. Hermanns (Ed.), *Psychoanalyse in Selbstdarstellungen, Vol.* 1 (pp. 147–202). Edition Diskord.

Kestenberg, J.S., Berlowe, J., Buelte, A., Hershey, M., & Robbins, E. (1971). Development of the young child as expressed through bodily movement I. *Journal of the American Psychoanalytic Association*, 19(4), 746–764.

Kestenberg, J.S., & Friend, J. (1954). Preliminary report on three infants. Presented at Arden House Conference, 8 May. Unpublished.

Kormos, J. (2021a). Kinaesthetic attunement, clashing and mismatches of early interactions and their influence in later development: Theoretical introduction to the

Kestenberg Movement Profile. *Imágó Budapest: Pszichoanalízis Társadalom Kultúra*, 10(1), 42–54.

Kris, M. (1942, January 12). Letter to Atkin [Letter]. In Training documents, Judith S. Kestenberg (1937–1999). A. A. Brill Library, Archives and Special Collections, New York Psychoanalytic Association and Society, New York, NY, United States.

Kris, M. (1959, January 21). Letter on training. Ernst Kris and Marianne Kris Papers, Correspondences, Box 36, Kestenberg, Judith S., 1959–1975, Manuscript Division, Library of Congress, Washington, DC, United States.

Kris, M. (1960, April 20). Letter to Ann Benjamin. Ernst Kris and Marianne Kris Papers, Correspondences, Box 36, Kestenberg, Judith S., 1959–1975, Manuscript Division, Library of Congress, Washington, DC, United States.

Kris, M., & Kestenberg, J.S. (1959–1975). Correspondence. Ernst Kris and Marianne Kris Papers, Box 36, Kestenberg, Judith S., 1959–1975, Manuscript Division, Library of Congress, Washington, DC, United States.

Loman, S. (1980). Dance therapy internship program: Attunement. *Child Development Research News*, 2(2).

Loman, S. (2016). Judith S. Kestenberg's dance/movement therapy legacy: Approaches with pregnancy, young children, and caregivers. *American Journal of Dance Therapy*, 38(2), 225–244.

Mahler, M.S. (n.d.). Notes to Kestenberg. Margaret Mahler Correspondences. Margaret S. Mahler papers (MS 1138), Series IX. Box 184. Folder 2530. Beinecke Rare Book and Manuscript Library. Yale University. New Haven, United States.

Naszkowska, K. (2023). Give me permission to remember: Judith S. Kestenberg and the memory of the Holocaust. In L. Henik & L. Aron (Eds.), *Contemporary psychoanalysis and Jewish thought: Answering a question with more questions* (pp. 197–217). Routledge.

New York Psychoanalytic Society & Institute. (1937–1945). 283rd Meeting of the New York Psychoanalytic Society, Scientific Session Program, Training Documents, Judith S. Kestenberg (1910–1999). New York Psychoanalytic Association and Society A. A. Brill Library, Archives and Special Collections. New York, NY, United States.

Paz, R.Y. (2014). A forgotten Kelsenian? The story of Helen Silving-Ryu (1906–1993). *European Journal of International Law*, 25(4), 1123–1146. doi:10.1093/ejil/chu078

Silberpfennig, I. (1933). Ueber Pseudotabes [About pseudotabes]. *Arbeiten aus der Neurologie. Institut Obserstainer-Marburg*, 35, 169–181.

Silberpfennig, I. (1936a). Die Klinik der medialen Akustikustumoren [The clinical presentation of medial acoustic tumours]. *Monatsschrift für Psychiatrie und Neurologie*, 92(3), 157–182. doi:10.1159/000154455

Silberpfennig, I. (1936b). Die Klinik der medialen Akustikustumoren (Schluß) [The clinical presentation of medial acoustic tumours (Conclusion)]. *Monatsschrift für Psychiatrie und Neurologie*, 92(4), 183–201. doi:10.1159/000154457

Silberpfennig, I., & Mahler-Schoenberger, M. (1938). Der Rorschachsche Formdeutversuch als Hilfsmittel zum Verständniss der Psychologie Hirnkranker. *Swiss Archives of Neurology & Psychiatry*, 40(2), 302–327.

Silberpfennig, I., & Urban, H. (1937a). Zur Frage der Hyperpathie [On the question of hyperpathia]. *Deutsche Zeitschrift f. Nervenheilkunde*, 142, 120–152.

Silberpfennig, I., & Urban, H. (1937b). Hemihyperpathie [Hemyhyperpathia of taste]. *Deutsche Zeitschrift f. Nervenheilkunde*, 68(4), 613–618.

Silberpfennig, J. (1938). Eye movements in insulin coma. *Confinia Neurologica*, 1(3), 188–200.

Silberpfennig, J. (1939). Recovery from bilateral gaze paralysis. *Confinia Neurologica*, 2(1–2), 15–31.

Silberpfennig, J. (1941a). Disturbances of ocular movements with pseudo-hemianopsia in frontal lobe tumors. *Confinia Neurologica*, 4(1–2), 1–13.

Silberpfennig, J. (1941b). Mother types encountered in child guidance clinics. *American Journal of Orthopsychiatry*, 11, 475–484.

Silberpfennig, J., & Birkmayer, W. (1938). Ueber zwei Faelle von Trigeminustumoren mit Zwischenhirnsymptomen [About two cases of trigeminal tumours with symptoms of the third ventricle]. *Archive F. Psychiatrie und Nervenkrankheit*, 103(2), 255–278.

Silving, H. (1988). *Helen Silving: Memoirs*. Vantage Press.

Sossin, K. M., Loman, S., & Merman, H. (1999). Remembering Judith S. Kestenberg, our mentor and friend. *American Journal of Dance Therapy*, 21(1), 53–55. https://doi.org/10.1023/A:1022890629390

State University of New York. (1964). Bulletin. Oskar Diethelm Psychiatric Library of the Weill-Cornell Hospital. New York.

Transcript of Records. (1929–1933). Judith Silberpfennig, University of Vienna Archive, AT-UAW_Med_Nat_SS_1929–1933_Judith_SILBERPFENNIG.

Woltman, H.W., & Wilder, R.M. (1929). Diabetes mellitus: Pathologic changes in the spinal cord and peripheral nerves. *Archives of Internal Medicine*, 44(4), 576–603. doi:10.1001/archinte.1929.00140040114010.

WPV/01/228. (1937). Training Report on Judith S. Kestenberg (n.d.). Anna Freud Papers. Freud Museum London Archive. London, United Kingdom.

WPV/01/230. (1937). Training Report on Judith S. Kestenberg (n.d.). Anna Freud Papers. Freud Museum London Archive. London, United Kingdom.

Chapter 2

Moving Concepts, Bodies in Mind

The following discussion of Judith S. Kestenberg's work adopts a somatic orientation, with particular focus on her developmental movement studies and psychodynamic theory of movement. She developed the core of this work between the 1940s and the mid-1970s, within the professional milieu of the New York Psychoanalytic Society. This chapter situates her work within its intellectual context, examining earlier studies in related fields, prevailing schools of thought, and the figures who most influenced her conceptual development. First, Kestenberg's infant observation studies will be introduced in the context of contemporaneous direct observation studies in psychoanalysis. Then, psychoanalytic debates on female sexual development will be reviewed as these provide a backdrop to understand Kestenberg's propositions on the libidinal charge of internal organs and her *inner-genital* psychosexual phase. The discussion then turns to Kestenberg's psychodynamic vocabulary of movement, which will be contextualised within contemporaneous systematic studies of movement in psychoanalysis. Further on, Kestenberg's developmental framework will be introduced in full. Then, her movement-based developmental assessment framework, the *Movement Profile*, will be outlined. This section will introduce her methods of documenting, quantifying, and visualising kinetic constellations. The following section outlines the application of the *Movement Profile* at Kestenberg's child-guidance project, the Center for Parents and Children. Finally, the discussion turns to introduce Kestenberg's last major project, her psychohistorical studies of the Nazi Holocaust. Considering her Holocaust studies, I emphasise their developmental and somatic orientation, which continued and extended her earlier concerns.

Infant Observation Studies

At the heart of Kestenberg's first major project was the relationship between personality development, bodily sensation, and movement behaviour. She explored questions such as the libidinisation[1] of internal organs, the role of *inner-genital* sensations in sexual development, and the psychoanalytic interpretation of bodily movement. Her earliest investigations centred around

DOI: 10.4324/9781003559955-3

kinaesthetic manifestations of drives, leading to her proposals of early vaginal tensions, the *inner-genital* developmental phase (Kestenberg, 1945, 1956a, 1956b). She expanded this somatic focus to the psychoanalytic study of movement behaviour and mapped categories of movement on to the structural agencies of the id, ego, and superego.

Her psychodynamic vocabulary of movement was published across three articles in the 1960s (Kestenberg, 1965a, 1965b, 1967a). In "The Role of Movement Patterns in Development I: Rhythms of Movement," she dealt with the motor specificities of drive-derivative processes through her concept of *Tension-Flow* (Kestenberg, 1965a). In "The Role of Movement Patterns in Development II: Flow of Tension and Effort," she outlined the developmental progression from id-derivative to ego-controlled movement patterns (Kestenberg, 1965a, 1965b). In "The Role of Movement Patterns in Development III: Control of Shape," she introduced her categories of shaping associated with the emergence of object-relations.[2] She also proposed a grammatical organisation of bodily movement and explored how intersubjectivity is reflected in bodily movement (Kestenberg, 1967a). Kestenberg's developmental framework, as a whole, was published in 1971, in collaboration with the members of the Sands Point Movement Study Group (Jay Berlowe, Hershey Marcus, Esther Robbins, and Arnhilt Buelte), in the article entitled "Development of the Young Child Expressed through Bodily Movement I" (1971a). In the 1970s, Kestenberg (1974b) presented her work as a movement-based developmental assessment framework, which she called a *Movement Profile.* In 1985, she published a more comprehensive version and proposed it as an instrument for prevention and diagnosis in developmental psychiatry (Kestenberg, 1985).

Kestenberg grounded her formulations on observational data collected from a longitudinal developmental study involving three infants. The research began in 1953 and concluded in 1977, following the same three subjects over a 24-year period. As mentioned before, she recruited the three mother–infant dyads from the Vassar Brothers Hospital newborn nursery in Poughkeepsie (Kestenberg, n.d.b). The participants represented diverse ethnic and socioeconomic backgrounds (Kestenberg, 1953–1978).

Kestenberg observed and documented the movement behaviour of infants and their mothers and interpreted it within a psychoanalytic developmental framework, linking patterns of movement to temperament, modes of drive-discharge, defence mechanisms, object-relationships, and modes of thinking and learning (Kestenberg, 1965a). Several psychoanalysts and child psychologists collaborated with her in this research, namely Jacqueline Friend, Stephanie Librach, Sybil Escalona, and Florence Halpern. Movement specialist Irmgard Bartenieff supported her in crystallising her observations about specific movement features. Bartenieff also conducted repeated observations in Kestenberg's project between 1957 and 1960 (Kestenberg, 1957, 1965a).

During the first year of the study, Kestenberg conducted monthly home visits, followed by two to three visits per month until the fifth year of life.

Subsequently, observations were scheduled two to three times annually. Initially, she focused on the motor behaviour of the individual infants during feeding, play, and interactions with family members, primarily their mothers and siblings. In later life, she observed her study subjects in a broader range of interactional situations, such as talking with their friends at home (Kestenberg, 1953–1978). During her observations, she interacted with the mothers and the children. At times, she would initiate games with the children or ask them to draw. She used the children's verbal reports and drawings to provide information on psychic development, sense of psychic separateness, and the development of ego functions. She noted information about their everyday lives to understand any events that might influence their behaviours. She also incorporated the parents' reports on the children's behaviour at home and performance at school (Kestenberg, 1953–1978).

Kestenberg's infant observation study followed the broader trends of developmental observation and child guidance research conducted internationally between 1920 and the 1940s (Polat, 2021). The first large-scale, systematic observational studies of infant development were carried out by Arnold Gesell and Charlotte Bühler in the early decades of the twentieth century. These studies aimed to collect comprehensive normative data on development from typically and atypically developing children. Gesell's studies focused on both individual differences and broader developmental trends of motor skills, intelligence, language, and relational behaviour (Polat, 2021, p. 286). He presented these developmental norms using both quantitative measures and qualitative case vignettes. His behavioural interviews consisted of standardised tests using basic everyday objects, which were given to the children repeatedly at different ages. These tests were designed to generate an active response from the infants, reflecting their behavioural repertoire and competencies. In addition to behavioural tests, he also collected data from parental notes and observations of parent–infant interactions. Gesell's studies compiled an extensive and comprehensive catalogue of child behaviour. Various components of these studies have been incorporated into later developmental tests such as the Bayley Scale of Infant Development and the Denver Developmental Screening Test (Thelen & Adolph, 1994).

Charlotte Bühler's observational studies were similarly influential in child and adolescent psychology. Together with her collaborator, Hildegard Hetzer, she devised standardised developmental tests that came to be known as the Baby Tests (Schenk-Danzinger, 1963). These were standardised performance tests that addressed domains of bodily control, mental ability, social development, and object manipulation (Bühler, 1930, pp. 193–195). Bühler's research was grounded in extensive direct observational data gathered from infants in their everyday environments. Observers were instructed to remain neutral and avoid contact with the children. They recorded the exact time and circumstances of new behaviours, sometimes with minute-level precision. The team analysed the data from various perspectives. Temporal analysis examined the timing and duration of behaviours, while interpretative analysis examined the meaning of the recorded data in relation to the broader developmental sequence during the first year of life (Bühler, 1930, p. 8).

Kestenberg was knowledgeable about the developmental assessments of Gesell and Bühler and used them while working in the Child Psychiatry Department at the Bellevue Hospital. At the same time, she found their classificatory system limited (Kestenberg, 1975a). She explained that:

> the lack of classification of infantile and adult qualities of movement made it difficult to compare early and later forms of motor behaviour. Motor development has been primarily appraised by tests of specific achievements such as grasping or sitting, rather than of qualities or sequences of movement. (Kestenberg, 1965a, p. 4)

Instead of cataloguing discrete units of movement in her developmental research, Kestenberg recorded motor patterns based on their underlying qualitative features. Each discrete movement – for example, lifting the right arm – can be executed in numerous ways. Kestenberg focused on how a movement is performed and how these qualitative features relate to development. She nonetheless applied infant intelligence tests and the Gesell Developmental Schedules during her own infant studies (Kestenberg, 1953–1978).

Drawing closer to psychoanalysis, Kestenberg's developmental research was situated within the tradition of psychoanalytic infant observation – an approach that emerged in the early twentieth century and became a significant line of inquiry by the middle of the century. She engaged with the work of early baby watchers, Hermine von Hug-Hellmuth (1871–1924) and Sabina Spielrein (1885–1942) (Kestenberg, n.d.d),[3] and extensively drew on the contributions of Anna Freud (1895–1982) and Margaret Mahler (1897–1985).

Most of Freud's psychoanalytic developmental concepts were based on the reconstruction of childhood experiences, derived from his adult patients' reports. However, Midgley (2013) pointed out that Freud actively sought empirical grounding for many of his central developmental formulations and encouraged his colleagues to collect observations of their own children. As early as 1905, at a meeting of the Vienna Psychoanalytic Society, he emphasised direct observation of children as a viable and vital method for psychoanalytic inquiry (Midgley, 2013, p. 85). However, it was not until later that Hermine von Hug-Hellmuth conducted the first systematic psychoanalytic infant observation, which she published in her book, *A Study of the Mental Life of the Child* in 1913 (Geissmann & Geissmann, 1998a). She intended to illustrate the Freudian psychosexual development model using material drawn from her direct observations and notes from other parents. She highlighted the importance of play in assessing drive-organisation and emotional development in children. Hug-Hellmuth asserted that cutaneous and muscular eroticism are central forms of infantile sexuality and suggested that a *muscular sense* dominates the activities of children in the first year of life. She linked this muscular sense to fetal movements practised in the womb (Geissmann & Geissmann, 1998a, pp. 43–47). Hug-Hellmuth's concept of muscular sense appears to anticipate Kestenberg's theories concerning fetal movements and muscle *Tension-Flow*. Although Kestenberg reviewed Hug-Hellmuth's work and annotated her article on child psychology (Hug-Hellmuth, 1914), she did not explicitly relate these concepts to Hug-Hellmuth (Kestenberg, n.d.d).

The legacy of another important early psychoanalytic infant researcher, Sabina Spielrein, comprises approximately 34 contributions to child development, many of which were based on observations of her daughter (Noth, 2015; Naszkowska, 2024a). As Naszkowska (2024b) explained, Spielrein's (1922/2015) concepts on language development were strongly somatic in their orientation. Spielrein viewed the intimate nature of bodily experiences between mother and infant as the foundation for the emergence of communication and language. She associated the rhythmic structure of an infant's sucking during breastfeeding with the movements of the lips and the temporal pattern of preparatory sounds such as mö-mö-mö and pö-pö-pö, which precede the articulation of the words Mama and Papa (Naszkowska, 2024b, p. 575). Spielrein also emphasised the collaborative and intersubjective dimensions of mother–infant relationships. Kestenberg made detailed notes on Spielrein's papers published in 1922 and 1923, dealing with the development of the concept of time in the unconscious (Kestenberg, n.d.d). There are striking resonances between Spielrein's embodied orientation to the development of language, through her emphasis on the rhythmicity of sucking, and Kestenberg's *Sucking Tension-Flow Rhythm*. Despite the conceptual echoes, Kestenberg did not make explicit connections between her work and Spielrein's.

Anna Freud's approach had the most significant influence on Kestenberg's developmental studies. Freud's work exemplified how observational data could inform and enrich psychoanalytic technique, which was a focal point of Kestenberg's ambition. Anna Freud argued that systematic observation of children had the potential to deepen understanding of the origins and development of psychological functioning. At the same time, she regarded traditional scientific methods, such as measurement, experimental controls, and statistical analysis, as inapplicable to psychoanalysis and developed a tailored methodological approach. She suggested that psychoanalytic inquiry should adopt a threefold focus on the dynamic, historical, and genetic aspects of behaviour. The dynamic dimension concerns the interplay of forces that constitute a specific behaviour, the historical focus traces its development, and the genetic perspective examines its initial function (Midgley, 2013, p. 84; Freud, 1951, p. 126). She further stressed the equal importance of external and internal reality, conceptualising it through her notion of *developmental lines*. These could be understood as markers of change across various domains of functioning over the course of development, accounting for interactions between the id, ego, and superego processes and environmental factors

(Midgley, 2013, pp. 132–134). In her infant observation studies, Kestenberg precisely focused on the dynamic interplay between id, ego, and superego processes and external environmental forces, as expressed in movement behaviour. Accordingly, she devised a psychodynamic vocabulary of bodily movement with the objective of aiding psychoanalytic theory and practice.

Working at the Hempstead War Nursery and then at the Hempstead Clinic with large numbers of children traumatised by the war, Anna Freud came to recognise that the existing, largely descriptive, symptom-focused psychiatric assessments were limited and potentially misleading. She argued that the same manifest symptoms in children could arise from a range of different underlying factors, depending on the child's developmental level and overall mode of functioning (Midgley, 2013, Chapter 9). She added that the same symptom could have different meanings for different children. Therefore, in the 1950s, together with her collaborators at the Hempstead Clinic, she set out to devise a systematic psychoanalytic assessment framework to guide clinicians in diagnosing and treating children. This work culminated in the development of her *Diagnostic Profile*. It was a psychoanalytic, developmental assessment framework that organised observational data into categories such as drive and ego development, interactions between id and ego processes, and aspects of frustration tolerance, social adaptation, and moral development. It also recorded intrapsychic conflicts that may govern the child's behaviour (Midgley, 2013, Chapter 9; Green & Joyce, 2017). At Hempstead, observational data were collected during play sessions with children that functioned as diagnostic interviews. These assessments also included notes from school reports and parental information, as well as incorporating cognitive and projective tests. In the 1960s, the *Diagnostic Profile* was extended beyond childhood, adapted for adolescents (Laufer, 1965) and for adults (Freud et al., 1965). The *Adult Profile* was used as a metapsychological assessment of adult personality when both the parent and the child were in treatment at the clinic. Corresponding sections of the adult and child profiles were compared at the clinic to provide a more comprehensive picture of the parent–child dyad.

The Well-Baby Research Group at Hempstead, established by W. Ernst Freud[4] in 1967, further adapted the *Diagnostic Profile* (Freud, 1967; Freud & Freud, 1976). They developed a *Baby Profile* to aid the metapsychological assessment of infants (Freud & Freud, 1976; Lupke, 2008). The Well-Baby Clinic operated as an independent research facility within the Hempstead Clinic, offering parental support and treatment with a focus on mental hygiene and child guidance. Participating parents received specialised knowledge regarding child development. The *Baby Profile* collected data on aspects of early functioning such as sleep, feeding, and elimination routines. It recorded early motor behaviours such as sucking, rooting, arm and leg movements, and caregiver–infant interactions. It specifically gathered information on the expression of instinctual processes and object-relationships, as well as aggression and ego development. It also aimed to catalogue affective reactions, documenting possible forerunners of later fixations and conflicts (Freud & Freud, 1976).

In the late 1940s, in her review of Anna Freud's book entitled *The Psycho-Analytical Treatment of Children* (1946), Kestenberg (1947) praised the volume for clarifying the necessary differences in analytic work with children compared with adults. Reading this publication may have paved the way for Kestenberg to anchor much of her developmental theory and assessment framework in Anna Freud's work. Her *Movement Profile* followed the outline of Freud's *Diagnostic Profile*; its initial focus on infant development and later expansion to adults also show notable parallels with the *Adult* and *Baby Profiles*. These frameworks were all elaborated during the 1960s, reaching a more final form in the early 1970s. Kestenberg first presented the *Movement Profile* in 1971 and 1974, whereas preliminary considerations on the *Baby Profile* were first presented in 1967 and again in 1971 (Freud & Freud, 1976). Given Kestenberg's visit to the Hampstead Clinic in the mid-1960s (Kestenberg & Freud, 1955–1969), some degree of cross-fertilisation between these systems seems likely. According to Sossin (personal communication, 18 November 2025), Ernst Freud also visited Kestenberg's primary prevention centre and research nursery in the 1970s; however, my archival research has not yielded any direct correspondence between them. Specific convergences between Kestenberg's *Movement Profile* and the *Diagnostic Profile* will be discussed in detail later in this chapter.

Another mid-century pioneer in psychoanalytic infant observation and child guidance whose work significantly influenced Kestenberg was Margaret Mahler. Mahler's studies initially concentrated on symbiotic psychosis and early infantile autism, conceptualising these conditions as deviations from typical development. According to her observations, these children experienced specific difficulties in developing a sense of separateness, resulting in a prolonged period of psychic fusion with mother and the external environment (Mahler, 1952; Mahler et al., 1975, p. 11). During the 1950s, Mahler established the Masters Children Centre, a research nursery and therapy centre that offered infant–parent psychotherapy for children exhibiting autism and schizophrenia-like symptoms with the active involvement of their mothers (Geissmann & Geissmann, 1998b, p. 217; Coates, 2004, p. 587). To further investigate the components of symbiotic psychosis, Mahler and her colleagues redirected their research towards non-clinical populations of typically developing children. They created an observational nursery at the centre, equipped with a large playroom and one-way mirrors, to observe mothers and children in a naturalistic environment (Mahler et al., 1975, Chapter 1).

They devised behaviour rating frameworks that documented emerging ego functions, from which they inferred the child's experience of separateness from the mother. They inferred aspects of the child's separateness and the development of ego functioning from a wide variety of behavioural data, including nonverbal behaviour. They argued that observing the preverbal period of development provided a unique opportunity to examine the interplay between nonverbal behaviour and psychic development (Mahler et al.,

1975, p. 15). This principal route between the intrapsychic process and the kinaesthetic and motor pathways was predicated upon the consideration that bodily movement is the primary mode of drive-discharge, ego defence, and expression in the preverbal years. Thus, their observation categories included sensory functioning, environmental scanning, goal-directed behaviours, communicative use of the mouth, and the infant's ability to elicit responses from the caregiver (Wolfs, 2022; Mahler et al., 1975, p. 262). They also examined expressive movements between mother and child, recording them according to frequency, amplitude, timing, and intensity (Wolfs, 2022; Mahler et al., 1975, p. 15). Based on these observations, Mahler and her colleagues conceptualised the psychological birth of the self through a multi-stage process of separation-individuation. The central proposition of this model was the emphasis on bodily experiences and nonverbal interaction between the infant and the caregiver from which self and object-representations evolve (Mahler et al., 1975, Chapter 1; Mahler & Furer, 1966). Kestenberg anchored her own developmental theory in these formulations and, in particular, identified specific motor components that comprise the developmental process of separation-individuation. Kestenberg's reconsideration of Mahler's concepts will be discussed in detail when her developmental theory is presented later in this chapter.

I intended to show in this section that Kestenberg's approach to infant observation followed the broader traditions of developmental inquiry in the twentieth century and was closely aligned with contemporaneous studies in psychoanalysis, such as the work of Anna and Ernst Freud at the Hampstead Clinic, as well as Margaret Mahler's research. As the following chapters will show, Kestenberg regarded her own contributions as a continuation of these lines of inquiry.

Theorising the Insides

Debates on the Development of Female Sexuality

Kestenberg's earliest psychoanalytic investigations centred on the psychosexual development of women. She reconsidered the libidinal activity and passivity of internal organs and argued for the significance of *inner-genital* sensations in the development of sex-specific identity. Before turning to Kestenberg's formulation, I first contextualise her ideas on female sexual development by reviewing the psychoanalytic debates on the subject from the 1920s through the 1950s, the period in which she developed her theories.

Questions of female sexual development occupied a central place in international psychoanalytic debates between the 1920s and mid-1930s and resurfaced in the 1960s (Birksted-Breen, 1993). Several analysts, predominantly women (Deutsch, 1925, 1930; Horney, 1924, 1926, 1928, 1933; Müller, 1932; Klein, 1928; Lampl-de Groot, 1928; Bonaparte, 2018; Brierley, 1936;

Jacobson, 1937), revisited fundamental tenets of psychosexual development. Some, such as Helene Deutsch (1925) and Marie Bonaparte (2018), largely followed Freud's principle of anatomical determinism, expanding upon his views without much critique. Others, including Karen Horney (1924, 1926, 1928, 1933) and Melanie Klein (1928), challenged the Freudian view of female anatomy as a lack, emphasising the developing girl's positive relationship with her own body. In relation to the concept of penis envy, Horney (1924, 1926) supposed that the visibility of the male organ, as opposed to the relative inaccessibility of the vagina for tactile exploration, is responsible for the envious attitude of girl children. Horney (1939) explicitly argued that Freud's libido theory, with its heightened focus on the pleasure-principle,[5] should be superseded by a sociological perspective in which safety was a central motivating factor (Herzog, 2016, p. 26). Within these debates, Freud's (1964a) association of femininity with passivity and masculinity with activity was also widely contested (Birksted-Breen, 1993, p. 5).

In the Freudian framework, recognition of anatomical differences between the sexes is what shapes the development of femininity and masculinity. Yet Freud did not conceive of sexuality as purely biological; he introduced psychosexuality as a psychic process through which individuals negotiate anatomical givens, invest them with meaning, and integrate them into their body-image, ego, superego structures, and object-relations (Birksted-Breen, 1993, p. 3). His psychosexual developmental theory ties drives to object-relations and personality formation. Sexual (libidinal) drives,[6] arising from multiple parts of the body, become organised around particular erogenous[7] zones and differentiate over development towards specific satisfactions through specific aims and objects. These differentiations are classically described through oral, anal, and phallic configurations (Freud, 1953, pp. 125–245; Yadlin-Gadot, 2022; Passos-Ferreira, 2022). In the phallic phase of development, the resolution of the Oedipus complex is understood to unify component instincts[8] of infantile sexuality under the primacy of genital organs and initiate the formation of the superego; understood as emerging via the internalisation of familial, cultural, and social laws (Freud, 1953, pp. 123–246; Yadlin-Gadot, 2022; Passos-Ferreira, 2022). In the phallic phase, drive organisation centres on the phallic organ (clitoris for girls, penis for boys); children of both sexes are understood to engage in phallic masturbation and become preoccupied with anatomical sex differences. For boys, the recognition of anatomical difference carries the meaning that the penis can be absent and lost; for girls, it conveys that something is missing. In Freud's account, the phallus occupies a privileged place in the child's self-image, so any threat to it is experienced not merely as bodily danger but also as a profound psychological injury. The threat of losing the penis for the boy is linked to the prohibition of incest. The girl's lack of the penis leads to penis envy. The castration complex denotes a set of mental processes associated with the recognition of sex differences (Birksted-Breen, 1993, p. 2). Freud attributed distinct functions to the castration complex in each sex. In girls, it is considered to initiate the Oedipus complex, while, in boys, it contributes to its dissolution by enforcing a "prohibition on the maternal object" (Laplanche & Pontalis, 1973, pp. 56–57). The Oedipus complex is characterised by the child's libidinal attachment to the opposite-sex parent and rivalry towards the same-sex parent. Freud outlined different pathways to the resolution of the Oedipus complex in boys and girls.

For boys, the perception of the girl's lack of a penis precipitates castration anxiety, intensified by the fear that the rival father will punish his desire for the mother. The boy, therefore, renounces the mother as love-object and identifies with the father as his ego-ideal, a process that is presumed to support the formation of the superego and inaugurate latency (Freud, 1931; Mitchell & Black, 2016, Chapter 1 and Chapter 8; Laplanche & Pontalis, 1988, pp. 282–287). For girls, Freud described the situation as more complicated. The girl's recognition of difference results in her feeling castrated and inferior. Disappointed with the mother who did not "give" her a penis, she turns to the father as love-object who could offer her a penis. During this process, the girl relinquishes her desire for a penis and redirects it into a wish for a baby from the father. This shift is presumed to mark the initiation of female sexuality, which does not become consolidated until after the latency period, when the vagina becomes invested with libidinal energy in puberty, and adult female sexuality emerges. Freud did not recognise knowledge of the vagina on the girl's part until puberty. Thus, the girl's pathway to femininity, in his view, involves two major transitions: a shift in the leading erotogenic zone from the clitoris to the vagina, and a shift in primary love-object from the mother to the father (Freud, 1964a; Mitchell & Black, 2016, Chapter 1 and Chapter 8; Laplanche & Pontalis, 1988, pp. 55–59, 282–287, 309–310).

Freud (1957a) considered activity–passivity as one of the fundamental polarities that structure mental life, best understood as a feature of an instinct's aim (Laplanche & Pontalis, 1988, pp. 8–9). He proposed that instincts can change their aims from active to passive, such as in sadism and masochism or pleasure derived from "looking at" or "being looked at" (pp. 127–128). He linked the instinct for mastery, the drive towards control and agency, to active aims. Freud (1964a) proposed an opposition between phallic and castrated, male and female, which he brought in relation to sex-specific propensities for active and passive aims. He supposed a constitutionally greater activity in men and more passivity in women. However, he also posited the concept of innate bisexuality – that is, the constitutional endowment in everyone for both masculine and feminine sexual tendencies. These tendencies are thought to become visible in the tensions and struggles involved in taking up one's own sexual and gender identity. In other words, each individual is viewed as encompassing a combination of masculine and feminine characteristics (Laplanche & Pontalis, 1988, p. 52; Birksted-Breen, 1993, pp. 4–5).

As Borgos (2017, 2019) pointed out, Freud's (1925, 1932, 1953, 1964a, 1964b) concepts on psychosexual development were a confluence of reformist and conservative ideas. His concept of innate bisexuality represented a strikingly modern view. But his anatomical determinism in relation to sexual development and superego formation, along with his theories of the castration complex, penis envy, and the universal passivity of the girl, reflected strong patriarchal assumptions of his time. He often oscillated between normative arguments and more subtle propositions regarding sexual difference and gender identity.

As Birksted-Breen (1993, p. 6) argued, in the debates of the 1920s and 1930s, however, many of these subtleties were lost in the interpretations advanced by various Freudian analysts such as Helene Deutsch (1925), Jeanne Lampl-de Groot (1928), and Marie Bonaparte (2018). While Freud described feminine masochistic desires,[9] understood as the child's passive position towards the father and present in both sexes, these analysts, in their search for an 'essential feminine', cast masochism as the defining characteristic of femininity.

Deutsch argued that the active libido of clitoral cathexis[10] is turned into masochism, leading to childbirth being the fundamental gratification of female desire and the epitome of masochistic pleasure (Birksted-Breen, 1993, pp. 6–7). Lampl-de Groot (1928) asserted that the girl needs to overcome a double Oedipus complex where she introjects[11] (internalises) both parental imagos upon which her superego is formed, which in turn contributes to its less energetic, less unified quality compared with the boy's. However, she added that, in achieving this integration, the girl child also exercises her masculinity. She also reported having observed a considerable number of infants of both sexes who exhibited behaviours with both active and passive aims.

Central considerations in these debates addressed the notions of activity and passivity, the presence of early vaginal sensations, and the importance of tactile experiences in the vaginal zone for female psychosexual and, particularly, superego development. Deutsch (1925) suggested that female development includes a vaginal phase, in which the girl is seen as more passive than the boy who, in the phallic phase, is outwardly oriented and takes active pride in his penis. Horney posited that vaginal sexuality precedes clitoral sexuality. She contended that early vaginal sensations in infancy are repressed owing to the girl's fear of punishment and are subsequently transformed into clitoral sexuality (Thompson, 2003, p. 359). Bonaparte (2018), following Freud, argued the significance of anatomical differences and stated that the two pillars of femininity are passivity and bisexuality (Thompson, 2003). She contended that a woman's possession of two interrelated erotogenic organs, the clitoris and the vagina, determines her inherent bisexuality. According to Bonaparte, in the oral phase, infants of both sexes exhibit no difference in activity or passivity. However, in the anal phase, the boy's libido gets projected on to his active muscular system, whereas the girl's centres on her passive cloacal zone.[12] She maintained that, in the subsequent part of the anal phase, both sexes display active, masculine masturbatory behaviour investing the clitoris and penis, respectively, with libidinal energy, while the mother remains the primary love-object. In Bonaparte's view, the castration complex of the girl, arising from the anatomical reality of lacking the phallus, creates the first step towards becoming a woman by accepting the loss of the phallus-clitoris and entering the passive Oedipus complex with the father as the object. This is when the wish for a phallus is converted into a wish for a child. Bonaparte permitted the vagina to have some role in early development but argued that the girl infant does not differentiate between vaginal or clitoral sensations because the cloacal structure is the central organising force of her psychosexual development (Thompson, 2003, pp. 360–361).

Greenacre (1950), based on clinical data of women in psychotic states, also confirmed the existence of early genital tensions in girls. Greenacre (1948) discussed the process of superego formation in both sexes and argued that, although anatomy influences superego and character formation, cultural norms around gender also have neutralising or reinforcing effects. She explained that, in the Oedipal period, children's loosening of their Oedipal attachments to the parent of the opposite sex is reinforced by social pressures and identification with the same-sex parent (Greenacre, 1948). Greenacre linked the genesis of ego and superego development to somatic sensations during the first 18 months of life. In the subsequent phases of habit training, she viewed the toddler as developing further capacities to master bodily impulses and functions. She contended that "body is the greatest part of its own first environment, it seems justified to stress the influence of the reactions within and to it of the developing ego" (Greenacre, 1948, p. 636). She further argued that, in the first year of life, infants expect that the "somato-instinctive urges" arising from their own bodies will be returned on to them (Greenacre, 1948, p. 637). In her view, ego and superego formation are significantly influenced by infants' reactions to their own bodily impulses, including the difference in genital organs and muscular development between the sexes. She highlighted that the difference in superego formation between the sexes is also influenced by the visibility and tactile accessibility of the male genitalia as opposed to the vagina. Endogenous sensations and sensory appreciation intensify awareness of an organ, which, in turn, becomes a more stable part of the body-image. Greenacre (1950) noted that a girl's sense of mystery about her genitalia often persists, at least to some degree, throughout her life. She contested the Freudian view that clitoral sensitivity precedes vaginal sensitivity, arguing that, although vaginal sensations are often too diffuse to elicit masturbatory behaviour, they nevertheless foster vaginal awareness and become incorporated into the female body-image. Greenacre (1950) imagined that these diffuse, early vaginal sensations provide an intuitive knowledge of the vagina as opposed to the tactile and visually concrete experience of the penis for boys. She added that the girl's emotional attachments are also more complicated than the boy's from early childhood onwards. Boys tend to remain firmly attached to the mother until the Oedipal crisis, when the process of renunciation and deferment of libido on to female love objects ensues, and the identification with the father sets in. However, the girl needs to turn from her mother to her father as her main love-object while remaining dependent on the mother's care to fulfil her bodily needs. The girl's love-attachment to the mother and sharper attraction to the father create a continuous division of attachment owing to which her Oedipus complex is less firmly resolved than the boy's. Greenacre (1948, p. 646) also linked the greater affinity for social skills and appreciation of social relationships in girls to this double attachment to the mother and father. Greenacre (1950) asserted that the boy's castration fear facilitates a more complete resolution of the Oedipus complex. In contrast, the girl's experience of penis envy and her denial of anatomical difference, expressed through the wishful hallucinatory assumption of the penis, disrupts her sense of bodily reality. She further suggested that the girl's deferred wish for a penis is redirected into a wish for a child, which may function as compensation for the invisibility of her sexual organ.

In her ideas on female sexual development, Kestenberg (1945, 1954, 1956a, 1956b, 1956c) drew upon the formulations articulated in these earlier debates but expanded them with her own concepts derived from observations of infants and reconstructions of adults. She began formulating her ideas on the subject in the mid-1940s. She presented these at the 283rd meeting of the New York Psychoanalytic Society on 18 December 1945, in her talk entitled "Early Reactions to Tensions" (New York Psychoanalytic Society & Institute, 1937–1945; Kestenberg, 1945). Then, she published her further-developed concepts in a series of papers in 1956, in which she posited early vaginal tensions as the biological basis of femininity and maternity (Kestenberg, 1945, 1956a, 1956c). Kestenberg aligned herself with the Freudian group in their reliance on anatomical determinism, contending that maternity and childbearing constitute the essence of true femininity. Her concept of an *inner-genital* developmental phase closely echoed Deutsch's (1925) notion of the vaginal stage. The influence of Greenacre (1950) is also evident in Kestenberg's work through her emphasis on the tactile accessibility of the genitals, inner vaginal sensations, and the girl's bodily dependence on the caring mother.

Kestenberg's Inner-Genital Phase

> It is true that there are a few isolated reports of early vaginal sensations as well, but it could not be easy to distinguish these from sensations in the anus or vestibulum; in any case, they cannot play a great part. (Freud, 1964a, p. 118)

Kestenberg critiqued the classical Freudian view of feminine development for overlooking the role of the inner genital organs, such as the ovaries and uterus, in psychosexual development, in contrast to its emphasis on the external genitals, namely the clitoris (Kestenberg, 1985). Her position is captured in the following quote:

> The psychoanalytic phase hierarchy conspicuously omits the female phase, while claiming that both sexes pass through the phallic phase, in which the penis or clitoris is the primary erotogenic zone. Femininity is assumed to develop during the positive Oedipal period. This means that the girl must pass through a masculine phase before she can become feminine. (Kestenberg, 1985, p. 117)

Through her focus on bodily sensations and movement, Kestenberg re-examined the psychoanalytic notions of organ activity, argued for the existence of early vaginal tensions, and introduced the idea of an *inner-genital* developmental phase.

Kestenberg (1956b, 1956c) challenged the classical psychoanalytic theory for its lack of precision about what organ activity and passivity mean and how these processes influence psychosexual development. She outlined that, in psychoanalytic theory, an organ is considered active when it is represented as initiating or acting, and passive when it is represented as receiving or acted upon. Organs are understood to acquire psychical prominence through cathectic investment of their psychical representations; where such investment is absent or withdrawn, the organ-representation may remain undeveloped or lose psychical prominence. She added that, at the somatic level, energetic investment and withdrawal are modelled through muscular activity: "Complete relaxation is generally used as a model for passivity. Contraction of muscles with its concomitant innervation and vascularisation serves as a model for activity" (Kestenberg, 1956a, p. 455). She elaborated with precision, reflecting her emerging interest in bodily specifics, that "reception is an active function of the living organism" because the release of muscular tension needed for relaxation and reception is itself initiated. [...] Passive reception is a quality of inanimate objects, determined by their shape" (Kestenberg, 1956a, p. 454). She further emphasised that many bodily organs, such as those involved in vegetative processes, are active continuously without corresponding psychic organ representations.

Kestenberg argued that children understand activity as something visible and movement-producing, such as a moving object. However, activity does not always produce observable movement, such as contractions of the perineal and laminal muscle groups. These become "real" activity only when the individual recognises the sensation as their own and is aware of having produced it. When muscular tensions have reduced activity, such as innervations, they may evoke sensations of pulling, swelling, or diffuse discomfort without the organ's activity being consciously recognised (Kestenberg, 1956a, p. 455). From an ego-psychology perspective, Kestenberg suggested that, in such cases, the organ can become alienated and may be experienced as passive, because these sensations take on the quality of an external force acting upon the ego.

She then inquired whether the vagina is to be considered a passive, uncathected, and psychically non-existent organ before its libidinal investment through manual or hormonal stimulation in puberty. Drawing on her clinical work with children, she maintained that the vagina is not experienced as an organ before puberty, but it exhibits activity well in advance. Like other organs that open to the outside, she argued, it is active from birth and is gradually incorporated into the body-image through ego development. She further proposed that pregenital girls react to vaginal tensions, and that, when such tensions lack a visually graspable locale, they remain without adequate mechanisms for discharge (Kestenberg, 1956c). She explained:

> Such seems to be the feeling arising from latent vaginal activity, prior to its acceptance as an organ, a part of one's own body: a sensation of something being inflicted upon the ego, an inability to discharge tension (identified with an aggressor) and a yearning for relaxation (identified with passive dependence). A swelling of the mucous membranes, a muscle contraction or both create a persistent need for release. (Kestenberg, 1956a, p. 456)

Kestenberg contended that, as a resolution to this problem, the ego, in its struggle for mastery over bodily pressures, seeks mastery over people, through which it gains satisfaction and relaxation of these urges. This manifests in the young girl's wish for a baby and the emergence of maternal behaviour in doll play. These inner genital tensions latently dominate the world of the developing girl. "Yearning for passivity dominates her, but true passivity is only attained with the experience of complete relaxation of genital tension in adulthood" (Kestenberg, 1956a, p. 456). Kestenberg hypothesised that these vaginal tensions could be linked to the infant's body being flooded with maternal hormones in the first month of life, resulting in swelling of the *inner-genital* organs (Kestenberg, 1956c).

In terms of psychosexual stage development, she argued that these early vaginal tensions become absorbed into stage-appropriate developmental drives and add to a general discomfort. She further elaborated that, as girls have less tactile or visual access to their genital organs, they develop organ-constancy later than boys, who discover pleasant sensations arising from the handling of their penis during the first year of life (Kestenberg, 1956a, p. 459). Kestenberg highlighted that the anal phase of the boy is concluded with cathecting his penis, which is demonstrated by the games he plays while peeing. At the same time, in the absence of a fully coherent organ-imagery and organ-concept, the girl projects her libidinal attachment on to an imaginary penis, the doll. She expressed that:

> In the process of experimentation during the anal stage, the girl seems to get a somewhat hazy idea of inside pressure unrelieved by anal manoeuvres. This unrelieved pressure is projected upon the baby at the end of the anal phase. (Kestenberg, 1956a, p. 461)

Building on these formulations, Kestenberg proposed an early maternal stage of development, occurring between approximately 2½ and 4 years of age, in which *inner-genital* sensations are projected on to the baby, which is equated with the body's interior. She described this stage as marked by identification with the mother, extending to boys as well, who may develop nurturing, parental attitudes and show interest in playing with dolls unless such behaviour is explicitly discouraged by the social environment (Kestenberg, 1956a, p. 462). Kestenberg (1956c, pp. 283–285) presupposed abdominal sensations in boys too, arising from the *inner-genital* organ of the prostate, similarly investing the baby doll. She stated that, in boys, the wish for a baby is first directed towards the mother, then towards the father, before transforming into the wish to give a baby to the mother. Kestenberg (1956b, 1956c) further noted that girls often take narcissistic pride in actively caring for a doll and present like busy mothers. She added that, in the *inner-genital* phase, children work through the losses of earlier pregenital phases while integrating bodily changes and their relations to objects. During this time, they become aware of diffuse *inner-genital* tensions that are transient and seem to produce no tangible outcome. By externalising these inner tensions, she suggested, children revive their own lost babyhood by creating a baby of their own.

In her account of the phallic phase in girls, she proposed that inner genital tensions associated with the cathexis of the inner-genital organs are displaced onto the external genitals, such as the clitoris. She described this phase as involving increased masturbatory activity, heightened aggression towards the mother, play with urination, urine retention, and penis envy, alongside the emergence of the negative Oedipus complex in which the father's capacity to please the mother is idealised (Kestenberg, 1956c). According to Kestenberg, this reconciles the girl with the mother, and she comes to compete with the father for her attention. In the next phase of the positive Oedipal phase, sexual drives are redirected towards the father, and masochistic fantasies emerge about being taken by him. During this phase, Kestenberg (1973a, 1956c) described the vaginal region as being treated as non-existent or inanimate; argumentativeness and verbal outbursts function as channels for discharging genital excitations. The girl expects the father to assume responsibility for her longings by seducing her and satisfying her wish for a baby. The father's failure to meet these expectations brings her Oedipus complex to a close. Kestenberg (1956c, p. 471) further suggested that "the girl then enters latency, disappointed in both parents but somewhat less so in the mother"; she therefore identifies with her while retaining her independence. Drawing on her own resources, she is said to seek identification through peer relations with other girls, in groups defined by the exclusion of boys.

Kestenberg (1956c) argued that puberty in girls, marked by the onset of menstruation, reactivates earlier conflicts concerning castration, injury, or the death of the baby (equated with the internal genital organ). As menstrual blood passes through the vaginal opening, she maintained, the vagina can no longer be denied and is fully discovered. She further suggested that menstrual cramps and penetration during intercourse intensify sensations in the vaginal walls, through which the vagina acquires clearer boundaries. In her view, pregnancy and childbirth then serve to compensate for the difficulties involved in mastering the vagina (Kestenberg, 1956c). Kestenberg concluded that the mechanisms underlying the rejection of the vagina and the development of penis envy can be traced to early childhood. She further proposed that maternal feelings are grounded in early, diffuse vaginal tensions, in the limited sensory and perceptual access to their sources, and in the consequent need to transform these urges and project them on to the baby (Kestenberg, 1956b, 1956c). The resolution of these struggles, she contended, relies on the integration of urges from the entire genital region and the acceptance of early bisexuality without shame. Furthermore, Kestenberg (1956a, p. 475) proposed that acceptance of bisexuality serves as a precursor to tolerance and social adjustment between the sexes, as masculine sublimations in women and feminine wishes in men establish the possibility of love and understanding towards the opposite sex, free from guilt and fear.

During a 1964 presentation to the Child Analytic Division of the Washington Institute for Psychoanalysis, Kestenberg expanded on her concept of the *inner-genital phase* and the hormonal changes she proposed underlie this stage (Kestenberg, 1967b). She drew on contemporaneous endocrinological findings suggesting sex-specific hormonal secretion by immature gonads and measurable differences in hormone levels between girls and boys during childhood (Kestenberg, 1967b, p. 579). She supposed an adult-like hormonal state in the neonate, followed by a period when no significant growth occurs in the reproductive organs. She observed that the pregenital phases involve rapid growth of bodily and brain structures, in contrast to the more gradual maturation of the gonads. She then proposed that the subsequent *inner-genital phase* is associated with neurohormonal changes and a degree of psychic instability. Its resolution, she argued, contributes to the integration of pregenital as well as inner- and phallic component drives (Kestenberg, 1967b, p. 587). She posited an increase in androgens during the phallic phase and divided this phase into two subphases: growth and differentiation. She described latency as a period in which drive-discharge becomes more firmly consolidated and inhibitory functions predominate, despite the increased steroid production she associated with this stage. She further proposed that prepuberty begins with the reactivation of the *inner-genital* organs and the emergence of secondary sex characteristics; here, a diffusion of psychic functions coincides with rising sex-specific hormone production. Then, puberty follows with the maturation of the gonads (Kestenberg, 1967b).

In "Outside and Inside, Male and Female" (1968), Kestenberg elaborated on the interplay between the inside and outside of the body in relation to the development of sex-specific identity. She proposed that, for both sexes, early diffuse *inner-genital* sensations generate anxiety and are managed through processes of externalisation, denial, or projection. In boys, development is characterised by a shift from these unsettling visceral experiences towards an outwardly directed, phallic orientation that supports differentiation, ego control, and adaptation to reality. In her view, male sexuality, therefore, becomes organised around externalisation, muscular activity, and the visible phallus, with *inner-genital* sensations largely repudiated or displaced. By contrast, she described female sexuality as inwardly oriented, grounded in diffuse, visceral, spreading vaginal sensations. Kestenberg (1968) argued that women's mature genital organisation requires substantial early priming and, in adulthood, synchronisation with a partner to integrate inner and outer genital drive configurations. In her view, orgasm, for both sexes, entails a temporary dissolution of boundaries between inside and outside, self and object, but, still, she supposed that women are more vulnerable to ego dissolution owing to the more diffuse quality of their *inner-genital* sensations. Kestenberg framed male development as moving towards external mastery and continuity of control. In contrast, female development culminates in the acceptance of inward orientation, with the balance of inner and outer genitality shaping sexual fulfilment, partner relations, and the integration of adult identity.

Kestenberg (1973a) also associated specific affective states in women with the unsuccessful neutralisation of *inner-genital* drives, drawing on her analysis of three adult women. She identified recurring patterns of nagging, excitement, and argumentativeness in interactions with men, which she attributed to childhood experiences of swelling and throbbing *inner-genital* sensations. She proposed that these so-called "feminine moods" correspond in their intensity contours to the kinaesthetic intensity contours of *inner-genital* tensions, which originate during the transitional stage between pregenital and phallic development. In her view, nagging reflects efforts to manage persistent inner tensions; the spreading of excitement corresponds to sensations of swelling and uncontrollable waves of arousal experienced as threatening to bodily integrity; and argumentativeness is linked to the projection of forbidden wishes and guilt on to men. She (Kestenberg, 1973a, p. 297) argued that, in adolescence, renewed genital sensations and revived Oedipal fantasies intensify these moods and may persist into adulthood despite greater integrative capacities.

Psychoanalytic Studies in Movement

Besides her concepts on the developmental significance of *inner-genital* sensations, Kestenberg's significant contributions were her psychodynamic vocabulary and theory of movement. Her project was special in its methodology, which she borrowed from dance studies; however, her specific interest in movement studies was not entirely unprecedented within psychoanalysis. Several psychoanalysts examined aspects of bodily movement; but, these efforts never coalesced into a unified psychoanalytic approach to movement behaviour until Kestenberg's work.

In early psychoanalytic thought, movement behaviour was conceptualised in various ways, such as an expression of sexual drives (Abraham, 1913; Freud, 1953; Reich, 1945; Ferenczi, 1952a, 1952b, 1955, 1994a, 1994b, 1994c); as an executive function of the ego (Freud, 1925, 1957a); as an instrument of defence (Deutsch, 1947, 1952; Reich, 1945); as both a vehicle and potential source of aggression (Freud, 1957b; Hartmann et al., 1949); and as a means of overcoming anxiety by converting passive experience into active engagement (Freud, 1975). The issues of tension, excitation, and discharge occurred often in Freud's writings, with not only their neuropsychological underpinnings but also accompanying movement data (Breuer & Freud, 1895/1955; Freud, 1925, 1953, 1961). Changes in muscle tension observable in body movements and their relation to affective and ideational states were within the focus of Breuer and Freud's *Studies on Hysteria* (1895/1955). They examined activity types and attributed individual differences to constitutional variations in the nervous system and temperament (Breuer, 1895/1955, p. 198). Without a systemic focus on movement, Freud made several significant contributions to the psychoanalytic interpretation of motility. Observing his grandchild, he interpreted the movements during play as attempts to turn his passive experience of separation from his mother into an active one (Freud, 1975, pp. 14–16). In *Three Essays* (1953), he wrote that "children feel a need for a large amount of active muscular exercise and derive extraordinary pleasure from satisfying it" (p. 202). He also highlighted the close relationship between movement and aggression in his following statement: "One of the roots of the sadistic instinct would seem to lie in the encouragement of sexual excitation by muscular activity" (1953, p. 203). In *The Ego and the Id*, he stated that the ego "is first and foremost a bodily ego" and assigned the "control over the approaches to motility" to the structure of the ego (Freud, 1961, pp. 25–26). He also discussed shadow movements, small, fidget-like actions performed on the body or on clothing as symptomatic acts (Freud, 1960).

Ferenczi (1994c) considered the function of tics to be a motor defence, an active flight from unbearable external stimuli. He also assumed a connection between muscle tension and emotional expression. Ferenczi (1952a, p. 231) observed the links between motility and ideational process, noting that people inhibit movement to think, while others may increase motility to deal with the overflow of ideas. He (1952b) also associated motor behaviour and the formation of the infant's gesture-language with the development of the ego, the sense of reality.

Contemporaneously with Kestenberg, in the 1950s, a few psychoanalysts took to the systematic study of movement behaviour. Their work not only expanded theoretical understanding of bodily movement and its therapeutic relevance but also proposed methodologies for its analysis. Felix Deutsch (1952) published case studies on changes in postural behaviour observed during long-term analytic therapy. He contended that "postural pattern appears as signal and symbol during the analytic process, preceding, substituting or accompanying verbal expressions" (1952, p. 197). He added that the movement observer must recognise that motor reactions in specific body parts are reflected throughout the entire body and become integrated into overall functioning. According to Deutsch, a psychic stimulus pressing for discharge activates muscular movement, which may in turn produce changes in posture. He understood these changes as completing the psychic process. Deutsch (1952) contended that voluntary musculature is synchronised with the demands of both the conscious and unconscious ego, and that asynchronous postural patterns signal a loss of ego control. He argued that the motivation for movement is inseparably linked to unconscious innervations, which generate proprioceptive stimuli that trigger movements subsequently regulated by the ego, which determines whether they are carried out or not. He added that the timing and manner of execution are specific expressions of ego control.

Margaret Fries and Paul Woolf (1954) investigated the relationship between congenital activity types and personality development. They defined congenital activity type as "a descriptive term, referring to the amount of activity a newborn infant shows in response to certain stimuli" (Fries & Wolf, 1954, p. 47). They stated that some aspects of the excitability of the neuromuscular system are the result of inheritance and intrauterine life, and other aspects are shaped by temporary bodily changes during birth, growth, emotional state, and parental emotional attitudes towards the infant. These combine into a "congenital rather than an inherited tendency to react to the environment in a characteristic manner which may be described according to activity type" (Fries & Woolf, 1954, pp. 47–48; Fries, 1944). In their view, *Congenital Activity Type* is a constitutional factor that plays an important role in the discharge of drives and in the development of the ego and superego. In relation to drive-discharge and id processes, they argued that, throughout development, different parts of the body become cathected to varying degrees, which may account for differences in libidinisation later in life. According to their observations, the *Congenital Activity Type* significantly shapes a child's approaches to reality testing and mastery, thereby affecting ego development.

Bela Mittelmann (1899–1959) examined normal and abnormal development of motility and its influence on psychosexual development (Schur, 1960). He argued that tactile, visual, and motor exploration of the body serves the mastery and differentiation of self-and-not-self in infancy (Mittelmann, 1960). He added that the influence of movement development on psychic development is most significant during the first 2 years of life and, to a lesser extent, remains until the age of 10. The first years of life, he argued, are characterised by a surge in self-assertion and aggression, gradually growing independence, and the translation of impulses into activity, reflected in affectomotor patterns of joy (clapping hands together), the predominance of motility-based language in communication, and, lastly, motor identifications with others. He further asserted that the second year of life is the motor phase of ego and libidinal development, as movement is the most dominant mode of mastery and pleasure-seeking (Mittelmann, 1957).

Mittelmann (1960) proposed a classification of movement patterns according to their psychic functions. He distinguished between id-derivative patterns, including those associated with object-relations and pleasure-seeking; ego-derivative movements, serving reality testing, mastery, communication, and integration; and superego derivatives, related to the formation of conscience and ideals. He argued that voluntary movements are among the most important means of reality testing and are, thus, an essential indicator of ego development and functioning. Mittelmann (1960) distinguished between adaptive and non-adaptive forms of motility. He further divided the non-adaptive category into reflexes, random movements, expressive movements, affectomotor patterns, and autoerotic movements. According to him, non-adaptive motility predominates during intrauterine life and the first 6 months after birth. Within this category, he identified autoerotic movements, such as rhythmic rocking, bouncing, or jumping, as forms of primary-process motility aimed at gratifying instinctual urges (Mittelmann, 1960, p. 113). Mittelmann considered non-adaptive motility to be the basis upon which voluntary movements develop, such as the "grasping reflex is a precursor of later voluntary grasping" (1960, p. 109). He further noted that random movements, which often occur in the limbs, have their antecedents in intrauterine motility and serve pleasure-seeking through the satisfaction of motor urges. These patterns are gradually displaced by more advanced patterns, such as turning, crawling, object manipulation, and expressive gestures. Mittelmann (1960) linked the category of expressive movements to changes in voluntary muscles associated with experiences of pleasure and displeasure, such as crying or smiling. He emphasised that these responses display considerable individual variation from a motor perspective. Mittelmann (1960) stressed that observation of bodily movement can reveal underlying motivational forces, such as aggressive or libidinal drives, and may reflect organisation of defences, immediate affective responses, and regressions.

Kestenberg built on classical psychoanalytic perspectives from Freud (Breuer & Freud, 1895/1955; Freud, 1925, 1953), Ferenczi (1952a, 1952b, 1955, 1994a, 1994b, 1994c), and Abraham (1913), who linked pleasure-seeking, drive-discharge, defences, ego development, and movement behaviour. Kestenberg incorporated Deutsch's (1947, 1952) clinical data on parallels between psychic and postural change; Fries and Woolf's (1954) notion of congenital activity types; and Mittelmann's (1957, 1960) formulations on the motor urge, the connection between rhythmic movements and drive-discharge, ego and motor development, and some of his classifications of movement behaviour. Sossin (personal communication, 18 November 2025) noted that Kestenberg greatly respected Mittelmann. They were both affiliated with Bellevue Hospital, though a few years apart. Despite their shared interest in the psychoanalytic study of movement, no correspondence between them has been found, possibly owing to Mittelmann's untimely death in 1959. While Kestenberg's (1965a, 1965b, 1967a, 1967b) work on movement is closely aligned with Mittelmann's, her project adopted a significantly different approach to classifying movement. Kestenberg applied Rudolf von Laban's movement theory and categorised bodily movement by its dynamic, structural, and qualitative features, as opposed to Mittelmann's method of function-based categorisations.

Laban's Movement Theory

When Kestenberg began her infant observation studies (Kestenberg, n.d.a, 1965a; Kestenberg & Freud, 1955–1969), she did not have a method to record changes in bodily movement. In the early 1950s, she devised her own method to document changes in muscle tension, which she called the *Tension-Flow Curve* (this will be discussed in detail in the section on her methodology). However, she felt the need to undertake further training in movement studies. Following the recommendation of dancer Maria Pescator, she began studying Labanotation, a movement notation technique developed by Rudolf von Laban (1879–1958). She initially learned this system from Irmgard Bartenieff, a Laban-trained German émigré dancer who later became a pioneer in American dance/movement therapy. In 1961, she continued her training through a correspondence course with Warren Lamb, a London-based management consultant, movement researcher, and former student of Laban (Kestenberg, n.d.b, 1975a, 1992a). In 1965, accompanied by Bartenieff, Kestenberg visited Lamb in London and pursued additional training with another London-based Laban disciple, Marion North.

Kestenberg also developed an interest in body-awareness techniques. Between 1967 and 1978, she trained in the Alexander Technique,[13] yoga, shiatsu,[14] and the psycho-tactile therapy of Volkmar Glaser (1912–1997) in Germany (Kestenberg, n.d.b). These studies attest to her strong determination to acquire an in-depth understanding of bodily movement. It also marked her move beyond the professional circles of psychiatry and psychoanalysis into the world of movement research and dance, a shift that would later yield some of the most fruitful collaborations of her career. To further contextualise Kestenberg's approach to bodily movement, it is necessary to briefly review Laban's movement theories, on which she grounded her conceptualisations.

Laban, an Austro-Hungarian dancer, choreographer, and dance thinker, devised a dance notation system, Labanotation, in the first decades of the twentieth century. He aimed to equip dance with a standardised means of inscription comparable to a musical score. He anchored this notation system in his movement theories that stressed the reciprocity of body and mind, proposing that movement not only expresses inner states but can also shape and transform them. Laban contended that bodily engagement with abstract physical forms, tensions, efforts, and spatial dimensions activates unconscious psychic work that generates movement ideas and elicits feelings. The elicited somatoaffective state is the manifest result of the unconscious impulse that produced the gesture, which not only affects the mover but also has an influence on others through its expressive quality (Ruprecht, 2015, p. 29). Laban further maintained that gestures directly influence another person's nervous system and viewed dance as curative not only at the individual level but also at the collective, societal level (Laemmli, 2016, pp. 41–42).

Ruprecht (2015, p. 28) characterised Laban as a theorist of gestural flow, a flow that he derived from a continuous current of vibratory energy. His vitalist approach understood gesture and expressivity not as confined to isolated body parts but as belonging to the body as a whole and as extending to the wider dynamism of all living phenomena (Ruprecht, 2015; Laemmli, 2016, p. 41). Laban's thinking drew on early twentieth-century psychophysical research, including Bell's distinction between sensory and motor nerves, Lange's (Lange & James, 1922) studies linking specific emotions to specific physiological changes, and Langley's[15] (1921) work on the autonomic nervous system (Laemmli, 2016, p. 35). Bell[16] proposed a reciprocity between motor nerves and emotionality based on his observation that the same motor nerves are activated during fast breathing and states of anxiety. He contended that sensory nerves provided information about the material world, informing cognition, and motor nerves were the instruments of emotional expression (Laemmli, 2016, p. 33). Lange[17] likewise proposed that emotions are accompanied by distinct bodily markers, such as the narrowing and widening of blood vessels (Lange & James, 1922). Laban synthesised these ideas with Langley's division of the autonomic nervous system into sympathetic and parasympathetic branches. As sympathetic activity was associated with heightened arousal (e.g., increased heart rate, reduced digestion, increased blood flow), Laban linked it to defensive, differentiating, or withdrawing actions; conversely, he associated parasympathetic activity with expansive, expressive, outwards-oriented movement (Laemmli, 2016, pp. 36–37).

These psychophysiological considerations informed his concepts of *Free* and *Bound Flow*, which referred to the continuous flow of activity and energy in the muscles during movement. In *Free Flow*, the movers appear (and through the principle of reciprocity also experience themselves as) mobile, active, outwardly oriented, and expressive. In *Bound Flow*, the mover seems to focus on stabilisation, disengagement, and self-discipline. Laban distinguished between *Choreutics* (movement pathways in space) and *Eukinetics* (movement dynamics), the latter forming the basis of his *Effort* theory (Laban, 1950, 1954, 1926/2008; Fügedi, 2015). Laban related his notion of *Effort* to the German term *Antrieb*: the organism's drive to make itself known (Bartenieff & Lewis, 2013, p. 51). Laban's system of *Effort* was defined by four motion factors, *Flow, Weight, Time*, and *Space*, which essentially represent the basic qualitative parameters of human movement. He proposed that each motion factor encompasses a spectrum of opposing qualities, such as *Free* and *Bound*

Flow, Light and *Strong Weight, Sustained* and *Quick Time*, and *Indirect* or *Direct Space*. These qualities described how the mover engaged with the physicality of action and served as key descriptors of bodily movement. Laban related *Flow* to the movers' qualitative investment in continuity, *Weight* to the movers' use of gravity and their own body weight, and *Space* to the movers' attention to their bodily and external space; *Time* denoted the movers' use of time and periodicity during movement (Laban & Lawrence, 1947; Wahl, 1984, pp. 93–97). After emigrating to Britain in the late 1930s, Laban began experimenting with new applications of his movement theories and notation. He applied these in the field of workflow optimisation for large factories struggling with a labour shortage of men during the war (Laemmli, 2016, p. 91, 2022). Lamb extended Laban's ideas into his systems of *Effort–Shape* analysis, which focused on how *Effort* qualities relate to spatial *Shaping* patterns in bodily movement. He argued that individuals exhibit consistent preferences in *Shaping* and *Effort* within their movement repertoires, which he viewed as revealing characteristic individual attitudes (Laban & Lawrence, 1947; Lamb & Watson, 1979; Wahl, 1984; Laemmli, 2016).

Kestenberg drew extensively on these concepts while formulating her developmental theory of movement. From Laban, she adopted the category of *Efforts* and his spatial theory organised around the three spatial planes. Kestenberg expanded Laban's concept of *Flow* through her own categories of *Attributes* and *Rhythms of Tension-Flow*. From Lamb, she took the principle of affinity between *Shaping* and *Effort* and applied it to the relationship between her categories of *Shape-Flow* and *Tension-Flow*. Her system thus integrates Laban's *Effort* theory with Lamb's *Effort–Shape* analysis, grounding and refining both through her infant-observation data. Kestenberg developed her category of *Shape-Flow* in parallel with Bartenieff, who was working on her own expansions of Laban's system (Bartenieff & Lewis, 2013). By integrating these movement concepts with psychoanalytic developmental theory, Kestenberg formulated her psychodynamic vocabulary of movement, which I introduce in detail in the following sections.

Kestenberg's Psychodynamic Vocabulary of Movement

The Flow of Muscle Tension

> Although both academic and psychoanalytic developmental psychology are based in good part on observation of motor behaviour, no systematic study of rhythms of motor discharge has been attempted. (Kestenberg, 1965a, p. 3)

Kestenberg's engagement with movement was shaped during her internship at the Adult and Child Psychiatry Department of Bellevue Hospital from 1937 to 1939, where she worked under the supervision of Paul Schilder (1886–1940). Schilder's research on body-image and the development of perception and thought, especially his focus on the relationship between psychic and organic processes, had a significant impact on Kestenberg's concepts (Schilder, 1942, 1950/2013). Schilder (1942, p. 85) argued that, owing to the close connection between the vestibular labyrinth (the sensory organ in the inner ear that controls balance and spatial orientation) and the autonomic nervous system (which regulates involuntary bodily functions), shifts in psychological states are reflected in changes in vestibular sensations, muscle tone, and posture. Schilder (1942) also proposed that rhythmic tendencies in movement and muscle tone reflect instinctual processes that belong to the realm of the id (pp. 28–29). Kestenberg conceptualised this connection within her category of *Tension-Flow*.

Drives in psychoanalysis are somatically based, need-derived forces that generate tensions in the mind (Csabai & Erős, 2000). Kestenberg sought to specify the qualitative, motor aspects of these pressures as expressed in the qualities and rhythms of muscle tension flow (Kestenberg, 1965a, 1965b). She formulated her concept of *Tension-Flow* as a synthesis of the Freudian life and death drives and Laban's notion of *Free* and *Bound Flow* (Freud, 1975; Kestenberg, 1965a, 1985). As discussed before, the *Flow* factor in Laban's theory pertained to the lack of constraint and the freeing of energy that mobilises the body, creating a continuous flow of movement. Consequently, binding *Flow* refers to the introduction of restraint, producing contained, stabilising movements or interruptions in the continuity of movement. Kestenberg (1965a) further clarified that *Free* and *Bound Flow* in muscle tension refer to the level of activation and interplay between agonist and antagonist muscle groups throughout movement. She explained that, at rest, there is a balance between agonist and antagonist muscles. Movement begins when this balance is disrupted. Increased participation of antagonistic muscles results in greater opposition and restraint of movement – which is perceived as inhibited – which denotes *Bound Flow*. Conversely, reduced simultaneous contraction of antagonistic muscles – perceived as realising unhampered movement – is referred to as *Free Flow*. Therefore, *Free Flow* is defined as the contraction of agonist muscles, allowing mobilisation; *Bound Flow* is the simultaneous contraction of agonist and antagonist muscle groups, enabling restraint and stabilisation in movement (Kestenberg, 1965b). She considered these the most fundamental qualities of muscle tension and equated *Free* and *Bound Flow* with Freud's concepts of pleasure and unpleasure, as well as with the life and death instincts. Freud (1975) argued that life instincts are binding forces and death instincts are unbinding forces. Similarly, for Kestenberg, *Free Flow* of muscle tension embodies the vital quality of organic life, oriented towards survival through opening, mobilising, incorporating, and connecting with the external world. In contrast, *Bound Flow* represents the pursuit of survival through withdrawal, separation, differentiation, and immobilisation in the face of overwhelming threat (Kestenberg, 1965b). Consequently, Kestenberg linked the release of tension in *Free Flow* with serving libidinal aims and the concentration of tension through *Bound Flow* with attending to the aims of the sadistic, aggressive drive. Kestenberg and Sossin (1979) later clarified that purely sadistic manifestations of drive-discharge in movement do not exist. Those that are termed sadistic are instead a mix of sadistic-libidinal tendencies, with the predominance of the aggressive drive-discharge.

Freud (1964b, p. 160) argued that pleasure and unpleasure could not be defined solely by changes in the quantity of tension but rather by qualitative changes. He emphasised that developing a method to measure this qualitative aspect of tension would represent a significant advance for psychology. He (1964b) further contemplated that the specific factor of tension, which qualifies it as pleasure or unpleasure, may lie in the rhythmic properties of its increase or decrease in intensity, or in the temporal factors of its rise and fall. This is precisely the question that Kestenberg addressed through her concepts of Tension-Flow *Attributes* and *Rhythms* (Kestenberg, 1965a).

In addition to the basic motor patterns of pleasure and unpleasure, *Free* and *Bound Flow*, Kestenberg devised further attributes of *Flow* pertaining to various qualitative dimensions of the changes observable in muscle tension. These conveyed the frequency, the rate of change, and the degree of intensity. These dimensions of the *Attributes of Tension-Flow* denote the qualitative features through which Kestenberg describes the binding or release of muscle tension. Degree of intensity refers to the level of intensity in the muscle tension without describing its quality (Kestenberg, 1965b). For instance, a *High Intensity Tension-Flow Attribute* may characterise the intensity contour of heightened states of anger as well as joy. Frequency of change denotes high fluctuation in muscle tension, named *Flow Adjustment*, or a low amount or absence of fluctuations, named *Even Flow* (when the tension in the muscles is held evenly during movement). Rate of change connotes the temporal factors involved in changes in tension, which could be embodied in *Abrupt* or *Gradual* changes in muscle tension (Kestenberg, 1965b). This dimension reflects the temporal contour of affect. *Graduality*, for example, indicates a progressive trajectory of increase or decrease, as experienced, for instance, during mourning or in the steady build-up of arousal before going on stage. Kestenberg interpreted the *Attributes of Tension-Flow* as reflecting temperament and basic affective responses to pleasure and displeasure. They do not denote discrete emotions but, rather, the subtle physiological-affective states that underlie them (Kestenberg, 1965b). In other words, Kestenberg's *Tension-Flow Attributes* are qualities of affects. *Free Flow* represents a carefree state as opposed to the degree of inhibition in *Bound Flow*; the quality of *Even Flow* accompanies consistent states, as opposed to the *Adjusting Flow* of changing attitudes; *High Intensity* refers to a heightened state of affect (such as elevated states of joy or anger), whereas *Low Intensity* signifies a low-key, perhaps disinterested, state; *Abrupt* denotes a sudden, as opposed to a *Gradual*, change in affect. To these basic attributes, Kestenberg and Sossin (1979) added *Neutral Flow*, defined as a diminished vitality in the flow of muscle tension, commonly observed in fatigue, illness, altered states of consciousness, and dissociation.

Kestenberg (1965b) observed that the *Tension-Flow Attributes* she identified seem to occur in specific constellations in movement, and, when their co-occurrences show distinct periodicity, she argued, they constitute *Tension-Flow Rhythms.* She identified characteristic configurations of these rhythms during periods of excitation, gratification, and relaxation (Kestenberg, 1965a, 1965b). Furthermore, she observed that certain *Tension-Flow Rhythms* become dominant at particular stages of development. Synthesising these observations with Freudian psychosexual phases,[18] she linked rhythmic patterns to oral, anal, and phallic component drives. Kestenberg (1965b) suggested that the various *Tension-Flow Rhythms* are the motor expressions of basic needs and drives across psychosexual development.

The earliest iteration of Kestenberg's *Tension-Flow Rhythms* included oral *Sucking* and *Biting Rhythm*, the *Anal Sphincter Play* and *Anal Defecatory Rhythm*, and the *Phallic* (masturbatory-type) *Rhythms* (Kestenberg, 1965a). She defined the oral *Sucking Rhythm* as the smooth, continuous alternation between *Free* and *Bound Flow* seen in breastfeeding and thumb-sucking behaviour of neonates. The oral *Biting Rhythm* refers to a rhythmic pattern with a sharp accent seen in the biting, chewing, or clapping of a baby. *Anal Sphincter Play* rhythms are characterised by the repetition of *Adjusting and Low Intensity* muscle tension and are observable in spine-rotation movements during crawling or floor shuffling, as well as in squiggly, comfort-seeking movements, such as snuggling up to the caregiver. She suggested that *Anal Defecatory Rhythms* are characterised by tension changes in the abdominal muscles during defecation, such as *Abrupt* changes between *High* and *Low Intensity* and *Evenly* held plateaus in between. Phallic masturbatory rhythms, she noted, utilise *Abrupt* changes between *Low Intensity Free Flow* and *High Intensity Bound Flow* of muscle tension and are visible in masturbatory jumping, hopping, and pelvic thrusts (Kestenberg, 1965a). Based on her observations of the three infants, Kestenberg concluded that individual preferences for modes of drive-discharge are reflected in preferences for rhythmic qualities of *Tension-Flow* in infancy. She highlighted that maturational processes and environmental factors can alter rhythmic preferences, and that early developmental disturbances may result from conflicts between the rhythmic preferences of mother and infant. She cautioned against assuming that the study of rhythmic movement alone could account for the role of motility in development, suggesting that early adaptive responses to physical aspects of reality, such as *Space, Weight*, and *Time*, modify early rhythmicity (Kestenberg, 1965a). Recognising how external reality shapes bodily movement and alters the rhythmic expressions of drive-discharge, she developed her concepts of *Efforts.*

From Tension to Effort, From Id to Ego

In her early publications, Kestenberg (1946, 1950, 1953) considered the movement-based indicators of basic ego functions and the transition from primary- to secondary-processes.[19] In her paper, "Early Fears and Early Defences" (1946), she drew attention to patterns of movement that can be linked to the development of defences. She posited that the two most basic forms of defence were increasing (*Free Flow*) and inhibiting (*Bound Flow*) muscle tension (Kestenberg, 1946, pp. 65–66). She added that this preliminary motor control, manifested in the ability to contract muscles, later allows for the execution of goal-directed movements (Kestenberg et al., 1971, pp. 750–755). In "*Notes on Ego Development*," Kestenberg (1950, 1953) described a dynamic interplay between ego functions and the formation of the earliest defence mechanisms, tracing the transition from id to ego and from primary- to secondary-processes. She argued that bodily movement reveals an observable developmental line from id to pre-ego and ego and, with this formulation, she challenged a central concept in ego-psychology at the time: Hartmann's autonomous sphere of the ego. Deviating from Freud's (1961) proposition that the ego, structurally, is a differentiated part of the id emerging from the conflict between wish-fulfilment and the demands of reality, Hartmann et al. (1946) proposed that the ego and the id emerge from an early undifferentiated state in postnatal life, and that the ego has an inborn basis. This grounds the ego's primary autonomy, as it is not brought into existence by dynamic conflict with instinctual forces. Hartmann (1958) further posited that the ego's autonomous sphere encompasses perception, motility, and memory, which, once differentiated, form the ego's main control apparatus.

Kestenberg (1953) argued that primary-processes dominate the earliest forms of defence and belong to the pre-ego. In contrast, basic ego functions operate under secondary-processes and are, therefore, assigned to the ego. She explained that, in the classical view, the id consists solely of free energy, while the ego can bind or release energy. She, however, argued that the id may contain precursors of binding insofar as it functions as a reservoir that stores archaic heritage. The key distinction, as Kestenberg (1953) explained, is that the ego exercises selective control over what to bind and what to discharge. She further elaborated that inertia is a defining feature of the id as it stores unrepressed material – such as inherited modes of response to somatic stimuli (reflexes) – that never presses for discharge and remains disconnected from, and does not function under, its control. Kestenberg concluded that such inertia of the id is, in fact, the foundation of the ego's inhibitory function. These propositions were supported by her clinical data, which indicated that the body, "including the nervous system, not only generates tensions within the id but also provides the basic motor apparatus for the pre-ego's control functions" (Kestenberg, 1953, p. 117). Freud (1957b) viewed the motor apparatus of the id as consisting only of organic reflexes. Kestenberg (1953) added that inhibition plays a central role in basic reflexes, suggesting that somatic imprints of rudimentary inhibitory patterns are present in the id and carry forwards into the ego. She proposed that these early motor patterns are gradually transformed by maturation and external demands, giving rise to the basic ego function of repression. Thus, Kestenberg maintained that the ego is an extension of the id (a proposition for which Heinz Hartmann reportedly labelled her neurotic) (Kestenberg, 1953, 1992a, p. 183).

In her description of the transition from primary- to secondary-processes, Kestenberg noted that, initially, infants respond to unpleasant stimuli with nonspecific discharge (e.g., crying, increased motility), nonspecific withdrawal (e.g., sleep), or displacement. These are reactions characteristic of the primary-process. However, as external reality intervenes, it introduces new opportunities for gratification that interrupt the free flow of mobilising energy from nonspecific discharge and direct it towards specific aspects. This shift enables the development of specific discharge to specific stimuli, better adapted to the demands of reality. Kestenberg (1953) further elaborated that external demands compel the infant to engage in specific actions to obtain gratification, necessitating the binding of energy. This process involves the emergence of basic ego functions belonging to secondary-processes. She exemplified this by arguing that the mother turning the baby's head towards the breast to take in food becomes a prototype for later specific reactions with a quality of 'taking in' such as turning towards love objects and opening arms in anticipatory gestures towards others. Kestenberg further suggested that condensing different aspects of a gratifying situation into a psychosomatic unit, such as a bodily movement, may constitute the infant's earliest attempt to bind energy. Over time, the child gradually relinquishes this rudimentary form of condensation and transforms it into ideation. Kestenberg (1953, p. 120) clarified that, through contact with reality, condensation evolves from an unspecific fusion to specific conceptualisation. Based on these formulations, she identified the motor-specificities of ego development and the transition from the predominance of primary-processes to secondary-processes in development through her concepts of *Pre-Efforts* and *Efforts* (Kestenberg, 1965b, 1967a).

As mentioned previously, Kestenberg designated muscle *Tension-Flow Rhythms* and *Attributes* as vehicles of drive-discharge and affects. She observed that, with maturation, initial rhythmic behaviour is incorporated into more complex movement patterns (Kestenberg, 1965b). She suggested that the motor patterns used in the regulation of drives to meet the demands of reality are closely related to the ego (Kestenberg, 1965b). She termed these ego-derived patterns *Pre-Efforts* and *Efforts.* She argued that these patterns are observable when muscle tension flow is controlled to meet a specific goal-directed, adaptive aim. Kestenberg clarified that, in *Pre-Efforts* and *Effort*, the dominance of the reality principle[20] becomes observable through the mover's clearly discernible orientation or engagement with physical aspects of reality. These physical dimensions of external reality were: *Space, Weight*, and *Time* (Kestenberg, 1965b). A movement dealing with these aspects of reality meant for Kestenberg that the action employed advanced temporal structures, negotiated aspects of weight (of the mover's body and objects), and traversed space along a specific constellation of pathways. For example, when throwing a ball to someone, a person needs to keep the (muscle) *Tension-Flow* in their arms *Bound* and *Even* to keep their arm on course, aiming at a specific point in space. Channelling (*Pre-Effort* element) in space is the external goal for which the quality of muscle-tension (*Bound Flow* and *Even Flow*) is selectively chosen, thus adapted. In other words, adaptations to physical aspects of reality (*Space, Weight*, and *Time*) lead to careful selection and regulation of *Tension-Flow Attributes*, and the qualitative aspects of actions, such as how a movement is executed, become adapted to questions of "where, what and when" (Kestenberg, 1967a, p. 378).

Kestenberg (1965b, 1985) understood *Precursors of Efforts* to reflect emergent ego-functions learning to mediate between inner impulses and the external demands of reality. She contended that these patterns are most often used in unfamiliar situations, when one still needs to learn to master the given task. *Tension-Flow Attributes* regulate affective internal states, but, when a situation requires adaptation to the external world, especially in an unfamiliar situation, *Precursors of Efforts* come to regulate the *Attributes of Tension-Flow*. She argued that these situations demand simultaneous internal focus and external goal orientation – for example, a child learning to write cursive or trying to regulate overwhelming emotions in a situation where their expression would not be accommodated (in both, one may discern the physical expression of internal concentration alongside an awareness of an external situation or goal). Kestenberg explained the transition from emergent ego functions to mastery through the progression from *Pre-Efforts* to *Efforts*. Once mastery of a task is achieved, *Effort* qualities come to dominate the execution of the task, which she understood as motor patterns reflecting advanced mechanisms of coping, personal styles of learning, and problem-solving (Kestenberg, 1965b, 1967b, 1985).

She considered *Precursors of Efforts* less adaptable than *Efforts* because they remain more beholden to internal states than to external demands. For instance, when hurrying because of anxiety, a person may use the *Pre-Effort* quality of *Suddenness*. Yet abrupt movements only create the feeling of being fast; alone, they may not resolve the problem of limited time. A more mature sequence, in Kestenberg's view, would involve the *Effort* quality of *Deceleration* (measured as slowing down), organising thoughts and planning, followed by controlled *Acceleration*, leading to more adaptive management of time constraints. Thus, for Kestenberg, *Pre-Effort* denotes rudimentary attempts at coping, while *Effort* qualities represent advanced adaptive strategies. Kestenberg (1965b) outlined the developmental and structural relationship between *Tension-Flow* and *Pre-Effort* and *Effort* in the following way:

> The various rhythms of tension flow seen in the neonate become differentiated in such a way that pure rhythms serve localised drive-discharge and modified rhythms are used in drive-derivative functioning as apparatus of secondary autonomy. Methods of flow regulation derive their style from the elements and attributes of rhythms from which they evolve. Selectivity in flow becomes differentiated with progressive

> development of the ego's control over expression of affect. [...] Developmental trends overlap and interact in such a way that patterns of tension-flow reflect changing constellations of drives, while patterns of Effort subordinate the flow of tension to their adaptive aims and reflect transitory and permanent ego attitudes to the world in which we live. (Kestenberg, 1965b, p. 544)

The structural relationship between id-derivative (*Tension-Flow*) and ego-controlled (*Pre-Efforts* and *Efforts*) patterns rests on Kestenberg's rule of affinity or harmony. The adaptive selection of an affined (harmonious) muscle *Tension-Flow* quality for a given external aim denotes harmonious intrapsychic functioning, whereas clashes between activated *Tension-Flow* and *Pre-Effort–Effort* patterns within a single movement reveal intrapsychic conflict[21] between drive aim and the ego's adaptive mediation of it according to external demands. Kestenberg's rule of affinity postulated that drive-derivative *Tension-Flow* patterns were classified as libidinal or sadistic (depending on their aims), while ego-derivative patterns were distinguished as indulging or aggressive.

Thus, sadistic *Tension-Flow* patterns are considered affined with aggressive *Effort* elements, and libidinal *Tension-Flow* is compatible with indulging *Pre-Efforts* and *Efforts* (Kestenberg & Sossin, 1979). For instance, *Even Flow* of *Tension* corresponds with *Direct Effort* in *Space*, as when holding muscle tension evenly to create a direct line towards an external target in reaching for an object. *Tension-Flow Adjustment* aligns with *Indirect Effort* in *Space*, observable in fine motor tasks such as beadwork or in dreamy psychosomatic states where attention drifts between tasks. *High Intensity Tension-Flow* is affined with *Strong Effort*, necessary for deliberate and committed actions such as stamping the feet, while *Low Intensity Tension-Flow* harmonises with *Light Effort*, as in the delicate hand movement of carefully picking up broken glass. *Abrupt Tension-Flow* corresponds with *Accelerated Effort*, evident in hurried movements driven by time pressure, and *Gradual Tension-Flow* aligns with *Decelerated Effort*, seen in slowing down and relaxing (Kestenberg, 1965b, pp. 546–548). Kestenberg observed that preferred modes of drive-discharge (expressed in qualities of *Tension-Flow*) foreground preferred modes of adjustment to demands of reality (expressed in qualities of *Pre-Effort* and *Effort* movements), which remain relatively constant within an individual's movement repertoire throughout life.

Flowing Shapes of Self-and-Other

Kestenberg (1967a) proposed that early *Shape-Flow* patterns provide the somatic basis for reaching towards or withdrawing from the world of objects. Whereas the *Tension-Flow* apparatus functions as the motor instrument of drive-discharge, the *Shape-Flow* system enables drive gratification through expressive interactions with objects. *Tension-Flow* allows for drive differentiation, while *Shape-Flow* enables the differentiation of self and other (Kestenberg, 1967a, p. 357). In other words, *Shape-Flow* serves as the instrument of phase-specific drive satisfaction by engaging the phase-specific objects through which the drive's aim is fulfilled. In movement terms, the qualities of muscle tension denote specific need-based and affective qualities, and the shapes that the body makes throughout movement enable the expression of these affective qualities towards others.

In Kestenberg's framework (1965a, 1965b, 1967a), early reflexes are classified as *Shape-Flow* movements and are understood as somatic precursors of object-relations. More broadly, *Shape-Flow* encompasses both outwards-oriented movements directed towards the environment and inward-oriented movements directed towards the self (Kestenberg, 1967a). Movements towards the self express either a need to withdraw from external stimuli or a need for self-directed engagement. The two basic attributes of *Shape-Flow* are *Growing* and *Shrinking*, representing the fundamental dynamics of attraction and withdrawal. Kestenberg identified further elements of *Shape-Flow*, such as *Widening* and *Narrowing* horizontally, *Lengthening* and *Shortening* vertically, and *Bulging* and *Hollowing* sagittally. *Shape-Flow* patterns are observable, for instance, in the rooting reflex as the infant's body grows and lengthens towards the nipple, then shrinks and narrows away from the breast once satiated.

Kestenberg defined *Shape-Flow* as movements characterised by trunk activation, which generally involve whole-body engagement to assume a specific bodily shape. For example, *Shape-Flow* is visible when the baby shrinks into a ball shape before dozing off to sleep, disengaging from the environment. Conversely, in initiating contact with the external world, they might use a horizontally *Widening Shape-Flow*, extending their arms, and *Bulge Forward* to welcome an embrace.

Kestenberg (1967a) posited that kinaesthetic experiences arising from *Shape-Flow* patterns generate affective images of self and other. These images are subsequently integrated into self- and object-representations, exerting a significant influence on the development of body-image and self-and-other schemas. She differentiated between *Bipolar* and *Unipolar Shape-Flow*. *Bipolar* patterns involve symmetrical changes in the torso and are associated with globalised experiences of comfort and discomfort, embedded within self-and-other schemas. These patterns originate from early kinaesthetic experiences, such as the rise and fall of the chest during breathing, the spreading of arms to embrace, withdrawal from discomfort, or hollowing of the torso in response to hunger. Such experiences serve as foundational elements for body-image and self–other representations (Kestenberg, 1985). In contrast, *Unipolar Shape-Flow* reflects asymmetric bodily reactions to specific stimuli, exemplified by early grasping or reaching movements.

In addition to elements of *Shape-Flow*, Kestenberg identified a separate category, *Shape-Flow Design*, which described the spatial design of movement. Its two basic elements are centripetal, towards the body, and centrifugal, away from the body. Further design factors describe how the movement traverses these spaces, such as in *Loops* or *Lines*, with *High* or *Low Amplitude*, and with *Angular* or *Rounded Reversals*. She argued that the regulation of these factors reflects the specific pathways through which the ego distributes libidinal and aggressive drive-discharge between self and object in the pursuit of equilibrium (Kestenberg & Sossin, 1979, p. 154).

Kestenberg (1967a) explained that, as development progresses, just like *Tension-Flow* patterns come under the control of the ego-derived patterns of *Pre-Efforts* and *Efforts, Shape-Flow* also becomes subordinated to mature patterns of *Shaping*. As children adapt more effectively to aspects of external reality, their movements become increasingly differentiated. Instead of responding with a whole-body activation (*Shape-Flow*), they learn to respond with precision, reaching out with a single arm, for example, to grasp an object. These localised and purposeful responses, often combining two spatial directions, formed what Kestenberg termed *Directional Shaping* patterns. These *Directional Shaping* patterns, she argued, also serve as a defence against external stimuli, as does a learner narrowing focus on a book while using the torso and arms to create a physical barrier. Kestenberg (1967a) further clarified that *Directional* and *Dimensional* patterns create bridges between self and other by extending body-boundaries into space and establishing differentiated relationships with objects and the external world. *Directional Shaping* erects vector-like bridges between self and objects; *Dimensional Shaping* organises movement into two- or three-dimensional forms, giving the relationship a more complex structure. The patterns provide the dimensional scaffolding for expressing the complex design of relationships.

Kestenberg (1967a, pp. 397–398) also formulated psychodynamic interpretations of the three spatial planes based on their roles in development. The oral phase is mostly spent with experiences in the *horizontal* dimension – taking in (feeding), learning the foundations of proto-communication through a give and take between mother and infant. Therefore, Kestenberg suggested that movements in the horizontal plane relate to the regulation of communication and attention. By narrowing the shoulders and arms horizontally, one turns to focus on a single person or issue (such as in a gesture accompanying concentrated thinking); by expanding the arms outwards, one adopts a broader, open bodily attention to the external environment. She added that the horizontal plane facilitates the exchange, acceptance, or rejection of ideas, as in turning away from noxious stimuli. The use of the *vertical plane* comes to dominate during the anal phase as the child stands up and gains control over balance and body weight, coinciding with the beginnings of verbal language. Thus, Kestenberg suggested, the vertical dimension conveys intentionality, self-presentation, and autonomy. She explained that vertically rising hand gestures often signal self-assertion or leadership, while descending gestures suggest yielding and humility. Strong feelings of pride may be expressed by 'standing up tall' and conviction by 'standing one's ground'. She further added that doubt often emerges through alternating rises and descents, such as eyebrow lifts or hesitant shoulder shrugs. Kestenberg (1967a) proposed that the *sagittal plane* is activated with the emergence of walking, signalling the child's growing independence. Movement patterns in the sagittal plane embody complex actions that traverse the space forwards and backwards. One advances or retreats, accelerates or decelerates, leads or follows. These actions have complex, prolonged temporal progressions; therefore, she associated sagittal movements with planned action, future orientation, and anticipation.

Somatic Syntax

Kestenberg (1967a) contended that movement behaviour is organised according to a specific grammar. She introduced a syntactic framework for bodily movement in which dynamic, affective (*Tension-Flow*) and ego-derived, cognitive (*Pre-Efforts and Efforts*) aspects are structured through expressive, intersubjective features (*Shape-Flow* and *Shaping*). Kestenberg suggested that this kinetic grammar reveals the inter- and intrasystemic dynamics of psychic processes, such as conflict or harmony between psychic agencies of the id, ego, and superego (intersystemic), or conflict or harmony within a single psychic structure (Kestenberg & Sossin, 1979). Kestenberg grounded her somatic grammar in her concept of affinity (following Laban's (1950, 1954) propositions). She outlined affinities (inherent links or correspondence) and clashes between the elements of her categories of *Tension-Flow, Pre-Efforts* and *Efforts*, and the *Shape-Flow-Shaping*.

In terms of drive and early object-related categories, Kestenberg considered sadistic *Tension-Flow* patterns to be affined with aggressive *Shape-Flow* patterns. Thus, the need for separation and withdrawal is affined and structured through closing shapes. In contrast, libidinal *Tension-Flow* corresponds to the indulging *Shape-Flow* of open shapes, directed outwards to engage with the environment. In this view, *Tension-Flow* expresses the feeling tone or drive aim (predominantly libidinal or sadistic), while *Shape-Flow* constitutes its accompanying spatial design corresponding to the drive object. Kestenberg viewed *Tension-Flow*, in combination with *Shape-Flow*, as conveying the "affecto-motor qualities of object-relations" (Kestenberg, 1967a, p. 369). In other words, *Tension-Flow* reflects the emotional content, for which *Shape-Flow* provides an expressive scaffolding that supports discharge of phase-specific drives towards phase-specific objects. Correspondingly, ego-controlled patterns of *Pre-Effort-Efforts* are structured through the expressive patterns of advanced *Shaping* (*Directional* and *Dimensional*) to convey mature object- and reality-related ideas, attitudes, and aspirations bound by external demands and cultural codes. Kestenberg (1967a, p. 396) illustrated this by likening *Effort* patterns to words, which carry meaning adapted to the context and to the person being addressed, and *Shaping* to sentence structure, which is adapted to the language being spoken and its communicational context.

Kestenberg proposed that the motor expression of superego processes is reflected in gesture–posture schemas and in the *Effort–Shape* affinities utilised within these sequences. Postures and whole-body movements that involve a clash between simultaneously used *Effort* qualities are understood to reflect intrasystemic conflict within the superego. A clash between *Dimensional Shaping* patterns is viewed as a conflict within the ego ideal. By contrast, clashes between *Effort* and *Shaping* in gesture–posture mergers indicate intersystemic conflict between the ego and the superego.

Kestenberg's principle of affinity was a didactic proposal to provide an embodied baseline for understanding which movement qualities naturally complement one another physically, rather than prescribing rigid normative combinations. She argued that several complex combinations between *Tension-Flow* and *Shape-Flow, Efforts* and *Shaping*, may be present in an individual's movement repertoire. However, Kestenberg (1967a) emphasised the need to evaluate whether the expressive pattern of movement provides adequate structure to convey affective content effectively. Table 2.1, in the later section on methodology, visualises Kestenberg's rule of affinity through the horizontal alignment of all affined/harmonious elements in each category.

Intersubjectivity in Movement

Kestenberg (1965a, 1965b, 1967a) observed that congenital preferences for patterns and modes of drive-discharge are expressed as preferences for specific *Tension-Flow* and *Shape-Flow* patterns within infants' movement repertoires. She examined how infant–caregiver interactions shape and modify these preferences. Kestenberg (1965a, p. 6) also suggested that the onset of psychopathology could be detected by observing early rhythmic movement interactions between mother and child.

Kinaesthetic attunement and kinaesthetic identification were key concepts in Kestenberg's work (1965b, 1967a). She defined attunement between mother and child as the creation of a shared state of affect through the embodiment of the same *Tension-Flow* and/or *Shape-Flow* patterns. Through attunement to each other's need-based motor patterns, ideally initiated by the caregiver, a sense of somatic and psychic communion is established within the dyad. She proposed that the kinaesthetic memory of sharing the same psychosomatic state provides the foundation for the emotional bond, upon which the process of kinaesthetic identification with the caregiver can develop. It is also through these kinaesthetic attunements to the caregiver's movement repertoire that the infant is gradually introduced to more advanced, ego-controlled movement patterns (Kestenberg, 1965b, 1967a).

Within this process, the caregiver first functions as an auxiliary ego of the infant, providing templates of coping that the infant internalises into their own repertoire of functioning. The caregiver's own constitutional preferences thus shape the infant's congenital preferences for the discharge of drives. Kestenberg (1965a) warned that overwhelming external interference with the infant's individual affective, rhythmic tendencies could significantly hinder development. She stressed the importance of the caregiver recognising the infant's temperament through these innate preferences expressed in the *Tension-Flow* and *Shape-Flow* repertoires. She further argued that, if the caregiver's *Tension-Flow* repertoire is narrow or markedly different from the infant's, opportunities to establish kinaesthetically shared affective states, essential for psychosomatic communion, are constrained. In such circumstances, infants may suppress their own congenital preferences to attune to the caregiver's patterns, which could be detrimental to the child's emotional development. Kestenberg explained that, even though early congenital preferences for *Tension-Flow* and *Shape-Flow* patterns are gradually modified by maturation and environmental influences, when these processes unfold without significant environmental disruption, they become enduring and discernible characteristics of the individual's movement repertoire and remain relatively constant aspects of personality throughout life.

In 1965, Kestenberg presented her paper entitled "Attunement and Clashing in Mother–Child Interaction" to psychiatry residents of the Kings County Hospital in New York. She discussed various patterns of nonverbal interaction between mother and infant that denoted different affective responses (Kestenberg, 1975b). Her formulations suggested that the more fully the mother and infant are attuned across modes of perception, sensory thresholds, and innate patterns of tension, the more symbiotic their relationship becomes. Conversely, the greater the disparity in these areas, the more likely everyday clashes will occur, potentially leading to developmental issues due to the lack of maternal containment. However, Kestenberg clarified that the process of normal development includes attunement and clashes within complex sequences. She formulated that each phase of development is governed by harmonious and conflictual aspects of the mother–child relationship that provide the foundations for mental life. Attunement provides the basis for shared states of affect, and clashes initiate separation, adjustment, and re-attunement, thereby sustaining the resilience of their relationship. Kestenberg differentiated between complete attunement, one-sided attunement, partial attunement, and selective attunement and generalised clashing, partial clashing, and selective clashing (Kestenberg, 1975b).

Complete attunement she defined as engaging in the same *Tension-Flow* patterns. Prolonged periods of such attunement extend the symbiotic phase, which, according to Kestenberg, can significantly hinder the development of ego boundaries and may lead to affective disorders. She argued that, in these circumstances, infants do not learn to differentiate their own needs from those of others, nor do they develop adequate frustration tolerance. Kestenberg identified one-sided attunement as a dynamic in which only one partner persistently adjusts to the other. She further noted that mothers with a heightened ability to recognise their infant's needs and attune to the corresponding *Tension-Flow* rhythms may predominantly assume the role of initiating attunement, thereby establishing a one-sided dynamic. Their seamless responsiveness, while adaptive in the moment, leaves little opportunity for the infant to initiate. This imbalance could affect the process of separation and the development of the child's ego functions. She further noted that, when the mother's needs and preferences dominate the dyad's interactions, infants become highly dependent on the mother's moods and affective tone, which may lead to a later preference for more object-centred rather than need-centred functioning (Kestenberg, 1975b, p. 162). In cases of partial attunement, Kestenberg observed that the infant and the mother managed to stay connected through using affined, similar qualities of tension and shape, with slight personal adjustments and preferences. This means that the needs of the infant–caregiver dyad could be met without complete attunement. According to Kestenberg, this configuration allows for individuality while remaining connected, thereby enabling the development of frustration tolerance. Kestenberg (1975b) viewed generalised clashing as occurring when partners exhibit opposing patterns of *Tension* and *Shape-Flow*, which are typically associated with conflictual situations.

She further noted that partial and selective clashing are strategies frequently employed by mothers to redirect and regulate the child's state. For instance, when the infant is in a heightened state of affect, the mother may partially match the baby's *Abrupt Tension-Flow* but not its intensity. By introducing *Low Intensity Tension-Flow*, she can initiate a gradual decrease of intensity in the child's tension. Kestenberg (1975b) observed that attunement initiates symbiosis, whereas clashing promotes separation; however, she further added that an omnipresence of attunement can trigger fears of engulfment, just as an excess of clashing can lead to overwhelming separation anxiety and fears of annihilation. She proposed that early somatic interactions often resemble an improvisational dance, unfolding through rounds of harmonisation, sequencing, and complementary phrasing between mother and child (Kestenberg, 1975b).

Kestenberg's Developmental Framework

With Kestenberg's psychodynamic vocabulary of movement having been introduced, this section turns to the discussion of her developmental framework as a whole. Kestenberg's developmental movement theory is an integration of Freud's dual drive-theory and structural model, and of Mahler's developmental ego-psychology and object-relations perspective. Kestenberg also drew upon several of Erikson's concepts.

As previously noted, Kestenberg diverged from the classical psychosexual stage model by proposing the *inner-genital phase* (Kestenberg, 1956a). She further posited a urethral developmental phase, arguing that urination and defecation are distinct bodily functions, accompanied by distinct postures and rhythms, and that control over them is acquired sequentially[22] (Kestenberg, 1966). Her observational data supported this differentiation as she explained in the following statement:

> Children who have already tamed their anal impulses to a considerable extent enjoy playing with their urine and water, as well as 'running' and 'dribbling' games. (Kestenberg, 1966, p. 156)

Thus, the stages of Kestenberg's developmental movement theory are the *oral, anal, urethral, inner-genital*, and *phallic* phases (Kestenberg et al., 1971; Kestenberg, 1985). Kestenberg, drawing on Freud (1953), Abraham (1949), and her own infant observation data, divided each developmental phase into libidinal and sadistic[23] subphases, which denote the predominance of discharge patterns in the given subphase serving the aims of sadistic or libidinal drives (Kestenberg et al., 1971). In the libidinal subphases, functioning is considered to be oriented towards mobilisation, connection, and indulgence. The sadistic subphases are characterised by a tendency towards separation and differentiation.[24]

As discussed earlier, Kestenberg's developmental approach employed the Freudian structural model of the psyche, identifying categories of movement associated with the id, ego, and superego. Kestenberg also applied Erikson's (1950b) epigenetic principle in her developmental framework.

Erikson's developmental chart delineated eight successive stages, each representing a critical period in the human lifespan. He adopted an epigenetic perspective on development (Erikson, 1937, 1950a, 1950b), borrowing the term 'epigenesis' from biology to draw an analogy between ego development and intrauterine growth, where organ systems sequentially emerge until a complex physiological integration is achieved in the newborn. By analogy, Erikson conceptualised ego development as unfolding through a sequence of cumulative stages, each corresponding to a phase of drive maturation (Mitchell & Black, 2016, Chapter 6). His bio-psycho-social perspective described development as a process through which an emergent ego capacity gradually enables the individual to coordinate and synchronise bodily developmental schedules with the organization of sociocultural processes (Erikson, 1950a, pp. 246–247). Erikson understood the ego, or self, as a mediating structure that manages inner conflicts and negotiates between the person's bodily needs and the external world. This ongoing mediating process enables individuals to handle the multiple, often conflicting demands of everyday life within complex and changing social contexts (Kivnick & Wells, 2014). Similarly, each phase in Kestenberg's developmental framework is defined by a specific bodily zone, distinct drives, and unique developmental tasks, which accumulate progressively (Kestenberg, 1965b, 1967a; Kestenberg et al., 1971).

Highlighting the relationship between id and ego development, Kestenberg (1965a) also incorporated Erikson's (1950a, 1950b, 1959) concept of the *organ mode* or *mode of function*. Erikson's modes describe how phase-specific modes of functioning extend to additional domains and ultimately dominate overall functioning within a particular developmental phase. Through generalisation, these modes detach from their initial context, become autonomous modes of function, and are further influenced by the social environment, forming behavioural modalities that facilitate ego adaptation (Rapaport, 1959). Erikson (1950a, 1950b, 1959) identified the principal modes of function in the oral, anal, and genital phases as incorporative-inceptive, retentive, and intrusive, respectively. In his view, the oral phase is characterised by relaxation in the prone position and passive taking-in of the world. The anal phase coincides with secure sitting, finer motor differentiation, and often standing, during which phase the toddler enjoys selecting, organising, piling, and discarding objects with determination. In the genital-intrusive phase, the child's independent and forceful mobility fosters behaviours of intrusion, such as jumping at others, talking assertively, or displaying vigorous curiosity.

Kestenberg applied these ideas to zone-specific discharge patterns that generalise and come to dominate the infant's movement repertoire in each phase. For example, in the first 6 months, the oral *Sucking Tension-Flow Rhythm* expresses the receptive mode of passive incorporation (an Eriksonian concept). This rhythm is generalised across most of the infant's behaviours at this stage and appears as the dominant pattern not only in feeding but also in many other activities. In the second half of the first year, with the emergence of teeth, the *Snapping-Biting Rhythm* prevails in the active incorporative phase (an Eriksonian term that he also linked to biting actions), which is also evident in clapping and tapping behaviours (Kestenberg, 1965a, 1985; Erikson, 1950b, p. 68). Erikson linked the achievement of autonomy in the anal stage with the ability to stand firmly on one's own two feet. Similarly, Kestenberg identified physical mastery of verticality as the somatic precursor to a sense of autonomy and confidence. In the third year of life, Erikson emphasised the importance of experiences of continuity, an unbroken sequence of ideas and imagination, emerging in tandem with the child's increasing locomotion (walking, running) and expanding language. Kestenberg's urethral developmental phase encompasses these same connections between the sense of time, continuity, and discontinuity, as reflected in her descriptions of *Run-Walk* and *Start-Stop-Go Tension-Flow Rhythms.* Finally, Erikson's association between the intrusive genital phase and jumping behaviours is conceptualised by Kestenberg in her *Jumping Tension-Flow Rhythm* (Erikson, 1950b, pp. 77–77; Kestenberg et al., 1971; Kestenberg, 1985).

Kestenberg's integration of Erikson's modes of functioning is also evident in her linking drive expression to ego attitudes. She proposed that, in subphases dominated by sadistic drives, aggressive ego attitudes and defences also predominate. Kestenberg (1985) explained that an infant in the oral-sadistic phase who might bite (the oral-sadistic *Biting Rhythm* of *Tension-Flow*) would also withdraw into isolation as a defensive response, or engage in hair-pulling or pinching. By contrast, in the oral-libidinal phase, defences are indulging. The infant may turn away from noxious stimuli through engaging in gentler actions, such as softly patting pets or objects.

Another important anchor of Kestenberg's developmental framework was Mahler's separation-individuation process. She identified kinaesthetic and motor-specificities of several Mahlerian concepts (Kestenberg et al., 1971; Kestenberg, 1965a, 1965b, 1967a, 1971b). In her developmental ego-psychology, Mahler proposed that psychological birth does not coincide with biological birth but is a gradual developmental process. Through the vicissitudes of separation and individuation, children slowly come to regard themselves as a separate self, with their own body and self-boundaries that are differentiated from others and the external world. This process of separation denotes the infant's emergence from an initial period of normal symbiotic fusion with the caregiver. The process of individuation brings about experiences of personal achievement through which the child comes to understand themselves as having their own individual characteristics and experiences. This view further proposes that the experience of separateness is the necessary basis for the creation of object-relationships, that is, an attachment to the caregiver as an external object of love. The intrapsychic process of separation leads to clear self- and object-representations (Mahler et al., 1975, p. 4). In this developmental model, the earliest sense of self of the baby is conveyed via internal bodily sensations that are called proprioceptive sensations (sensations about the body's position in space, movement, and efforts via feedback sent from specialised receptors in the muscles, tendons, and joints) (Mahler & McDevitt, 1982, p. 829). With the emergent functioning of the sensori-perceptive organs, the infant begins to receive a surge of external stimuli, which only gradually come to be regarded as coming from the outside. This shift is predicated on an awareness of a body-self-boundary. In Mahler's view, the infant's life starts with a state of undifferentiation, which is without any concept or schema of self and other. This is the normal autistic phase, when the infant is relatively unresponsive to external stimuli and functions in a sleep-like state (which occurs during the first 4–6 weeks). It is followed by the normal symbiotic phase, characterised by the fusion between the infant and the caregiver without awareness of separateness or boundaries (lasting from 6 weeks to 5 months) (Gober, 2014, p. 13). The separation-individuation phase begins between 5 and 9 months of age, with the event of "hatching," which signals the emergence of body-self-boundaries (Mahler et al., 1975, p. 44). There is a shift of libidinal cathexis from internal bodily sensations on to the periphery of the body, and this awareness of the self (body) boundary engenders sensations to be registered as internal and others as external bodily perceptions. Self and other differentiation is engendered by this awareness of the body-boundary. This marks the emergence of the ego. "Infants start to organise their experiences as good or bad, pleasurable or painful, which also instates the storage of these experiences as memory traces" (Gober, 2014, p. 16; Mahler et al., 1975). What follows is the practising subphase of the separation-individuation phase, characterised by the child's greater independence from the mother, as motor development surges. In the subsequent rapprochement subphase, the child is seen as caught between the enjoyment of their independence and mobility and the fear of the increasing distance from the mother. During this period of crisis, the child is seen to frequently and suddenly seek the caregiver's proximity and emotional containment. In the following phase of object-constancy, the child becomes able to maintain a stable internal representation of the mother even in the mother's absence, leading to a greater ability to be alone (Mahler & McDevitt, 1982; Gober, 2014).

Kestenberg added specific kinaesthetic, spatial, and motor aspects to Mahler's concepts. She argued that self- and object-representations are initially organ-images and organ-object-representations. They are anchored in organ-object sensations, which are experiences of bodily contact between caregiver and infant (Kestenberg, 1971b). She further emphasised that the ways caregivers attend to the infant's needs become part of the child's body-image (Kestenberg et al., 1971).

Kestenberg (1967a) differentiated the space of early development into three zones: *Near Space* (close to the body), *Reach Space* (within arm's reach), and *Intermediate Space* (between the *Near* and the *Reach Space*), each providing a distinct context for evolving self-object-relations. She specified that, in the symbiotic phase, self and object are fused in the *Near Space*, and the infant's body-image incorporates the mother. The event of hatching instates *Reach Space*. As motility develops, the physical distance between caregiver and infant increases, and their interactional field expands into *general space*, signalling growing independence and greater physical and psychic separation (Kestenberg, 1967a). Kestenberg linked Mahler's (1968) concept of hatching to the infant's emerging capacity to activate the first motor control, *Bound Tension-Flow* (counteractivation of agonist and antagonist muscles). She proposed that, when the infant engages *Bound Flow*, the resulting contraction of surface muscles sharpens the awareness of the skin and the body-boundary, thereby initiating the earliest somato-psychic sense of separateness (Kestenberg et al., 1971, p. 752). *Bound Tension-Flow* also creates greater firmness of muscle tone, enabling self-directed movements such as grasping. Because these self-directed movements provide opportunities for expressing interest in objects and others, Kestenberg viewed *Bound Flow* also as the first motor expression of intentionality; the first manifestation of the emergent ego (Kestenberg et al., 1971, pp. 750–764). She further argued that a child's ability to stand forms the basis for developing a sense of a separate self, achieved through the sensorimotor experience of standing as a coherent, vertical, solid unit (Kestenberg et al., 1971). After reviewing the key developmental concepts that Kestenberg adopted and outlining the organising principles of her approach, I now turn to discussion of her developmental framework as a whole.

Oral Phase

Kestenberg's first phase is marked by the dominance of the oral mode of functioning, feeding, sucking, biting, and incorporating. The central developmental task of this phase is the establishment of communion and communication between the infant and the caregiver. The physiological event inaugurating psychic development in this phase, according to Kestenberg, is the sucking reflex and the intake of nourishment (Kestenberg et al., 1971). The incorporating mouth serves as the prototype of the oral body-image, and the libidinal *Sucking Tension-Flow Rhythm* employed in feeding dominates the infant's movements throughout the body, as seen in rhythmic movements of the hands and feet. The subtle and frequently pulsating muscle *Tension-Flow Rhythm of Sucking* not only enables feeding (biological need) but also fosters merging (developmental need) with the caregiver, as the tactile sensations of blurred body-boundaries generate a psychosomatic merger, psychic containment, and symbiosis. This embodied experience underpins the infant's emerging trust in the caregiver and in the environment. Teething introduces the first bodily and psychic separations as the infant bites the nipple and the mother pulls away; physical distance enforces psychic differentiation. In the oral-sadistic subphase, the *Biting and Chewing Rhythm* predominates, observable in the clapping and tapping behaviours typical of a 1-year-old. The emergence of *Biting Rhythms* coincides with the increased use of *Bound Flow* of tension in the muscles, both of which, Kestenberg argued, heighten tactile awareness of the body's enveloping tissue, thereby sharpening skin awareness and inaugurating the first sense of separateness – in Mahlerian terms, hatching (Kestenberg et al., 1971, p. 752). Kestenberg (1967a) contended that the initial phase of development is characterised by a state of "objectless autism" from which there is a transition to the "self-centred relation with the anaclitic object, the emergent body-boundaries are blurred, and the rudimentary body-image merges with a near object" (p. 358). This is followed by the somatic differentiation between self and object, marked by the emergence of *Reach Space* and *Shape-Flow* movements. The infant extends towards phase-specific, need-satisfying objects through the specific use of *Shape-Flow* patterns (Kestenberg, 1967a). In the oral phase, *Shape-Flow* patterns of libidinal horizontal *Widening* and sadistic *Narrowing* predominate as the infant embraces the mother's body, clings to her, opens to contact, or withdraws (Kestenberg et al., 1971). Kestenberg proposed that stable representations of self and objects (object-constancy) develop in successive stages aligned with concrete aspects of external reality: *Space, Weight*, and *Time* (Kestenberg, 1967a). During the oral phase, infants begin to establish spatial object-constancy by exploring the *Near* and *Reach Space* around their own and their mother's body. The realisation that objects remain stable within this immediate field, together with the growing sense of bodily separateness, is what lays the foundation for early communication (Kestenberg et al., 1971).

Anal Phase

The bodily change that inaugurates Kestenberg's anal phase is the profound morphological and functional maturation of the digestive system, particularly the rotation and elongation of the sphincter muscles. She proposed that the motor quality of these changes generalises, producing frequent rotational movements visible in various other age-specific activities such as spinal twists, facilitating turning over from one side to another (Kestenberg et al., 1971). Through the libidinal *Twisting Rhythm*, the infant learns to integrate the left and right sides of the body, establishing the foundation for the contralateral movement patterns essential for crawling and walking. According to Kestenberg, this exploration of left–right dynamics also serves as a somatic precursor to ambivalence, as the infant gains the capacity to shift perspective by turning from one side to the other. The sadistic subphase of the anal phase is marked by the dominance of the *Straining Rhythm* utilised during the passage of solid stool, but can also be observed in typical behaviours of 2-year-olds, such as squatting and standing up, pushing heavy toys, or the rhythmic surges of temper tantrums. The use of *Straining Rhythm* is observable as the toddler strains with *Evenly* held *High Intensity* muscle tension in their legs to push away from the ground and then releases this tension *Abruptly* upon arriving at standing (Kestenberg et al., 1971). *Shape-Flow* patterns characteristic of the anal phase include vertical *Lengthening* and *Shortening* of the torso. These are the whole-body shaping patterns fundamental to crawling, squatting, standing, reaching, and climbing. Through differentiation of *Shape-Flow* elements, the child coordinates the upper and lower body, thereby grasping the somatic correlates of above and below. Kestenberg described the establishment in this phase of the prehension-release system between mother and infant. This enables grasping, holding, and letting go, understood both somatically and psychically. Kestenberg characterised the body-image in the anal phase as a weightful, solid, vertical unit (Kestenberg et al., 1971). Developmentally, the toddler achieves object-constancy in weight by exploring the weight of objects and learning to mediate their body weight relative to gravity.

Urethral Phase

Kestenberg's urethral phase is inaugurated through the mediation of tasks relating to urination. In its libidinal subphase, the focus is on letting go and releasing the muscle tension necessary to initiate urine flow, while the sadistic subphase concerns the ability to stop this flow on demand through increasingly complex muscular coordination. The organising bodily experiences of this phase are the acquisition of control over urethral muscles and the emergence of walking (Kestenberg et al., 1971). According to Kestenberg's observations, toddlers begin walking by "pouring" their body weight forwards like a fluid, allowing gravity to pull them off balance and thus propelling them into their first step. This early gait, described as a drift-type walk, is characterised by a forwards orientation of body weight, creating a continuous sense of drifting through space. Embodied by the *Run-Walk Tension-Flow Rhythm*, this quality of movement is mirrored in the child's attention, which often appears diffuse, absent-minded, and prone to losing sight of the caregiver. The body-image at this stage is fluid and uncertain, becoming more agile during the sadistic subphase (Kestenberg et al., 1971). As children gain mastery over drifting, they learn to slow down or stop on demand by shifting body weight backwards. The *Run-Stop-Go Rhythm* becomes dominant in this sadistic subphase, observable in games of tag, darting from place to place, and running purposefully towards specific goals in space. Kestenberg proposed that, through the somatic exploration of continuity via drifting and practising discontinuity embodied in the *Run-Stop Rhythm*, the child establishes a nascent sense of time, leading to object-constancy in time. The corresponding *Shape-Flow* patterns, *Bulging Forward* and *Hollowing Backward*, provide the shaping structures for traversing the sagittal plane. In this phase, the mother–infant dyad develops what Kestenberg termed the *mobilising-containing system*, which supports the child's growing independence and capacity for distance while still allowing for rapprochement, recharging, and containment (Kestenberg et al., 1971; Kestenberg, 1985).

Inner-Genital and Outer-Genital Phases

The following two phases in Kestenberg's developmental theory address the integration of pregenital drives and ego attitudes into a more coherent sense of self. At this stage, the toddler is considered to have achieved object-constancy in space, weight, and time but must still learn to integrate these dimensions into complex behavioural sequences that reflect differentiated ego attitudes (Kestenberg, 1967a).

Kestenberg's *inner-genital phase* involves consolidating control over pregenital drives and integrating them into an early form of infantile genitality, still expressed within the dyadic relationship with the primary caregiver. This phase precedes the triangulation of relationships that emerges with the

Oedipal situation. As discussed earlier, Kestenberg (1956a, 1956b) first introduced the concept of the *inner-genital phase* in the late 1950s, positioning it as a stage that precedes the phallic phase. She also considered this phase to mark the origins of later parental love. Initially, she proposed it as specific to girls, but later expanded it to include both sexes through the work of the Sands Point Movement Study Group. Esther Robbins and Martha Soodak "identified inner-genital rhythms in the scrotum of boys" (in Kestenberg Amighi & Loman, 1990, p. 24). Kestenberg hypothesised that an increase in gonadotropic hormone secretion contributed to wave-like *inner-genital* sensations and contractions, directing the child's attention inward and heightening preoccupation with conception and birth stories (Kestenberg, 1975c). An internal focus, creativity, and a strong identification with maternal, nurturing activities characterise this phase. While children of both sexes exhibit *Inner-genital Rhythms* of drive-discharge, Kestenberg observed that the phase tended to last longer for girls than for boys (Kestenberg & Sossin, 1979, pp. 5–8). Movement during this phase reflects attempts to integrate the multi-dimensionality gained in earlier phases, traversing the horizontal, vertical, and sagittal planes through a variety of undulating, wave-like patterns. The dominant rhythms of this phase include the libidinal *Undulating Rhythm*, which sweeps across left to right and up and down in complex patterns, and the sadistic *Swaying Rhythm*, characterised by *High Intensity* and *Gradual* flow of tension (Kestenberg, 1985). The latter rhythm can be likened to cramps and contractions during labour. Through its high intensity, it underpins sustained commitment to tasks such as nurturing a pet or caring for a doll. Retention activities also increase during this stage, signalling increased attention to the inside of the body. The developmental task of the *inner-genital phase* is the integration of pregenital experiences into a complex whole, marking both the end of toddlerhood and the transition into childhood (Kestenberg & Sossin, 1979; Kestenberg et al., 1971). In this process, the mother–child relationship becomes increasingly complex, as both partners develop awareness of their distinctive subjective inner worlds and psychic realities.

Following the *inner-genital phase*, children of both sexes enter the phallic *outer-genital* phase, when, according to Kestenberg, an influx of exhibitionistic tendencies, an interest in the external world, and identifications with the father figure come to the fore (Kestenberg, 1975c). The central somatic experience of the phase is the externalisation of drive-discharge on to the outer parts of the body and into the environment. The developmental task of this phase is to integrate heightened drives and expanding interests. The final subphase of this stage is marked by conflicting wishes and ego attitudes, which foreshadow the differentiation of psychic structures, particularly the ego and superego, during latency. Children delight in exhibitionism, expressed in the libidinal, penetrative *Jumping Rhythm*, while also testing their impact on the external world through the precise punches, kicks, and stamps of the sadistic *Leaping Rhythm*. The body is experienced as a whole, mobile, elastic, yet solid unit, capable of delivering complex, planned, and coordinated actions upon the environment. Developmentally, this phase supports the emergence of a sense of self-coherence and agency (Kestenberg, 1975c). Kestenberg argued that, with the resolution of the Oedipal conflict, the child transfers attachment away from the primary caregivers, a shift that consolidates the turn towards the external world, as teachers and peers increasingly become attachment figures.

Latency

Kestenberg argued that, before the consolidation of ego and superego structures, the child passes through various progressive and regressive periods (Kestenberg, 1975c). Kestenberg (1967a) added that, during latency, when *Tension-Flow* is controlled by *Efforts*, and *Shape-Flow* is regulated by *Shaping*, the consolidation of aim-directed intention with the most suitable spatial configuration is achieved. This consolidation is somatically reflected in the consonance between *Effort* and *Shaping* patterns, in accordance with the previously described rule of affinity. Children learn harmonious matches between *Effort* and *Directional* and *Dimensional Shaping* by imitating the adults around them, though their actions remain less complex. This is shown in their more limited range of *Effort–Shape* combinations. Latency brings in the enhanced differentiation of psychic structures as the superego develops through attempts to synchronise *Effort* with *Shaping*, reflected in increasingly varied gestural behaviour. Unlike the 'insatiable', drive-discharge-laden motility of a 2- or 3-year-old, the latency child expresses themself through symbolic actions such as gestures and words.

Adolescence

In adolescence, Kestenberg added, the cohesiveness of the ego is reflected in the ability to mobilise the whole body purposefully, in accordance with the awareness of personal identity within a group. Kestenberg contended that, although adolescence often brings some disorganisation in movement, this is counterbalanced by the maturation of motor systems that enable independent postural attitudes. Thus, young adults combine multiple *Effort* and *Shape* elements within a single action, whether in gestures or postures. Kestenberg defined gesture as a movement that concentrates in one part of the body, utilised as protection from overwhelming exposure to danger or as a means of thinking through and testing ideas. When gestures preceded postures, Kestenberg viewed these as examples of trial of ideas, and, when gestures followed postures, these were to test the limits of the idea or action (Kestenberg & Sossin, 1979, p. 142). Kestenberg viewed postures not as static positions but as movement constellations in which the whole body participates using the same qualitative pattern. In global postures, the entire body adopts a single qualitative constellation, whereas, in integrated postures, the whole body cooperates to support a pattern centralised in a specific body part. Kestenberg defined cases of gestures and postures utilising affined qualitative elements of *Effort* and *Shaping* as gesture-posture mergers, which she interpreted as a harmony between executive (ego) and supervising (superego) mental structures (Kestenberg & Sossin, 1979, p. 149). She observed the use of effort and shape combinations in young children and gesture–posture mergers in adolescents, which come to predominate the adult's movement repertoire.

Kestenberg added that the motor skilfulness of adolescents is most evident in contexts such as dance recitals or sports games, where they perform complex movements within the structured frameworks of choreography or game rules. In stark contrast, during unstructured breaks between classes, their movements often reveal clashing *Effort–Shape* combinations and disorganised rhythms. Such fluctuations illustrate the oscillation between progression and regression characteristic of this stage. Through these repeated cycles of drive and ego reorganisation, adolescence ultimately establishes a new order in which a stable repertoire of harmonious *Effort–Shape* patterns becomes embodied in the gesture–posture mergers of adulthood (Kestenberg, 1967a, 1975c).

The Development of Community Spirit

To diversify her developmental data through further observations, Kestenberg travelled to several collective settlements in Palestine/Israel, including Lahavot Bashan, Barkai, Kfar Blum, Hatzor-Ashdod, and Shamir Kibbutzim,[25] in the 1960s. Based on these visits, she formulated her views on the development of community spirit (Kestenberg & Robbins, 1975). Kestenberg argued that both social conscience and community spirit are incorporated into the structure of the superego and expressed in the mature *Effort–Shape* combinations. She viewed the sense of community spirit as something that protects individuals and their communities from excess drive-laden behaviours (Kestenberg & Robbins, 1975, p. 443). As explained before, Kestenberg believed that primary identification in infancy is anchored in rhythmic attunements between the caregiver and child, which later include mirroring of peers as well. She called these the early sensorimotor experiences of group life, the basis of the early sense of community. Kestenberg and Robbins (1975) further argued that these socio-sensorimotor experiences and rhythmic attunements lay the foundation for balancing the rhythms of needs for privacy, one-to-one peer relations, and group experience in adulthood. They emphasised the importance of early community life, similar to what surrounds the kibbutz child. They stressed that the community setting allows for diverse attunements, socio-sensorimotor experiences, and motor identifications upon which social conscience and community spirit can develop. They expressed concern over the increasing isolation of the nuclear family in modern urban settings. Kestenberg and Robbins (1975) concluded that the developmental task in adolescence is the ability to create intimate relationships within a stable framework of a sense of community. Kestenberg and Sossin (1979) observed that the movement repertoires of adolescents and adults become increasingly characterised by the blending and merging of various *Tension-Flow Rhythms* to express complex needs and affective states. Through attunement with partners and peers, individuals acquire rhythms that facilitate mutual satisfaction while preserving individual distinctiveness.

Charting Kinaesthetic Imprints: The *Movement Profile*

Kestenberg began her infant observation studies in the early 1950s, coinciding with a growing interest in case studies of developmental assessment at the Hempstead Clinic within the New York psychoanalytic community (Kestenberg, 1975a; Sossin, 2007). As the draft of Anna Freud's *Diagnostic Profile* (1962) began to circulate, the Sands Point Movement Study Group, led by Kestenberg, developed a movement-based assessment framework, the *Movement Profile.* It was designed to align with the *Diagnostic Profile* while also serving as an independent assessment tool (Kestenberg & Sossin, 1979). Kestenberg first introduced the concept of a *Movement Profile* in 1967, describing it as a method for quantifying and graphically visualising the qualitative aspects of an individual's habitual movement repertoire, comparable to the Rorschach test and other clinical assessment methods (Kestenberg, 1967a, 1985). She formally presented this method at the American Psychoanalytic Association meeting in 1971, the International Symposium of Non-verbal Aspects and Techniques of Psychotherapy in Vancouver, Canada, and the Dance Notation Bureau in New York in 1974 (Kestenberg, 1974b). An expanded version appeared in her 1985 essay, "The Role of Movement Patterns in Diagnosis and Prevention" (Kestenberg, 1985). The following section discusses Kestenberg's *Movement Profile*, along with her methods of quantification and movement visualisation.

Kestenberg (1985) argued that individuals tend to repeat their habitual constellations of expressive patterns. According to Kestenberg (1967a), an individual's characteristic modes of drive-discharge and adaptation to the external world are encoded in the specific combinations and sequences of movement qualities that constitute the movement repertoire. She further contended that these differences arise from congenital patterns and from kinaesthetic identifications with objects throughout development (Kestenberg, 1967a, p. 406). The absence of kinaesthetic memories for particular movement patterns is, therefore, reflected in their infrequent occurrence within an individual's movement repertoire. Infrequently used patterns may impede both the expression of affects associated with them and the capacity for attunement to others when these patterns are initiated by a partner. Kestenberg maintained that motor data obtained from direct infant observation possess predictive significance for psychological development (Kestenberg, 1965a; Kestenberg & Sossin, 1979).

Kestenberg (1985) recommended that observations should take place in naturalistic contexts – for example, a conversational setting for adults or play in a familiar environment for children. For adults, she prescribed a single observation period of approximately 1 hour whereas, for children, she advised several shorter periods of 10–20 minutes across different contexts. She noted that live observation could be further supplemented by analysis of film recordings (Kestenberg & Sossin, 1979; Kestenberg, 1985). Movement observation was grounded in Kestenberg's (1985) concept of the observer's kinaesthetic identification with the mover. Informed by dance practice and her Laban-based training, this approach foregrounded somatic attunement to the qualitative and patterned features of observed movement rather than detached classification. Her approach maintained that, when movement patterns resisted categorisation, the observer should physically enact them. Such embodiment functioned as a criterion of analytic clarity, with categories understood to arise from the movement experience itself.

According to Kestenberg, developmental movement data offer insight into preferred modes of drive-discharge, the impact of external factors on congenital tendencies, the developmental transition from id to ego processes, and early indicators of pathology stemming from mismatches between the child's and caregiver's preferences. She further emphasised that congenital preferences in infancy for specific modes of motor expression may have predictive capacity for later behaviour (Kestenberg, 1965a). Kestenberg and Sossin (1979) contended that, while external factors and maternal rhythms influence congenital patterns, conflicts between maternal and infant rhythms alone are not sufficient to predict future pathology. They explicitly revised Kestenberg's (1965a) earlier position that particular motor pattern constellations predict specific syndromes.

Kestenberg's *Movement Profile* is a developmental assessment framework that classifies observed structural and dynamic features of bodily movement using Kestenberg's psychodynamic movement vocabulary. Coded motor qualities are then quantified – to capture both their frequency and complexity – and displayed graphically. These graphs provide the basis for psychodynamic interpretation grounded in Kestenberg's developmental movement theory. According to Kestenberg, the *Profile* offers insight into intrapersonal processes associated with the id, ego, and superego. Additionally, she argued that comparing the profiles of infants and caregivers can reveal underlying interpersonal dynamics.

The *Profile* comprises 52 primary motion factors across eight categories. These are the previously reviewed: *Tension-Flow Rhythms* (expressing modes of drive-discharge and need satisfaction); *Tension-Flow Attributes* (reflecting temperament and affective responses); *Precursors of Effort* (associated with emergent ego functions); *Efforts* (pertaining to advanced coping and adaptive behaviours); *Bipolar Shape-Flow* (relating to global self-feelings and object-relational schemas); *Unipolar Shape-Flow* (expressing specific reactions to external stimuli); and *Directional* and *Dimensional Shaping* (reflecting complex relational patterns) (Kestenberg, 1985).

Table 2.1 Overview table of the *Movement Profile*

				Tension Flow Rhythms	**Tension Flow Attributes**	**Pre-efforts**	**Efforts**		**Bipolar Shape Flow**	**Unipolar Shape Flow**	**Direction al Shaping**	**Shaping in Planes**
				Needs, drives	Safety, Danger Temperament	Defences	Learning Coping		GlobalSelf-feelings	Relating to Specific Stimuli	Localizing Relating	Complex Modes of Relating
	Freudian Theory	**KMP Developmental Theory**		**System I: Tension Flow Effort System**					**System II: Shape Flow-Shaping System**			
				Id-Derivative		**Ego-Derivative**			**Early Object Relations**		**Mature Self-Other Schemas**	
0–0.6	Oral	Oral	Libidinal Indulging	Sucking	Flow Adjustment	Flexible	Indirect	Horizont al Space	Widening	Lateral Widening	Sideways	Spreading
0.6–1			Sadistic Fighting	Biting	Even flow	Channeling	Direct		Narrowing	Medial Narrowing	Across	Enclosing
1–1.5	Anal	Anal	Lib./Ind.	Twisting	Low Intensity	Gentle	Light	Vertical Gravity/ Weight	Lengthening	(L) Lengthen/ (S) Shorten *Up*	Up	Ascending
1.5–2			Sad/Fight	Straining	High Intensity	Vehement or Straining	Strong		Shortening	(L) Lengthen/ (S) Shorten *Down*	Down	Descending
2—2.5		Urethral	Lib./Ind.	WalkRun	Gradual	Hesitating	Decelerating	Sagittal Time	Bulging	(L) Bulge/ (S) Hollow *Anterior*	Forward	Advancing
2.5–3			Sad/Fight	Run-stop-go	Abrupt	Sudden	Accelerating		Hollowing	(L) Bulge/ (S) Hollow *Posterior*	Back	Retreating
3–3.5	Phallic	Inner genital	Lib./Ind.	Undulating	Free Flow	Free Flow	Free Flow		Growing	Growing	Growing	Growing
3.5–4			Sad/Fight	Swaying	Bound Flow	Bound Flow	Bound Flow		Shrinking	Shrinking	Shrinking	Shrinking
4–4.5		Outer genital	Lib./Ind.	Jumping	Neutral Flow							
4.5–5			Sad/Fight	Leaping								

Note: The table provides an overview of the most comprehensive iteration of the *Movement Profile* published by Kestenberg in 1985 (it does not pertain to any later development of the *Movement Profile* by Kestenberg's collaborators).
Source: Information compiled by the author based on Kestenberg (1985).

Table 2.1 represents Kestenberg's *Movement Profile* in its entirety. The left-hand column presents Kestenberg's stage theory, juxtaposed with the Freudian psychosexual development. Reading the table horizontally illustrates how the different movement categories build upon one another, while a vertical reading shows how elements within each category develop sequentially. The colour coding (ranging from light grey to black) highlights the syntax and organisation of movement behaviour as articulated in Kestenberg's rule of affinity between categories.

All patterns represented in horizontal alignment on the table are affined qualities through their libidinal/indulging or sadistic/fighting orientations (libidinal and sadistic relate to drive-derived and early object-related patterns; indulging and fighting label ego-controlled patterns of defences, coping, and self-and-other relations). One exception in the table is the *Unipolar Shape-Flow* category, in which anal and urethral elements with oppositional libidinal and sadistic orientations are depicted in the same rubric because, here, Kestenberg's categorisation grouped the elements developmentally according to spatial directionality (horizontal, vertical, sagittal). For example, vertically Lengthening Up and Shortening Up are placed in the same rubric even though their drive orientations are oppositional – libidinal and sadistic, respectively. For clarity, the drive orientations of these components are labelled next to them as L (libidinal) and S (sadistic).

Horizontal alignment of elements represents Kestenberg's developmental movement theory, as all elements in alignment are understood to come to dominance in the child's movement repertoire during the corresponding developmental phases represented to the left, or relate to those developmental phases in later development, in the case of more advanced patterns such as *Pre-Efforts, Efforts,* and *Shaping*. For example, oral *Sucking Tension-Flow Rhythm, Flow Adjustment Tension-Flow Attribute*, and *Widening Bipolar* and *Lateral Widening Unipolar Shape-Flow* patterns dominate the movement repertoire of the infant in the first 6 months of life. Nascent aspects of the developing ego and object-relations are present, expressed in goal-directed behaviours engaging with oral *Flexible Pre-Effort* and *Indirect Effort* elements and *Sideways* and *Spreading Shaping* structures, which gradually come to take dominance over *Tension-Flow* and *Shape-Flow* as development progresses. In adolescence and adulthood, these are considered oral ego-controlled, object-relations-associated patterns.

Reviewing the *Movement Profile* table highlights how closely it aligns with Anna Freud's *Diagnostic Profile*, especially when we examine their shared interpretative domains. Section V of Anna Freud's *Diagnostic Profile* encompasses instinctual development (including libidinal processes, phase-specific growth, and aggression), the development of the self and ego (such as self-functions, defence mechanisms, and reactions to danger), personality development (through mastery of developmental tasks), and the dynamic and structural evaluation of conflicts (Freud, 1965, 1962, pp. 151–153). These categories parallel Kestenberg's system: *Tension-Flow Rhythms* (phase-specific development and drive-discharge), *Tension-Flow Attributes* (elementary reactions to danger), *Pre-Efforts* (defence mechanisms), and *Efforts* (ego functions and coping strategies).

Anna Freud emphasised the importance of assessing intrapsychic conflicts from both dynamic and structural perspectives, an approach Kestenberg also integrated into her *Movement Profile*. Within Kestenberg's framework, the dynamic interplay among object-relations, affective states, and drives is traced. A structural perspective on personality emerges when she links movement categories to id and ego processes, focusing on how ego-controlled motility evolves from drive-derivative movement patterns, signifying either harmonious structural development or structural conflict. Another key correspondence between Anna Freud and Kestenberg lies in their shared allegiance to Freudian drive-theory, coupled with an emphasis on object-relations (cf. Midgley, 2013). Kestenberg further argued that instinctual drives related to phase-specific needs optimally discharge through a phase-specific object (Kestenberg, 1967a). The concept of developmental lines is embedded in the *Movement Profile*, which becomes evident when the chart is read horizontally. The developmental evolution of function is depicted in the succession from *Tension-Flow* categories related to instinctual processes and affective states towards the ego-directed categories of defence mechanisms and coping strategies that evolve from their mediation (*Pre-Efforts and Efforts*). Likewise, Kestenberg drew a developmental line from early generalised responses to environmental stimuli expressing general patterns of object-relations (*Bipolar Shape-Flow*) to differentiated reactions to specific stimuli (*Unipolar Shape-Flow*) to complex modes of relating through directional and dimensional spatial structures (*Directional* and *Dimensional Shaping*). Kestenberg clarified this in the following statement:

> In successive developmental phases regulations of tension-flow and shape-flow come under the control of the ego. Regulation of tension-flow aids drive differentiation; regulation of shape-flow contributes to the differentiation of self and objects. In later development, ego attitudes to space, gravity, and time, expressed through 'efforts', control the flow of tension. At the same time, shape-flow becomes subordinated to selective shaping of movement in the dimensions and planes in which transactions with objects take place. (Kestenberg, 1967a, p. 356)

Like Anna Freud, Kestenberg (1966) also stressed that development is a complex interaction of biological and psychological processes, which she saw less as hierarchical than as a continuous flow of progressions and regressions along different developmental lines.

Writing Tension: Reading Movement

When Kestenberg began her infant observation studies, she did not have an established method for documenting movement. Thus, in the early 1950s, she began experimenting with her own inscription technique on paper.[26] With her initial focus on the flow of muscular tension, she developed a system to record qualitative changes in *Tension-Flow*, which she called *Tension-Flow writing* or the *Tension-Flow Curve* (Kestenberg, 1953–1978, 1965a, 1985; Kestenberg & Sossin, 1979). Kestenberg also adapted this method of flow-writing to record pathways of *Shape-Flow-Design*.[27]

This method relied on freehand tracing to capture fluctuations in muscular tension across a movement sequence. Kestenberg's *Tension-Flow Curve* was designed to register the nuances of muscle *Tension-Flow* using the examiner's kinaesthetic attunement as a route into otherwise inaccessible somatoaffective states of the mover. She reconceptualised her observation that the infant–caregiver dyad communicates through kinaesthetic identification and attunement and turned it into a methodological intervention. She proposed that the movement observer must kinaesthetically attune with the mover's *Tension-Flow* qualities to document them accurately. Those attuned qualities are then channelled into the observer's hand and translated into the traced line on the page (Kestenberg, 1985, pp. 100–104).

Rather than assigning discrete symbols to qualities of tension, Kestenberg depicted changing qualities of muscular tension through a continuous line, emphasising the process-based nature of the flow of muscle tension during movement. She organised the paper around a horizontal midline. Movements employing *Bound Flow* were drawn below the line, while those expressing *Free Flow* were drawn above. Intensity was represented on the vertical axis, with *High Intensity* positioned further from the midline and *Low Intensity* closer to it, while time extended along the horizontal axis (Kestenberg, 1985). *Graduality* was illustrated by long, slanted lines marking extended transitions, whereas *Abruptness* appeared as sharp vertical shifts, forming mountain-like peaks or small triangular shapes. *Adjusting Flow* was rendered as a series of squiggly, worm-like repeating curves, while *Even Flow* was shown as a straight, unbroken horizontal line. An example of Kestenberg's flow-writing[28] is shown in Figure 2.1.

As mentioned earlier, Kestenberg studied Labanotation, a method for segmenting and systematically documenting bodily movement. Designed as a standardised method, much like a musical score, it allows movement sequences to be reproduced from written notation alone (Laban, 1950, 1954, 2008; Laban & Lawrence, 1947). It does so by assigning symbols to specific dynamic and

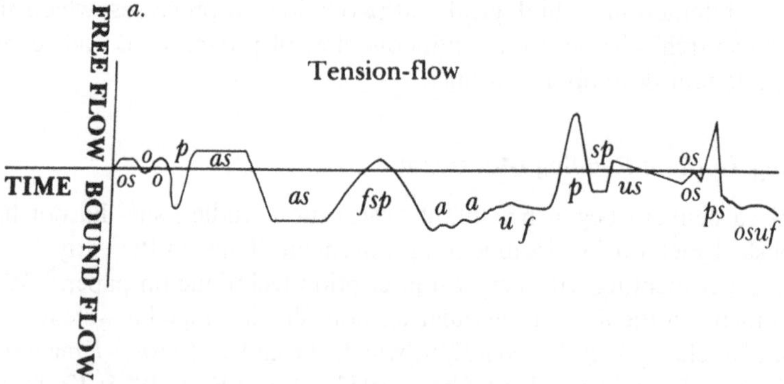

Figure 2.1 An example of Kestenberg's Tension-Flow Curve.
Source: Reprinted from Kestenberg (1985). Copyright 1985 by Human Sciences Press. Reprinted with permission.

structural aspects of the movement. These symbols can be combined into more complex clusters to indicate co-occurring qualities, forming a constellation analogous to how letters combine to form words (Kestenberg, 1985). To record movement patterns in categories beyond *Tension-Flow*, Kestenberg used these Labanotation symbols.[29]

Scoring the Soma

As mentioned previously, Kestenberg's *Movement Profile* entails the quantification of the qualitative aspects of movement recorded during observation. She adopted the scoring method from her movement notation teacher, Warren Lamb (1961; Berlowe & Kestenberg, 1972; Kestenberg, 1985).

Kestenberg's *Tension-Flow Curve* documents qualitative changes in muscular tension throughout a movement sequence. Quantification of these qualitative aspects is achieved by annotating segments of the curve with labels[30] corresponding to relevant *Tension-Flow Rhythms* and *Tension-Flow Attributes.* For *Tension-Flow Attributes,* Kestenberg annotated only changes in the constellation of qualities across successive movements; simple repetitions were excluded to emphasise the variety of *Tension-Flow Attributes* rather than the frequency of repeated elements. In all other movement categories, such as *Pre-Efforts, Efforts, Bipolar* and *Unipolar Shape-Flow,* and *Dimensional* and *Directional Shaping*, elements present in each action are annotated using Labanotation symbols. Annotations are subsequently tallied for each category to generate frequency counts of each element relative to the total number of actions in that category. This process indicates the extent to which each pattern was employed during observation. The final frequency counts for each category, therefore, represent the variety of elements utilised by the mover within that category (Kestenberg, 1985; Berlowe & Kestenberg, 1972).

As illustrated in Figure 2.1, the *Movement Profile* comprises eight individual movement categories. Each category includes three pairs of oppositional elements, such as *Free Flow* and *Bound Flow* (*Tension-Flow Attribute*) or *Direct* and *Indirect* (*Effort*). The *Tension-Flow Rhythms* category is an exception, containing five pairs of oppositional rhythms. According to Kestenberg's system, oppositional qualities cannot be embodied simultaneously within a single movement. For instance, a movement cannot employ, to the same extent, both *Free* and *Bound Flow* at once. Muscle tension flow in a single action is either unconstrained (*Free Flow*) or constrained (*Bound Flow*) (or has the tendency towards contraction or release). Kestenberg noted, however, that non-oppositional qualities within a category may combine in various ways, forming constellations. A movement may incorporate a single qualitative element, such as *Abrupt Tension-Flow*, or combine multiple elements, such as *Abrupt, High Intensity*, and *Bound Tension-Flow.* To address this complexity, Kestenberg calculated load factors for each category, thereby quantifying the extent to which bodily movement involves multiple co-occurring qualities and providing insight into the relative complexity of an individual's movement (Sossin, 1987). For example, a high load factor in *Tension-Flow Attributes* reflects frequent and complex combinations of multiple attributes, suggesting a broader range of affective modulation. The load factor is defined as the ratio of the total number of coded elements to the total number of actions performed by the mover within a given category. A greater number of co-occurring qualities within an action yields a higher load factor, reflecting increased movement complexity (Kestenberg & Sossin, 1979). As a maximum of three elements can be coded per action in each category, the load factor ranges from 33.3 per cent (one element per action) to 100 per cent (three elements per action). To further refine this measure, the range and the median are calculated. The range is determined by multiplying the load factor by 0.67 and dividing the result by 5. The median is calculated by dividing the total number of coded elements in a category by 3.[31]

For diagrammatic visualisation, the range is divided by this average and then multiplied by the frequency of occurrence for each component within the category. These calculations yield plot-point values for each coded element, which are subsequently used for graphical representation (Berlowe & Kestenberg, 1972; Sossin, 1987). The resulting graphs display the frequencies of all patterns, enabling comparison of their respective ratios. Furthermore, the graphs facilitate analysis of sadistic or fighting tendencies in relation to libidinal or indulging tendencies within the overall profile. Sadistic or aggressive patterns are shown on the left side of each graph, while libidinal or indulging patterns are shown on the right (see Figure 2.2).

Kestenberg conceptualised the graphs as visual representations of kinaesthetic imprints of personality, reflecting characteristic affective, relational, and adaptive tendencies. The interpretation process requires comparing the relative widths of graphs across categories to identify affinities or conflicts.

Balance was central to Kestenberg's interpretive framework. Within each category, she regarded a relatively even distribution across paired oppositional elements as desirable. In the *Effort* category, for example, comparable use of the indulging/Indirect and fighting/Direct elements would support flexible coping, allowing the individual to respond in ways that best fit the external task or situational demands. Consequently, Kestenberg treated a wide variety of patterns as desirable, suggesting a broader repertoire of socio-affective states and expressions, defences, coping strategies, and modes of object-relating. Graphically, a broad and evenly distributed profile, reflected in relatively similar frequencies across libidinal-sadistic and indulging-fighting elements, yields a wider graph. In turn, narrow graphs indicate reliance on a limited set of expressive and mastery patterns, which she regarded as less adaptable because they provide fewer motor patterns to embody the complexities of affectivity, ideation, and relating.

PROFILE 2–JOHNNY, 8 MONTHS OLD

Solid lines = Pure rhythms. Broken lines = Mixed rhythms. All subsequent broken lines (2–9) = Patterns observed in gestures, dotted lines = patterns observed in postures. These do not occur in infants (see diagrams 4 and 9 in profile 1). Load Factors = LF indicate how many qualities are used all at once in a single action (33% is lowest and 100% the highest LF). Horizontal lines on diagrams 2–9 indicate frequencies of variations. Horizontal lines on diagram 1 indicate frequencies of repetitions.

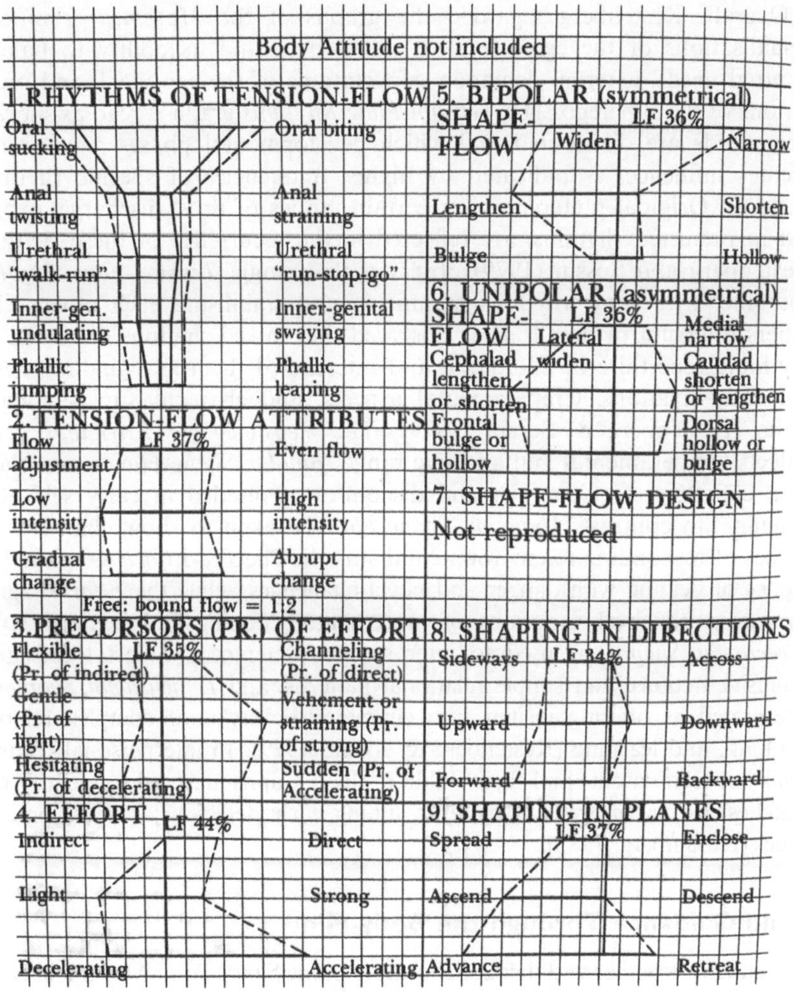

Figure 2.2 Graphs of the Movement Profile of an 8 month old child.

Source: Reprinted from Kestenberg (1985). Copyright from 1985 Human Sciences Press. Reprinted with permission.

Harmony across categories, such as between *Tension-Flow* and *Shape-Flow, Pre-Efforts* and *Directional Shaping*, and *Efforts* and *Dimensional Shaping*, is represented by roughly equivalent frequency distributions across affined patterns, as evidenced by similar plot-point values or graph widths. Kestenberg understood the lack of harmony between *Tension-* and *Shape-Flow* or between *Efforts* and *Shaping* to indicate difficulty coordinating drive-derived expression with adaptive functioning in relation to objects and reality (Kestenberg & Sossin, 1979; Kestenberg, 1967a).

Overall, Kestenberg regarded the graphs of the *Movement Profile* as visualisations of the ego's level of adjustment and its ability to balance internal needs, external demands, expectations of the ego-ideal, and prohibitions of the superego. The *Tension-Flow Rhythms* graph is read as showing how needs are distributed and which developmental phases have exerted greater influence, as indicated by higher frequencies of specific rhythmic patterns. Original preferences for certain modes of drive-discharge, expressed in preferred rhythms, are reflected in the recurrence of these rhythms. Kestenberg and Sossin (1979) observed that single *Tension-Flow Rhythms* combine, with some rhythms organising and stabilising each other, while others interrupt or derail. They observed that mixed rhythms dominate the rhythmic repertoire in adulthood and interpreted them as signalling developmental fixations, temperamental aspects, and characteristic personality traits (Kestenberg & Sossin, 1979). The *Tension-Flow Attributes* graph reflects temperamental and affective range. *Bipolar Shape-Flow* is associated with expressions of comfort and discomfort grounded in early self–other schemas. In contrast, *Unipolar Shape-Flow* is taken to show characteristic modes of responding to environmental stimuli. The *Pre-Efforts* graph reflects modes of dealing with danger and novel challenges, while the *Effort* diagram represents preferred variations of more mature coping and learning styles. *Directional Shaping* is used to infer spatial preferences, object localisation, defensive actions, and simple relational patterns, and *Dimensional Shaping* is interpreted as offering insight into characteristic styles of complex relating, thinking, and learning (Kestenberg & Sossin, 1979). In interpersonal comparisons between parents and their children, these graphs are used to identify mismatches in their movement patterns, aiding early detection of developmental issues (Kestenberg, 1985).

Child Guidance Through the Body-Mind

Kestenberg, together with her collaborators in the Sands Point Movement Study Group (Jay Berlowe, Hershey Marcus, Arnhilt Buelte, Esther Robbins, Marta K. Soodak) established an educational organisation, Child Development Research (CDR), which was incorporated by the University of the State of New York in 1970.[32] Its professional advisory board consisted of 14 professionals from the fields of psychiatry and movement studies, including Albert Solnit (1919–2002)[33] and Irmgard Bartenieff. Kestenberg also asked Margaret Mahler to serve on the board, but this did not come to fruition (Kestenberg, 1972b). CDR sponsored the *Center for Parents and Children*, the *Sydney L. Green Prenatal Project*, and later the *Jerome Riker International Study of Organised Persecution of Children* (ISOPC). Esther Robbins and Martha Soodak directed the Prenatal Project; Judith Kestenberg Arnhilt Buelte co-directed the Center for Parents and Children; Eva Fogelman and Helene Bass-Wichelhaus oversaw the ISOPC (Child Development Research, n.d.c).[34]

In an unpublished preliminary proposal from the late 1960s,[35] Kestenberg outlined plans for the establishment of a research nursery for typically developing infants, alongside an afternoon program for older children and a specialised babysitting service (Kestenberg, n.d.c). The project aimed to establish training opportunities for medical and psychiatric professionals, social workers, teachers, and anthropologists to conduct observational research on typical child development, an area reportedly underrepresented in medical and psychiatric training at the time (Kaplan, 1978; Reubens, 1978). Kestenberg contended that community mental health and child guidance practitioners lacked professional experience with typically developing children, which she sought to remedy by offering clinical placement opportunities. The project also intended to integrate knowledge of movement and psychological development by establishing a centre for developmental movement studies (Kestenberg, n.d.c). The proposal included a budget for the project, including paid staff such as a nursery school teacher, a social worker, a psychologist, a sociologist, an anthropologist, four part-time psychiatrists, and part-time creative arts teachers. Regarding the plans for the physical environment, the proposal listed a nursery room with a garden, a babysitting room, a recording room, and a consultation room. The establishment of the *Center for Parents and Children* marked the realisation of several elements of this earlier plan. It was introduced through an open meeting held on 18 October 1972 at St. Stephen's Church in Port Washington, Long Island, New York (Kestenberg, 1972a).

The centre functioned as a community-based initiative focused on primary prevention, child guidance, and research. Its objective was to study child development with the involvement of a multidisciplinary team of professionals as well as parents, with the goal of preventing childhood trauma and developmental disorders. This was achieved through early detection, utilising nonverbal observation and assessment methods, as well as movement-based corrective developmental interventions. One of the key focuses of research conducted at the centre was to examine how children separate from their parents in a community setting and how peer relations support this process, a line of inquiry Kestenberg considered to be a continuation of Mahler's work (Kestenberg, 1972a). The centre's objectives encompassed developing training curricula for professionals working with children across various disciplines, as well as providing psychoanalytically informed childcare training for parents. These initiatives sought to reduce alienation between children and parents, elevate the status of parenting, and strengthen parents' capacities as caregivers (Kestenberg, 1972a, 1972b). The centre was conceived as a demonstration project and pilot model for other community projects, integrating parenting support, training, and research (Child Development Research, n.d.c).[36]

The centre served a stable group of local middle-class families from the Long Island area. It was funded by private contributions, membership fees, and research grants.[37] Membership granted access to newsletters and discounts on publications issued by Child Development Research (Child Development Research, 1978). The newsletters[38] addressed specific topics relevant to child development, including creativity, humour, the role of grandparents, and the concept of a holding environment, and also provided updates on ongoing research projects. The newsletters also featured essays from parents about their engagement with the centre and their reflections on personal challenges such as parental guilt, separation, and balancing parenthood with professional responsibilities. The centre's ethos emphasised community development by integrating parent education with research focused on the critical early years of child development. Although it was primarily a prevention project, a structured referral pathway was established for cases requiring clinical intervention (Sossin, personal communication, 1 November 2022).

Among the parents who attended the centre were several mental health professionals interested in the embodied, somatic aspects of development and child guidance. They consented to be observed and filmed with their children by the research staff (Center for Parents and Children, n.d.a). Kestenberg often carried a camera to record children playing and interacting with their parents; she also set it aside during activities and noted their movement.[39]

A movement-based mother–infant assessment scale[40] was also developed and applied at the centre. In addition to observational data on movement, the instrument also collected information on how parents perceived and defined themselves in their parental role. Observations were conducted either live at the centre or through film recordings, with each session lasting a minimum of 2 hours. These observations were to be repeated over several years. Observer ratings were compared to determine inter-observer agreement. The resulting scores indicated the extent of harmony or discord between parents and their child's movement characteristics across domains of temperament, coping mechanisms, learning, and relational styles (Center for Parents and Children, n.d.d). Additional studies conducted at the centre examined the development of self and self-recognition, alterations in maternal body-image during pregnancy, and specific motor interactions between fathers and children (Sossin, 1978; Borowitz, 1978a, 1978b; Weinstein, 1978).

The centre provided internship placements for psychiatrists, psychologists, child care workers, and creative arts therapists. Child psychiatry fellows from the Division of Child and Adolescent Psychiatry at the Long Island Jewish Hillside Medical Centre completed a portion of their training at the centre to observe typical child development within a non-institutional environment (Kaplan, 1978; Reubens, 1978). Among the early trainees at the centre were psychology student K. Mark Sossin, who joined in 1976, dance/movement therapy trainees Susan Loman and Carol Fishman, who joined in 1978, and anthropologist Janet Kestenberg Amighi, the daughter of Judith Kestenberg (Sossin, personal communication, 12 April 2024). The centre became an official internship facility for dance-therapists accredited by the American Dance Therapy Association in 1979, with Loman as the supervisor. In 1988, this role was transferred to Beth Gonzalez-Dolginko, an art therapist. Loman, Sossin, Kestenberg Amighi, and Gonzalez-Dolginko went on to become lifelong collaborators of Kestenberg, playing central roles in further developing and disseminating her work (Kestenberg Amighi et al., 2018; Sossin, 2018; Sossin & Birklein, 2006; Birklein, 2018; Gonzalez-Dolginko, 1988, 2021). Sossin's doctoral dissertation in clinical psychology focused on the ontogeny of aggression, based on infant observation data collected at the centre. Sossin began co-teaching the *Movement Profile* course with Kestenberg in 1978, while also serving as the supervising psychologist at the centre (Sossin, personal communication, 1 November 2022; Kestenberg & Sossin, 1979).

Interns and trainees were required to participate actively for 1 or 2 years. Their training included movement notation and profile construction, which involved three intensive weekend courses at the Laban Bartenieff Institute for Movement Studies in New York City. Full certification in Kestenberg's *Movement Profile* required a weekly 3-hour class for 30 weeks, covering Kestenberg's developmental theory and movement notation techniques. Sossin remembered Kestenberg as a vigorous teacher who expected her students to read literature extensively from contemporaneous movement behaviour researchers, such as Albert Scheflen and Ray Birdwhistell on kinesics and context analysis, as well as Laban's and Lamb's work. Her teaching methods strongly incorporated embodied experiential aspects, as illustrated in the following quote from Sossin:

> Early on in the first class, participants (including those with backgrounds ranging across creative art therapies, psychiatry, psychology, social work, psychoanalysis, and child-developmental specialization) were told to get on the floor and lie on their bellies, and to then roll over, attending to what part of their bodies initiated the rotation (e.g. shoulder, pelvis, leg), and what parts followed. This was informative about early developmental processes, but further established the point that learning how to discern and notate the body movements of another required knowing those and related experiences in one's own body. Hence, the grounding principle of 'kinaesthetic identification' was in the very first lesson. (Sossin, personal communication, 12 April 2024)

Families had often engaged with centre staff already during pregnancy. The focus of parenting support was to aid harmonious interactions between children and parents, preventing the development of developmental disturbance and, later, personality disorders.[41] Centre staff provided expectant parents with psychoeducation on child development, with a particular focus on embodied approaches.[42] Weekly evening classes for parents offered opportunities to participate in movement tasks designed to address conflicts and disharmonies within their movement repertoires. Each session concluded with presentations on child development delivered by centre staff (Meehan, 1979). Additionally, qualified parents were invited to participate in ongoing research projects at the centre, thereby fostering a collaborative knowledge community and reducing distinctions between staff and parents (Child Development Research, 1985).

Parents affiliated with the centre were instructed to maintain systematic journals that documented their child's development, daily activities, and observed behaviours. These journals also included records of parental emotional responses and reflections on past family trauma. Traumatic events potentially affecting the child or the entire family were explored in collaboration with psychology professionals (Center for Parents and Children, n.d. c). Centre staff provided individual guidance to families, offered developmental interpretations based on the parental journals, and recommended child-focused interventions. Difficulties with nursing, eating, sleeping, sibling rivalry, family illness, or death were addressed using centre-based methods tailored to support coping and provide reassurance for the child (Sossin, personal communication, 12 April 2024). Staff at the centre also developed psychoanalytically oriented, educational booklets[43] for children to facilitate their overcoming traumatic events such as a parent being hospitalised (Center for Parents and Children, n.d.b).

Staff also observed and documented nonverbal interactions between parents and children. Based on these observations, they provided movement-based interventions known as *movement retraining* (Buelte, 1978). These interventions sought to harmonise parent–child movement repertoires and foster resilient cycles of attunement (Buelte, 1978, 1979; Loman, 2016). The interventions incorporated motor sequences that progressed from drive-derivative to ego-controlled patterns (from *Tension-Flow* to *Pre-Effort* to *Effort*), enabling parents to support their children's developmental transitions. *Movement retraining* further promoted the safe expression of aggressive drives and reinforced ego functions. Children engaged in playful movement and arts activities designed to facilitate the expression of aggression in modified forms, such as through songs or by directing it towards soft toys (Kestenberg, 1981b). A large, soft doll was designated for this purpose, and children were encouraged to kick and hit it at times when they felt angry[44] (Sossin, personal communication, 18 November 2025). The centre's programme integrated a range of arts-based approaches, including music, visual arts, and dance/movement therapy[45] (Loman, 1980). There were ongoing efforts to recruit musicians, musicologists, and illustrators to develop a music and art profile based on Kestenberg's *Movement Profile* (Kestenberg, 1980e). The foundations of an Art Profile were being laid by Beth Gonzalez-Dolginko (1985, p. 7, 2021). The children's drawings were archived, and both staff and Kestenberg analysed the depicted shapes using *Tension-Flow* notation and Kestenberg's developmental theory (Center for Parents and Children, n.d.c).

Fostering a sense of community was central to the project's pedagogical approach. Staff provided individual guidance to children and parents while prioritising collective needs (Kestenberg, 1981b). Active parental involvement was likewise emphasised, with parents expected to participate in everyday centre tasks to strengthen both parenting skills and community engagement.

The centre's physical environment was deliberately planned to support creative, tactile, and sensory exploration, with art supplies, a grand piano, and a range of small instruments and toys readily available. A large, custom-made staircase with a hollow interior offered an enclosed hiding space and often became the centrepiece of children's games. This design choice was intentional and echoed Kestenberg's developmental emphasis on exploring the insides and outsides of bodies and objects (Sossin, personal communication, 18 November 2025).

The focus at the centre was not only on the mother-infant dyad. Marcus and Sossin lead the Father Project, a primary prevention initiative to foster optimal father–child relationships, which also served as a research project (Sossin, personal communication, 12 April 2024). Home visits and initial interviews were conducted with the fathers to explore their experiences of fatherhood and their relationships with their own fathers (Center for Parents and Children, n.d.e). The Father Group convened ten times annually on Sundays, during which Marcus observed interactions between fathers and their children and assessed the development of paternal attitudes in boys from early childhood (Marcus, 1981; Kestenberg, 1980c; Bell, 1984; Sossin, personal communication, November 1 2022). Additionally, Marcus met with the fathers on five Monday evenings each year to discuss emotional topics, including separation, guilt, and protective feelings associated with fatherhood.

The centre ran two children's groups. The young group, from birth to age 2, met twice a week. The older group, for those between 2 and 4 years old, met three times a week. A typical day at the centre was organised around recurring scheduled activities such as Table Time, Gross Motor Play, and Snack Time. Table Time focused on calming, creative activity such as working with paint, clay, or sand or drawing. This was followed by Vehicles, which aimed to stimulate motor skills through encouraging children to drive toy vehicles and climb structures. This part of the day also often involved listening to music, playing the piano, or dancing (Bell, 1984; Sossin, personal communication, 1 November 2022). There was particular emphasis on smooth transitions between activities at the centre. Each transition was accompanied by a specific song that parents, centre staff, and children sang together. Kestenberg believed this served to regulate the children's emotions (Weinberg, 1981). Staff and parents compiled a list of these songs in a booklet of special songs

(Meehan, 1979; Center for Parents and Children, n.d.b). Snack Time also incorporated educational aspects. Kestenberg sat with the children at the large table and addressed each of them, initiating discussions about meaningful topics in their lives, such as the arrival of new siblings (Weinberg, 1981; Sossin, personal communication, 18 November 2025).

The centre's work received positive feedback from many parents, as evidenced by numerous personal exchanges documented in journal notes and letters. A parent letter to Kestenberg from 1976 expressed that her involvement with the centre facilitated the overcoming of child-rearing difficulties and traumatic experiences, ultimately resulting in a more harmonious family dynamic. Another letter, from 1973, reported the writer benefited from the centre's programme by acquiring specialist knowledge of child guidance and receiving support to address the emotional challenges inherent in parenting (Child Development Research, 1971–1987). In contrast, one parent letter also indicated that some parents perceived the centre's daily regimen and the professionals' hands-on approach as rigid and somewhat intrusive (Child Development Research, 1974).

The CDR also sponsored the Sidney L. Green Prenatal Program, which supported expectant parents through educational films and lectures on childbirth and early development. Kestenberg led this project together with Loman and Buelte, introducing somatic exercises that encouraged mothers to attune to their unborn children through fetal-movement notation. A well-baby clinic was established at Long Island Jewish Hillside Hospital, where Kestenberg and her colleagues observed about 20 infants and their parents, integrating research with child guidance that emphasised somatic aspects of development (Lanzkowsky, 2012; Kestenberg, 1992b). CDR staff liaised between parents and medical professionals throughout pregnancy and birth and often attended deliveries. Sossin filmed several births for movement study (Sossin, personal communication, 12 April 2024). Additionally, Kestenberg and Sossin periodically consulted on cases at the Weill-Cornell Hospital infant physiotherapy rehabilitation centre. According to Sossin, her interventions were frequently unconventional but yielded immediate results.

> I remember one infant at the post-Neonatal Intensive Care Unit, who was deemed muscularly rigid, showing no flexibility or rotation, nor early crawling patterns, despite her age, and we were asked to observe and consult, as standard habilitation methods were not facilitating progress. So Kestenberg asked to talk to her mother, who was a musician [...] and asked the mother to sing to her child in front of us, carry along and then transition the sustained note with a flow-adjustment tension-flow attribute. It was very dramatic because the baby softened, relaxed, and showed pelvic rotation, which they were not able to elicit with all the hands-on, joint-focused, vestibular and proprioceptive kinds of input they were employing in their interventions. (Sossin, personal communication, 1 November 2022)

Later Expansions

Between the late 1970s and the 1990s, drawing on work conducted at the *Center for Parents and Children*, Kestenberg and her collaborators revised several of her earlier concepts, placing increasing emphasis on mutuality and object-relatedness. During this period, they also revisited questions of innate bisexuality and the development of sex-specific behaviours and their influence on parental attitudes, and formulated new ideas about fetal movement patterns (Kestenberg & Marcus, 1979; Kestenberg et al., 1994; Kestenberg, 1976, 1980a, 1980b, 1980c, 1987, 1989, 1990). The following section discusses these developments.

Transcending the Self, (Trans)Sensing the Other

Drawing on their work at the *Center for Parents and Children*, Kestenberg and Buelte (1977a, 1977b) turned their attention to the nonverbal components of mutuality in early caregiver–infant interaction. They argued that the coordinated way in which mother and infant support, contain, and adjust to each other's bodies, through attunements in *Tension-Flow* and *Shape-Flow*, provides the somatic foundations for the physical and psychological capacity of "holding oneself up." They contended that the infant is not only held but also "holds" the caregiver through their own qualities of muscle tension and postural patterns. They argued that, in an optimal holding environment, the caregiver's mature movement patterns interweave with the infant's innate motor tendencies. They specified that the mutual synchronisation of *Tension-Flow* patterns forms the embodied core of empathy, allowing mother and infant to resonate affectively with one another, whereas reliable adjustments in *Shape-Flow* constitute the sensorimotor basis of trust, enabling infants to anticipate that their needs will be met (Kestenberg & Buelte, 1977a).

Kestenberg and Buelte (1977b) further noted that early failures of adequate mutual holding may distort the infant's body-image, compromise the emergence of basic trust, and interfere with the ability to become genuinely self-supporting. They suggested that, in the absence of reliable holding from the caregiver, the child may develop rigid movement patterns, overusing certain muscle groups as a way of "holding oneself up." They suggested *movement retraining* interventions for the systematic synchronisation between the mother's and baby's *Tension-Flow* and *Shape-Flow* patterns (Kestenberg & Buelte, 1977b). They extended their model of mutual holding to the analytic situation, proposing that therapist and client co-create a holding environment that reactivates and transforms early bodily memories of attunement. They suggested that certain habitual body attitudes in adults, such as chronic bracing in the neck, back, or shoulders, reflect early experiences of insufficient holding. Analytically exploring these postural patterns can, in their view, uncover links between muscular overuse and underlying anxieties about both physical and psychic disintegration (Kestenberg & Buelte, 1977b).

Kestenberg further expanded the object-relations perspective embedded in her concept of *Shape-Flow* by engaging with Winnicott's (1958, 1960) ideas on maternal holding, transitional phenomena, and the intermediate zone. She addressed these themes in two essays published in 1978 in a collection of texts honouring Winnicott's legacy (Kestenberg, 1978; Kestenberg & Weinstein, 1978). In her paper, "*Transitional Objects and Body-Image Formation*," Kestenberg focused specifically on somatic experiences of transitional phenomena and distinguished three types of transitional objects: intermediate, supplementary, and transitional (Kestenberg & Weinstein, 1978). She viewed food and bodily fluids associated with experiences of gratification as intermediate objects. Supplementary objects, she argued, denote experiences that substitute for bodily interactions with the caregiver, often somatic experiences with other close persons. She added that transitional objects both evoke and replace satisfying bodily experiences with the primary caregiver.

Kestenberg (1978) integrated Winnicott's notion of the intermediate zone with Volkmar Glaser's concept of *transsensus*. Although she firmly aligned her developmental theory with Mahler's normal autistic and symbiotic phases (Kestenberg, 1967a; Mahler et al., 1975), in these later formulations she gestured towards primary object-relatedness expressed in patterns of *Shape-Flow*. Yet this concept of *transsensus* remained underdeveloped and was never integrated into her developmental framework.

She proposed that the *Bipolar Shape-Flow* movements of reaching, stretching, and grasping, which are present at birth, demonstrate the fundamental tendency of infants to engage with external objects, seeking to merge with, incorporate, and grasp the external world. Kestenberg (1978) expanded Balint's concept of primary object-relatedness to include environmental objects, such as air and light, that the infant registers very early on, rather than only discrete love objects. She further contended that her observational data revealed neonatal movement reactions indicating comfort or discomfort, security or unease responses that are inherently relational insofar as they reflect an attitude towards the environment. Based on parental reports, she added that infants seem to notice their primary caregivers based on the tone of their voice or outline of their body as early as 4 weeks after birth. Kestenberg (1978) believed that these early psychosomatic interactions between mother and infant are anchored in the activation of gamma motor neurons through the caregiver–infant dyad's holding and touching of each other's body surfaces. She posited that actions such as stretching (expanding the body's outline through muscular elasticity, such as while inhaling) or reaching with the arm represent a primary tendency towards outgoingness, serving as a prototype for a wish to incorporate others. To conceptualise this notion, she employed Volkmar Glaser's[46] concept of *transsensus*, which she understood as the psychophysiological foundation of basic trust between caregiver and infant. She added that this may also serve as the somatic basis of transference and countertransference in therapy (Kestenberg, 1978).

Glaser's theory claimed that human beings are oriented towards contact and communication (Behrens, 1997). He equated health with being in touch with the external world, and this primary tendency towards connectedness is reflected in people's involuntary movements. He believed that breathing and the muscular system are essential organs of communication, as they fulfil their task by involuntarily engaging with the world through meaningful action. He viewed disturbances in breathing, posture, and movement as having a communicative dimension that could be addressed through bodily contact. At the core of his theory was the concept of *transsensus*, understood as the embodied basis of intentionality. With *transsensus*, he was referring to a somatic intention and awareness of the external world that he thought was present in every movement, even in breathing. He contended that every intention, whether outwardly directed in perception or action or inwardly engaged with objects of thought or imagination, involves involuntary muscular activity expressed in shifts in posture, movements, and breathing. Glaser believed that, through these involuntary actions, posture changes, and embedded breathing patterns, people organise their relational space (Behrens, 1997). He further elaborated that the continuous flow of muscle tension between contraction and release has a gestural character, with a tendency to extend beyond the body's boundaries into the external world. Glaser argued that external space is never neutral but vitally charged with people's intentions. He further theorised that there were elementary movements of social behaviour corresponding to the meridian channels described in Chinese medicine (Schmincke, 2012). He asserted that the flow of vitality and tension along these meridian lines ensures the interconnectedness of all parts of the human body and its organs, while mediating interaction with the environment through involuntary movements. Glaser's psychosomatic respiratory therapy incorporated breath-work and compassionate physical contact with the patient's body (Schmincke, 2012). He applied touch along meridian lines, instructed patients to breathe into the affected area, and encouraged them to imagine that his hand was an extension of their own body (Kestenberg, 1978, p. 67).

Kestenberg (1978) conceptualised *transsensus-outgoingness* or the "trustful stretching toward" the environment not purely as a reaction to stimuli but as a total sense of being-in-relation, already present in the movement repertoire of the newborn. She described this with an evocative metaphor of seeking out or melting into the external world of objects (Kestenberg, 1978, p. 66). She viewed this as a state of mutually expanded body-boundaries of the mother–infant dyad, each containing the other. Kestenberg distinguished *transsensus-outgoingness* from expressive movements, contending that these movements originate in tension travelling along meridian lines during nonverbal interactions in the early nursing situation. She further proposed that, when a mother places the infant's head in the crook of her elbow, she stretches the meridians inside her arm as well as activating the frontal middle meridian in the infant's body. When infants reach to embrace the mother's back, the meridians in their inner arms receive tactile stimulation (Kestenberg, 1978). Kestenberg explained that it is through the psychophysical imprints of *Shape-Flow* movements (reaching, grasping, clinging) in this expanded, dually containing body-image in the near (body) space that infants discover the body-boundaries of the mother as well as their own. She contended these explorations are the building blocks of later body-image formation (Kestenberg, 1978).

Parental Attitudes

Between the late 1970s and the mid-1990s, Kestenberg, together with her collaborators from the Sands Point Movement Study Group, developed her formulations of parental attitudes (Kestenberg, 1980a, 1980b, 1980c, 1981c; Kestenberg & Marcus, 1979; Kestenberg et al., 1994).

Building on Freud's concept of innate bisexuality (Freud, 1953), Kestenberg and Marcus (1979) proposed an adaptively bisexual model of parental identity and critiqued rigid cultural norms that advance a monosexual gender identity. Their model conceptualised the biological and cultural basis of bisexuality as a continuum between masculinity and femininity, as well as activity and passivity, that supports the development of distinct maternal and paternal behaviours (Kestenberg, 1980a, 1980b, 1981c). Kestenberg and Marcus (1979) argued that both feminine and masculine tendencies are evident throughout development in children of both sexes. They associated early paternal attitudes with innate capacities for activity, whereas they linked precursors of maternality to desires to be held and contained by another.

Kestenberg adopted Benedek's (1952, 1959, 1970) view that parenting attitudes are shaped by the reproductive drive and extended Bonaparte's (2018) and Deutsch's (1944, 1945) notion of maternal instinct by arguing for a biological basis of the reproductive drive in both sexes. Kestenberg associated this reproductive drive with a universal quest for continuity, creation, and self-renewal inherent in human existence, while also acknowledging the role of culture and learned patterns in its inhibition (Kestenberg, 1980a, pp. 63–65). In this context, Kestenberg et al. (1994) problematised the increasing availability of intimacy for young people through the use of contraception, citing its potential to delay the drive towards parenthood. Turning to developmental implications, Kestenberg (1981c), in line with Benedek (1952), argued that parenthood constitutes a distinct developmental phase of adulthood owing to the unique constellation of erotic and sadistic drives, specific phantasies, and altered self- and object-representations that reorganise psychic structures. She identified particular libidinal orientations towards children, expressed as deep concern for their well-being and adoration, alongside sadistic drives manifesting in phantasies of ejection and separation. She maintained that this phase is characterised by drives towards satisfaction in reproduction, creation, and nurturing and further argued that these drives, in sublimated form, also fuel artistic creation, community development, and caring orientations, thereby extending her model to include childless adults. She further contended that this phase – like other psychosexual phases – reorganises prior psychic structure through regressions associated with reproduction, gestation, anticipation, creation, and nurturing of the child (or analogous passionate, creative pursuits). These regressions offer opportunities to address unresolved conflicts from infantile development, including issues related to early care, the Oedipus complex, self- and other-representation, ego defences, and coping mechanisms. Kestenberg accounted for variations in adult parental attitudes as resulting from the divergent reproductive developments of boys and girls stemming from the integration of *inner-genital* (feminine) and *outer-genital* (masculine) developmental drives with parental identifications and prevailing cultural norms. Collectively, these factors contribute to distinct sex-specific identity and parental attitudes in adulthood (Kestenberg, 1965b, 1980a, 1980b, 1980c, 1981c; Kestenberg et al., 1971, 1994).

In relation to the formation of adult sex-specific identity in women, Kestenberg (1980b) outlined what she presented as the three versions of femininity, each associated with phases of psychosexual development in girls. According to her developmental model (Kestenberg, 1956a, 1956b, 1956c), the *inner-genital* phase is characterised by cryptic and diffuse inner-genital sensations that promote an internal focus and a gestational, nurturing attitude, which she described as early maternal tendencies. As these tensions build, discomfort arises in the second part of this phase, leading to wishes to expel or destroy the illusory baby. This shift marks a transition into the *outer-genital*, phallic phase (which she also termed the negative Oedipal phase). In this phase, she suggested that girls become goal-directed, outwardly oriented, and assertive, often competing with male figures such as fathers and brothers. The subsequent subphase of the *outer-genital*, phallic phase (the positive Oedipal phase), she characterised by a pronounced external orientation, denial of inner-genital tensions, and the emergence of wishes to be penetrated by the father. She described the girl as developing admiration and passionate feelings towards the father. The phase culminates in the repression of the girl's Oedipal wishes, including both aggression towards the mother and desires related to the father, and leads to the differentiation of the feminine superego. Through the relative quiet of latency, and the later reactivation and reorganisation of these phases in adolescence, this developmental sequence leads to what Kestenberg called the "three faces of femininity": the caring mother, the career-oriented achiever, and the sensual wife (Kestenberg, 1980b, p. 333).

Kestenberg (1980c, 1981c) proposed that sex-specific parental attitudes manifest in distinct movement behaviours. She argued that fathers are generally more active and physically separate during interactions with infants, while mothers tend to exhibit containing and merger-oriented behaviours. She specified that smooth, flexible *Tension-Flow* qualities and open *Shape-Flow* patterns, fostering connection and union, are characteristically more feminine. By contrast, a more masculine movement repertoire was described by more frequent aggressive, sharp *Tension-Flow* qualities and closed, self-focused *Shape-Flow* patterns. However, she maintained that the presence of feminine components in men, such as indulging *Tension-Flow* and open, incorporating *Shape-Flow* patterns, provides the necessary basis for receptivity, whereas masculine components in women promote self-containment and stability, enabling them to care for and safeguard their children (Kestenberg & Marcus, 1979). Kestenberg (1980c, p. 78) contended that "pure maleness and femaleness" are inadequate for effective parenting, suggesting that optimal parental attitudes emerge from borrowing characteristics from the opposite sex. She further contended that it is the experience of *inner-genital*, maternal and *outer-genital*, paternal identifications in both sexes that enable individuals to identify with their spouses and with their children of the opposite sex.

Kestenberg and Robbins (1975) extended these claims to the contemporary cultural domain, linking the widespread use of contraceptive pills to what they perceived as a reduction in sex-specific behaviours among women. They posited that, as girls become "*less feminine*", their capacity to counterbalance boys' aggressive tendencies in society diminishes; this, they argued, contributes to "unisexisation" and, ultimately, impairs child-rearing skills (Kestenberg & Robbins, 1975, p. 452). Relatedly, Kestenberg (1980b, p. 320) critiqued the emergence of new sex research that contributed to the clitoris gaining recognition as a legitimate female sexual organ. She contended that this recognition fostered greater acceptance of phallic sexuality in women and encouraged women to seek equality with men. Kestenberg problematised these developments, suggesting they conflicted with traditional expectations of motherhood and the necessity of a heterosexual relationship (Kestenberg, 1980b).

Drawing upon direct observational data from expectant mothers at the Center for Parents and Children and notes from analysts working with pregnant women and from clinicians at the Neonatal Unit of Long Island Jewish Hillside Hospital, Kestenberg (1976) proposed that pregnancy should be viewed as a new *inner-genital* phase of development in which certain regressions to pregenital phases occur. She suggested that regression during the three trimesters of pregnancy follows the first three phases of psychosexual development, revisiting oral, anal, and urethral conflicts. She proposed that, in the first trimester, oral incorporative wishes foster attachment (psychic and physical) to the fetus. In the second trimester, anal drives support the conceptualisation of the fetus as a separate being that, in the third trimester, turn into urethral patterns of letting go, preparing the mother for birth.

Turning to maternal attitudes, Kestenberg and Javaid (1983) examined *maternal entrancement* and its development across the first postpartum year. Their research utilised observational data and interviews with mothers and young children. They defined entrancement as a profound sense of love between parents and the newborn, marked by admiration and intense engagement with the infant's development. They further specified maternal entrancement as the somatoaffective component that ensures the newborn's survival by counteracting potential aggressive urges activated during labour. They observed that maternal entrancement with the newborn leads to estrangement from the older children. They stressed the father's supportive role in caring for and nurturing the older siblings' disappointments, thereby also reducing the mother's guilt over her diminished attention to them (Kestenberg & Javaid, 1983). They also emphasised the relevance of child guidance work to foster the development of maternal entrancement when the process may have been hindered by postpartum depression or negative birth experiences. Their model emphasised the positive effects of the mother witnessing others' admiration for her baby. They also proposed assisted somatic exercises of mother–infant attunement (Kestenberg & Javaid, 1983).

Fetal Movements

Around the end of the 1980s, Kestenberg (1987, 1989, 1990) expanded her developmental formulations to the prenatal period. Drawing on contemporaneous research on fetal movement patterns, intrauterine development, and pre-birth memory, Kestenberg and Borowitz (1990) challenged the classical psychoanalytic view that the fetus is in a constant state of zero tension and without capacities to react to external stimuli (Comparetti, 1981; Verny, 1981; Birnholz et al., 1978). Kestenberg and Borowitz (1990) reported that ultrasound studies revealed spontaneous fetal movements as early as 7–10 weeks of gestation. These developed into independent limb movements by 10–12 weeks. By 24 weeks, self-soothing behaviours such as sucking were also observed. In considering primary fetal motor patterns, Kestenberg and Borowitz (1990) drew on Comparetti's distinction between *Primary Motor Patterns* and *Primary Motor Actions*, proposing that the former anticipate the emergence of id-derivative movement patterns, while the latter function as precursors to ego-controlled movements *in utero* (Kestenberg & Borowitz, 1990, p. 25). Based on sonogram records and expectant mothers' reports of fetal movements, they argued for the existence of prenatal experiences of pleasure and unpleasure, as well as comfort and discomfort, demonstrated in the fetus's use of *Tension-Flow* and *Shape-Flow* patterns.

Kestenberg emphasised the importance of fostering trust and empathy between the expectant mother and the fetus, which could be achieved through fetal movement notation (Kestenberg, 1989, 1990). She argued that mothers' visualisation and embodiment of the fetus's *Tension-Flow* and *Shape-Flow* patterns enhance the formation of an individualised emotional connection to their unborn child. Kestenberg proposed that early aspects of the baby's temperament may be reflected in these prenatal *Tension-Flow* expressions, and that their exploration could support parents in developing tolerance and acceptance of their future child's personality (Kestenberg, 1990, pp. 120–121). To this end, she taught expectant mothers her *Tension-Flow* notation to document the fetus's movement patterns. Kestenberg further asserted that, during pregnancy, basic trust can be cultivated by the mother responding to the fetus's kicks and punches through *Lengthening* or *Widening Shape-Flow.* She also encouraged mothers to breathe into the area to facilitate tissue stretching and create additional space for the fetus. She proposed that mothers' exploration of their vertical alignment during pregnancy gave the fetus the sense of being actively held and embraced in the womb (Kestenberg, 1990, p. 123). Additionally, she emphasised the importance of sound, recommending singing or humming during birth to alleviate tension.

Holocaust Studies

This section discusses Kestenberg's final major project. In the late 1960s, she embarked on a new research direction, the psychohistorical study of the effects of the Nazi Holocaust. Later, with her husband, Milton Kestenberg, and colleagues at Child Development Research, she went on to conduct one of the largest international studies of the Nazi Holocaust, the Jerome Riker International Study of Organised Persecution of Children. Across Kestenberg's life-work, a significant shift of interest is palpable between her two principal projects: developmental movement studies and psychohistorical studies of the Nazi Holocaust. Although these topics appear dissimilar, a closer examination uncovers a consistent somatic and developmental orientation. In what follows, I orient my analysis to explicating the relationship between her earlier movement studies and later Holocaust research by tracing the embedded somatic threads.

Attention to the psychological effects of the Nazi Holocaust gradually began to emerge in psychoanalysis during the 1960s. A few reports started to circulate in psychiatric journals addressing the mental health of Holocaust survivors. Henry Krystal organised conferences and seminars for professionals in social services and doctors on the effects of massive psychic trauma (Jucovy, 1985; Fogelman, 2019). In 1966, the Israel Psychoanalytic Society organised a symposium on the pathological effects of the Holocaust and the treatment of survivors (Bergmann & Jucovy, 1982). The issue gained international attention when the Congress of the International Psycho-Analytic Association entitled "Psychic Traumatisation through Social Catastrophe" was held in 1967. In the coming years, pioneering works on the psychoanalytic study of the effects of the Holocaust were published by Krystal (1968) and Niederland (Krystal & Niederland, 1971). Interest in survivors' children also gradually grew as analysts began documenting specific psychological patterns among the second generation (Trossman, 1968; Sigal & Rakoff, 1971; Anthony & Koupernik, 1973).

Initially, there was less focus on the experiences of child survivors. The prevailing view among many psychiatrists and even within the survivor community was that children were either too young to have been significantly harmed or resilient enough not to have been affected. Child survivors rarely spoke openly about their experience in the postwar years. Many of them did not fully remember what had happened to them and did not perceive themselves as real victims of the Nazi Holocaust (Jucovy, 1985; Herzog, 2019; Stein, 2009; Kangisser Cohen et al., 2019). It was not until they grew older and sought help for emotional difficulties that mental health professionals began to focus on their specific needs (Jucovy, 1985, p. 32; Herzog, 2019). The first focused study on child survivors was Yaffa Eliach's oral history project, launched in 1979 (Kangisser Cohen et al., 2019; Fogelman, 2017; Herzog, 2019). Despite the growing awareness of the psychological complexities of Holocaust trauma, it was not until the 1980s that survivor syndrome was added under the category of Post-Traumatic Stress Disorder in the *Diagnostic and Statistical Manual of Mental Disorders* (Stein, 2009, p. 35; Herzog, 2019).

Kestenberg's interest in the Nazi Holocaust was sparked in 1968 by the case of a patient in analysis. She was a child of a survivor, who, although never having personal experience of the Nazi Holocaust, according to Kestenberg, "looked like a concentration camp prisoner" (Kestenberg, 1992b, p. 188). Surprised by the patient's presentation, Kestenberg began to wonder how other psychoanalysts approached what appeared to her as a distinct form of traumatisation. She became fully engrossed in research on the Nazi Holocaust. She was determined to uncover every little detail about deportations and concentration camps, from their overall layout and the placement of bunk beds to the routines of daily life in the camps (Naszkowska, 2023). This was substantiated by my archival research in Janet Kestenberg Amighi's private collection of her mother's work, where I found numerous boxes of maps of concentration camps and photos of Jewish ghettos.

Kestenberg sent a questionnaire to about 320 psychoanalysts worldwide, asking about their analytic work with second-generation survivors of the Nazi Holocaust (Jucovy, 1985; Fogelman, 2017, 2019; Kangisser Cohen et al., 2019). She received only a few responses, which she interpreted as indicative of both widespread indifference and the underrepresentation of second-generation survivors in analytic treatment (Jucovy, 1985). At the time, and even later in the 1970s, many psychoanalysts were reluctant to address the Nazi Holocaust in analytic work or to link their patients' difficulties to the persecution their parents had endured (Krystal, 1984; Eickhoff, 1989). A well-known example is Heinz Kohut's (1913–1981) discussion of his frequently cited patient (Mr A), in which he omitted key details about the patient's forced separation from his father and subsequent displacement during the Nazi control of Germany. Kohut also explicitly rejected linking the patient's difficulties to the effects of the Holocaust (Kestenberg & Kestenberg, 1982, p. 41; Krystal, 1984). The small number of psychoanalysts interested in the transgenerational effects of the Nazi Holocaust attempted to establish a study group within the American Psychoanalytic Association but encountered substantial resistance. As a result, they organised ad hoc meetings at psychoanalytic conferences to discuss the topic (Fogelman, 2019, p. 84).

Drawing on her questionnaire data, Kestenberg and her collaborators convened a workshop at the 1970 Congress of Child Psychiatry, held in Palestine/Israel, followed by another at the 1971 joint meeting of the American Psychoanalytic Association and the Association for Child Psychoanalysis in New York (Bergmann & Jucovy, 1982; Kestenberg, 1973b, 1974a). In 1973, Kestenberg organised a session at the fall meeting of the American Psychoanalytic Association on the effects of the Nazi Holocaust on survivors' children and grandchildren. The subsequent meeting took place on 19 May 1974 at the Kestenbergs' home. Minutes from these early gatherings set out their initial agenda (Kestenberg, 1973b, 1974a). Kestenberg noted that many analytic treatments with second-generation survivors ended prematurely because patients discontinued therapy. She attributed these disruptions to the difficulty of confronting unconscious dimensions of their parents' Holocaust trauma. Meeting participants noted a particular resistance among some survivor parents, who opposed their children's treatment or engagement in discussions related to the Nazi Holocaust. Bergmann raised concerns about countertransference among therapists, noting that feelings of restitution and the sublimation of personal guilt could affect their work with second-generation victims.

Participants stressed that the project's success depended on establishing clear inclusion criteria. They debated whether to include cases involving children of survivors who had not been in concentration camps but had endured other forms of atrocity, such as separation from their parents or living in hiding. The group emphasised the need to broaden the study's scope to include the children of Nazi persecutors. Kestenberg encouraged several psychoanalysts, including Edith Buxbaum, Margaret Fries, and Marianne Kris, to join this project and sent them the meeting minutes. However, Kestenberg's correspondence and later project documentation suggest that this never came to fruition (Kestenberg, 1973b, 1974a).

Based on these informal meetings, in 1974, Judith and Milton Kestenberg, along with Milton E. Jucovy (1918–1999) and Martin S. Bergmann (1913–2014), officially established the Group for the Psychoanalytic Study of the Effect of the Holocaust on the Second Generation. The group's work was sponsored by the Fund for Psychoanalytic Research of the American Psychoanalytic Association (American Psychoanalytic Association, 1976, 1978a, 1978b; Bergmann & Jucovy, 1982, p. xi). The study group met eight to ten times per year for approximately 15 years to discuss cases of survivors they had been treating (Jucovy, 1985, p. 33; Fogelman, 2017; Kangisser Cohen et al., 2019). Several other clinicians joined the group throughout the years. The study group also corresponded with German analysts about cases of children of Nazi prosecutors (Bergmann & Jucovy, 1982, p. 29). With their inclusion of children of persecutors, the group members saw an opportunity to explore the relationships between trauma and the mechanisms of memory and identity from a broader perspective (Jucovy, 1985, pp. 33–34). Their inquiry essentially focused on the effects of untold family trauma on the psychic development of the next generation and on the mechanisms of transgenerational trauma transmission (Jucovy, 1985). They defined a child survivor of the Nazi Holocaust as any Jewish child who was 13 years old or younger at the onset of persecution in their country and who managed to survive in German-occupied Europe through various means, including hiding, joining partisan groups, residing in ghettos, evading capture, or enduring internment in concentration camps. The definition of war child referred to non-Jewish children who lived in Germany or any other country occupied by the Third Reich (Kangisser Cohen et al., 2019). Bergman and Jucovy published the group's results in the anthology *Generations of the Holocaust* in 1982. The volume included chapters from several members that covered the first 6 years of work, 34 cases in total (21 involving children of survivors, with the remainder a mixed cohort of child survivors, individuals displaced in childhood, and children of Nazi persecutors).

Somatisation and Transposition

Kestenberg (1980d) examined how the manifest and latent messages of survivor parents are taken up, transformed, and expressed in the inner lives of their children, and how the parents' experiences of the Nazi Holocaust reverberate in the patient material that second-generation survivors bring to analysis. Drawing on a range of analytic accounts (Winnik, 1968; Laufer, 1973; Furman, 1973; Rosenberger, 1973), Kestenberg (1980d) emphasised the heterogeneity among these patients. Differences pertained to their manifest symptoms, family background, parental histories, and pre-Holocaust personality organisation, as well as to the severity, timing, and context of the original traumatisation and post-liberation conditions (Keilson & Sarphatie, 1979; Porter, 1979). Nevertheless, she identified recurring features across multiple cases. Parent–child relationships often appeared to be influenced by the persistent threat of annihilation facing the entire Jewish population. Rather than positing a 'survivor's child syndrome', which would imply a specific pathology, she emphasised that aspects of Holocaust trauma impact people differently, at times contributing to both vulnerability and strength. Kestenberg (1982) observed that somatisation was a symptom for both first- and second-generation survivors. She argued that child survivors' deprivation during persecution would have contributed to regressions to the oral phase, which may have left them vulnerable to physical manifestations of illness in later life. She stressed that the second generation often seemed to be deprived of responsive maternal containment, which leads to a risk of later developing psychosomatic symptoms (Kestenberg, 1982, 1998a). One of Kestenberg's (1980d, 1982) most influential contributions to the mechanisms of transgenerational trauma transmission was a concept related to somatisation, which she termed *transposition*.

Kestenberg (1980d) presented the case of a second-generation survivor who sought analysis in late adolescence owing to marked disturbances of bodily functions and profound inhibition in social and academic performance. Her patient, Rachel, reportedly ate very little, sometimes to the point of near starvation, retained stool for prolonged periods, and suffered from severe insomnia. Kestenberg explicitly distinguished this case from psychosis and personality disorders, contending that the client's symptoms were closely associated with a persistent internal sense of danger originating in her father's Holocaust experience. Kestenberg (1980d) added that, unlike in cases of narcissistic grandiosity, Rachel had a profound devotion and commitment to her family and friends. She proposed that Rachel lived in the past of her father's life as she withdrew from social relations and spent most of her life in hiding, as her father had done outside the camp. Kestenberg (1980d) suggested that Rachel's 'grandiose dissociation' from her bodily needs was an attempt to represent the horrors her father suffered during the Nazi Holocaust. She interpreted that Rachel's body had been invested with meanings derived from her father's experience of persecution.

Based on Rachel's reports, her father treated his and her bodies as emotionless machines, vehicles of omnipotence whose steeling against assault was understood as a precondition of both personal survival and the rescue of others. Bodily endurance was imbued with a quasi-messianic task of restituting the dead. Kestenberg (1980d) contended that Rachel's survival came to be linked to the idea of resurrecting the dead and perhaps contributed to her sense of herself as a reincarnation of relatives who did not survive. Kestenberg proposed that Rachel may have imagined that, when she ate, she was also feeding her murdered relatives, and perhaps all those who starved to death. At the same time, Rachel may have felt obliged not to eat to train her body. During analysis, Rachel became aware of her phantasy that, by starving herself, she was also starving those internal others. Kestenberg (1980d) interpreted that Rachel felt a bodily responsibility for all the Jews she carried within her.

Kestenberg (1982) explained that the massive trauma of the father, which he could not feel, mourn, or integrate, intruded into the psychic reality of the daughter through the process of transposition. Kestenberg viewed Rachel's symptoms as creative attempts by her as a second-generation survivor to undo the past, rescue those who perished, and compensate for the suffering of those who survived. Kestenberg (1982) further clarified that *transposition* went beyond the psychoanalytic concept of identification as it relied on bodily and psychic incorporation of the past. Second-generation survivors lived out the lives of dead children and lost relatives and often carried the mission to undo the losses of their parents and make their survival worthwhile (Kestenberg, 1998a, p. 59). Kestenberg also emphasised that *transposition* essentially happens on subsymbolic and somatic levels as ambivalent family trauma and secrets permeate the intersubjective space between generations of survivors.

Kestenberg asserted that the distinctive psychological effects of Holocaust trauma on survivors necessitate specialised clinical approaches. She maintained that analysts must possess a thorough understanding of the historical context of the Nazi Holocaust to formulate targeted questions and identify indications of unspoken or ambivalent family trauma. She viewed this as particularly important as she found that survivor parents frequently withhold, modify, or fragment narratives of their experiences when communicating with their children (Kestenberg & Kestenberg, 1982). Kestenberg and Kahn (1998) argued that, as repeated ruptures in survivors' lives led to a fractured sense of continuity of the self, treatment should aim to help survivors reclaim childhood memories that had been repressed or denied. They stressed the need for a specific, integration-focused approach rather than non-survivor-specific interventions that encouraged survivors to simply live in the present.

The Body Testifies

In 1953, West Germany passed a uniform indemnification law to compensate victims of Nazi persecution. "West Germany created treaties with allied countries of lump sum compensation, and these countries awarded their nationals for damages" (M. Kestenberg, 1982, 1985, p. 64). According to the indemnification law, only those whose earnings had been reduced by at least 25 per cent owing to persecution were eligible for restitution. However, the German government and psychiatrists frequently exploited this standard, assessing losses at 24 per cent or less or demanding extensive evidence that it was nearly impossible for claimants to provide (M. Kestenberg, 1985; Herzog, 2019). The process of filing reparations was itself rigorous; survivors were subjected to repeated questioning and required to produce detailed statements, which were examined by German-appointed psychiatrists.

Judith Kestenberg's husband, Milton, was an attorney who became well known for representing survivors of the Nazi Holocaust, especially child survivors, who fell through the loopholes of indemnification laws (Lambert, 1991; Kestenberg & Kestenberg, 1982). Milton argued that the restitution process was not only difficult but also potentially retraumatising, and it called for a special interviewing technique and an empathetic attitude on the part of legal professionals (Kestenberg & Kestenberg, 1982; Kestenberg & Kahn, 1998). He stressed that child survivors were especially disadvantaged. They often could not remember enough details of their persecution to construct a convincing narrative for their claims (M. Kestenberg, 1985). Additionally, German psychiatrists often dismissed the psychological suffering of children, arguing that, if they could hardly remember their experiences, they could not have experienced significant harm. Milton and Judith Kestenberg (1982) fought to establish psychological trauma as legitimate grounds for restitution, especially in cases of child survivors.

As discussed in detail earlier in this chapter, Judith Kestenberg attributed a significant role to somatic and movement-based experiences in psychic development. Based on these formulations, she devised a psychoanalytically oriented narrative interview technique that employed a kinaesthetic approach to support the recovery of inaccessible traumatic experiences. She employed this technique to help recover child survivors' early memories, both to support their reparations claims and as a therapeutic tool (Kestenberg & Kestenberg, 1982). She stressed that childhood memories differ from adult recollections, appearing in flashes and often devoid of meaning. In interviews, Kestenberg asked survivors to imagine crucial events from their childhood, including developmental milestones in movement (Kestenberg, 1988a, p. 562). She would direct the child survivor's attention to somatic memories of crawling, walking, and sleeping, as well as to parental interactions. By evoking these kinaesthetic memories, such as rhythms of movement, muscle tension, and bodily sensations associated with feelings of safety or danger, she attempted to aid the reconstruction of details of the survivor's narrative. In the case of a Hungarian child survivor, they managed to establish the survivor's age at deportation, a decisive factor in the reparation trial, by evoking somatic memories such as rhythms of crawling or being carried (Kestenberg, 1988a; Kahn, 1998). Another reason for Kestenberg to inquire about the movement memories of child survivors was to substantiate psychological damages as a basis for restitution. She aimed to assess potential delays in movement development based on survivors' reports, which she argued exerted a decisive influence on ego development. Kestenberg explained:

> The effect of persecution on the ego is manifold. The restriction of space with the ensuing inability to move freely, the breaking down of the children's sense of gravity with the ensuing inability to stand up or stretch, the loss of the sense of time, all represented an infringement on basic ego functions, acquired during early development. (Kestenberg, 1992, p. 374)

Through listening to kinaesthetic memories, Milton and Judith Kestenberg brought the body to trial. In their view, movement became evidence, and the body testified.

International Study of Organised Persecution of Children

In 1981, as an expansion of their previous projects, Judith and Milton Kestenberg launched the *Jerome Riker International Study of Organised Persecution of Children* (ISOPC) under the auspices of Child Development Research. The CDR revised its mission statement[47] to reflect and explicitly incorporate the work of the ISOPC. It declared itself to be an:

> organisation dedicated to restoring and preserving the mental health of children, especially those who suffered under the extreme trauma of organised persecution. This includes documenting patterns of normal child development and disruptions, distortions, and adaptations that occur in the aftermath of trauma. The organisation is dedicated to discovering and promulgating approaches that can ameliorate the long-term effects on victims of past, present, and future mass dehumanisation. One of our points of focus will be the nonverbal expressions of normal and disrupted child development. (Child Development Research, n.d.b)

Their 4R policy[48] articulated four action areas: *Remember, Record, Reflect, Recover*. Their updated goals were to prevent childhood disorders, particularly those linked to extreme trauma; to validate nonverbal methods of personality assessment and treatment; to collect interviews with child survivors of the Nazi Holocaust worldwide; to analyse the effects of organised persecution and examine mechanisms of adaptation and recovery in the aftermath of trauma; and to train mental health professionals to treat child survivors, with special emphasis on creative arts-based approaches (Child Development Research, n.d.a).

The ISOPC collected approximately 1,500 psychohistorical interviews from child survivors, children of survivors, and war children worldwide. Its research objective was to illuminate the tragic losses suffered by a diverse group of victims during the Second World War (Kangisser Cohen et al., 2019). The semi-structured interviews were designed to document personal experiences of the Nazi Holocaust for historiographical purposes and to support the processing of trauma among survivors (Kestenberg & Kahn, 1998). These testimonies were audiotaped and anonymised. Family members were not shown the footage, so the survivors could speak more freely about their experiences (Fogelman, 2017; Sossin, personal communication, 18 November 2025).

The project involved approximately 83 interviewers from around the world, most of whom were mental health professionals who were often survivors themselves (Child Development Research, n.d.d). In such cases, the protocol required that they themselves be interviewed first, before conducting interviews with others. Many participants in the ISOPC project spoke about their experiences for the first time and described the process as transformative, encouraging other survivors to take part (Fogelman, 2017). Kestenberg's kinaesthetic narrative interview technique was further applied in this project. Interviewers would ask about memories of anxiety or hunger, and whether the survivor could explore the physical environment safely or instead felt confined and restrained (Kestenberg, 1992, p. 379). The interview process also included a body-focused questionnaire, inviting survivors to attend to bodily sensations and to report which body parts were most clearly present in their awareness when recalling certain events (ISOPC, n.d.). Kestenberg also believed that transgenerational trauma, such as trauma of the Nazi Holocaust, could be identified in the bodily movements of the individual (Laemmli, 2016, 2021), and she notated the movements of interview subjects when other Holocaust researchers showed her video footage of interviews they conducted (Sossin, personal communication, 18 November 2025).

Testimonies collected during the ISOPC project were later digitised and placed in the Kestenberg Holocaust Child Survivor Archive at the Hebrew University of Jerusalem, with digitisation support from the Conference on Jewish Material Claims Against Germany, the Fondation pour la Mémoire de la Shoah, and Child Development Research. Results of the ISOPC project were published in the volume edited by Judith Kestenberg and Charlotte Kahn (1998) entitled *Children Surviving Persecution: An International Study of Trauma and Healing* and in another collection of papers, edited by Judith Kestenberg and Ira Brenner (1996a), *The Last Witness: The Child Survivor of the Holocaust.*

Judith and Milton Kestenberg not only devoted their later lives to studying the transgenerational effects of the Nazi Holocaust but also disseminated information about survivors' associations and self-help groups in the ISOPC newsletters, published between 1984 and 1998 (Child Development Research, 1990; Kestenberg & Kahn, 1998).[49] They were particularly interested in how artistic expression influenced trauma recovery and collected a large number of artworks of survivors[50] (International Study of Organised Persecution of Children Files, n.d.; M. Kestenberg, 1987). Their large collection of survivors' artwork now constitutes an integral part of the Kestenberg Papers in the Library of Congress.

Developmental Effects of Holocaust Trauma

Kestenberg's psychoanalytic studies on the effects of the Nazi Holocaust all sought to understand the intricacies of traumatisation – physical and psychological implications – and their long-term consequences. She and her collaborators explored how massive trauma affected psychic development ego and superego functioning. They argued that persecution often continued after the Holocaust in various psychosomatic and intersubjective forms (Kestenberg & Kahn, 1998; Jucovy, 1985; Kangisser Cohen et al., 2019; Caropreso, 2024a, 2024b; Naszkowska, 2023).

Kestenberg (1981a; Kestenberg & Kestenberg, 1987) analysed how punitive Nazi ideology invaded the psychic life of Holocaust survivors, arguing that its violence operated via psychosomatic and developmental registers. She contended that, in concentration camps, victims lost their bodily autonomy through the infantilising regimes of being confined, silenced, and fed at the oppressors' will, which resembled authoritarian parenting (Caropreso, 2024b). She further noted that the arbitrariness of camp rules, the impossibility of testing reality (e.g., time or seasonal changes), and reliance on information provided by the oppressors – often purposely deceptive – damaged ego functioning (Kestenberg, 1981a).

In relation to the superego development of child survivors, Kestenberg (1981a; Kestenberg & Brenner, 1986) emphasised the detrimental effects resulting from the breakdown of cultural norms and family values. She argued that the ego ideal and superego emerge from internalised cultural and parental proscriptions, which are embedded in recurring, habitual practices imbued with cultural meaning in which children participate. These practices provide the foundation for ideal self-representations and morality, and their consistency is essential for the formation and internalisation of stable systems of meaning. In the case of child survivors, Kestenberg asserted, the abrupt transition from parental independence and authority to powerlessness and vulnerability significantly disrupts processes of superego development. She also noted that cases in which, to ensure survival, previously law-abiding parents had to abandon their values and engage in theft may generate irreconcilable ambivalence and conflict in the development of their children's ego ideal and superego. Kestenberg (1981a) further argued that the necessary submission to the oppressors' violence leads to the internalisation of an aggressive parental imago. As a defence against its cruelty, survivors must identify with this parental ideal, which later operates through self-degrading prohibitions, contributing to irrational guilt over one's own liberation and leaving many survivors to live as if they were still persecuted (Kestenberg, 1981a, 1980d, 1988b; Kestenberg & Kestenberg, 1987; Kestenberg & Brenner, 1986, 1996b; Jucovy, 1985; Caropreso, 2024b).

A case Kestenberg and Brenner (1986) reported was a child survivor who, after liberation, received personal items that belonged to her beloved aunt, who had been killed. Although her mother allowed her to keep the aunt's pocketbook, she continued to experience intense anxiety and physical discomfort associated with this memory, linked to guilt about surviving and taking a cherished object from the dead. The authors further highlighted that hidden children, or those who survived by concealing their Jewish identity, frequently carried a persistent guilt over having had to abandon their cultural heritage. They also stressed that precocious awareness of the worst possibilities and the lack of parental guidance led child survivors to develop prematurely strong capacities for resilience. These were often intertwined with guilt and anger over deprivation and later manifested in specific forms of somatisation (Kestenberg & Brenner, 1986, 1996b).

The Nazi Superego[51]

Kestenberg's Holocaust studies were uniquely wide in scope. As mentioned earlier, from the work of the psychoanalytic study group to the ISOPC project, she viewed war children and the children of Nazi persecutors as victims of the culture of cruelty during the Third Reich. As part of the ISOPC project, Kestenberg and her collaborators collected testimonies from children of Nazi perpetrators, revealing the harmful psychic impact of concealed family secrets and the devastating effects of discovering the atrocities of their parents' past (Kestenberg, 1988b). Kestenberg argued that superego conflicts may arise from misalignment between the superego's punitive prohibitions and the ego ideal's aspirations, and from inconsistencies in authority figures' prohibitions. In case of children of former Nazi persecutors, she contended that the parents' denial of their actions as well as their Nazi ideology may simultaneously become incorporated into their children's superego, along with the child's secret knowledge of the parents' past, leading to disorganised superego development (Kestenberg, 1988b, p. 3). However, she poignantly highlighted the dual potential inherent in this conflict and argued that, because the superego is shaped by ancestral history, it possesses the capacity for both corruption and cultural transformation, as illustrated when a child chooses not to become like their parents (Kestenberg, 1988b, p. 2).

Across various late papers, Kestenberg (1981a, 1988b, 1992, 1998b; Kestenberg & Brenner, 1986; Kestenberg & Kestenberg, 1987) analysed the developmental and cultural dimensions of the Nazi superego from an economic psychoanalytic perspective. Building on Freudian drive-theory (and primal horde theory),[52] she argued that civilisation and its moral consciousness emerge from the renunciation and redirection of primal, aggressive drives. This is understood to occur through the introjection of parental and social proscriptions, and through the regulatory functions of the ego and superego. Kestenberg (1988b) assumed an intrinsic hostility between generations, particularly manifesting as parental aggression towards children. Under optimal developmental conditions, this aggression is transformed into concern for the child's well-being. When the Oedipus complex is successfully resolved during development, the emergence of the superego activates feelings of guilt regarding parental sadistic impulses (Kestenberg & Kestenberg, 1987). She added that, in the case of conflictual superego development, however, this renunciation fails, and sadistic urges remain untransformed, leading to cruel parental attitudes towards children. She identified this phenomenon as exemplified by the Nazi superego, which manifested as contempt for the weak and vulnerable.

Expanding these formulations with her developmental theory, Kestenberg (1988b) added that the superego does not arise solely from the Oedipus complex but follows its own developmental line. She maintained that stable superego structures depend on the successful fusion of nurturing, *inner-genital* drives with sadistic, *outer-genital* ones. In her developmental view, the child moves from the urethral phase into the feminine, *inner-genital* phase, then to the phallic, masculine, *outer-genital phase*, both of which serve psychic integration. She added that, with latency, pre-Oedipal taboos combine with the first resolution of the Oedipus complex to establish cultural safeguards against incest and murder. In adolescence, the Oedipus complex is reworked, and identifications with peers, siblings, leaders, and abstract ideologies are embedded into the superego (Kestenberg, 1988b, p. 10). When the maternal, *inner-genital* phase is overwhelmed by pregenital drives, the wish for a baby (which activates in children of both sexes) could transform into a wish to kill the child. She further stated that, in these cases, parental attitudes become infused with sadistic and punitive tendencies. Kestenberg argued that Nazi ideology embodied the sadistic parental superego by glorifying German motherhood but also expecting mothers to send their children to war, killing other children and mothers without remorse. She further proposed that sanctioned violence in the Third Reich extended even to German youth, who were sent to fight impossible battles. She concluded that the Nazis' child-hating superego was born of untamed *outer-genital* drives, and the wish to kill their own vulnerable children was displaced on to Jewish children (Kestenberg, 1988b, 1992; Caropreso, 2024b).

Kestenberg contended (1981a, 1988b) that an authoritarian state and a sadistic parent both exert a similarly corrupting influence on the ego, superego, and moral development. She suggested that the weakening of the ego prevents precursors of the superego from adequately regulating the id's temptations, leading to an overflow of infantile, pregenital drives. Infantile drives then fuse with the genital wish to eliminate the Oedipal rival and expand into a destructive desire to destroy anyone close to the mother (Kestenberg, 1988b, p. 4). She further proposed that, out of fear of paternal retaliation, these murderous impulses become displaced on to others and, together with the pre-Oedipal wish to degrade the mother, are projected on to vulnerable victims. She linked this mechanism to the Nazis' generalised contempt for the weak and to the eugenic narrative that viewed Jewish men as contaminators of German women.

In Kestenberg's psycho-cultural framework, based on drive-theory, the Nazi state is understood as a punitive and sadistic parent. In this view, those subjected to it (like children of a possessive, murderous parent) must identify with the aggressor while also remaining victims of aggression, which leads to the projection of their destructive desires on to others. She argued there was a distinctiveness of the "German superego" in the way Nazi ideology supplanted its internal morality with an authoritarian code of cruelty and loyalty (Kestenberg, 1981a, 1988b, 1998a, 1998b). She argued that Hitler came to embody a grandiose ego ideal, leading to the development of a corrupt superego. The hallmark of this corruption, she asserted, was its double morality, which openly legitimised violence and self-serving laws for the in-group while preaching religiosity and traditional family values (Kestenberg, 1980d, 1981a, 1988b, 1998a, 1998b; Caropreso, 2024b). Kestenberg (1988b) further supposed that Germans, through the internalisation of the tyrannical parental imago embodied by the state, developed an infantile mode of moral functioning (pre-cohesive and self-exempting) that led ordinary Germans to accept the mass dehumanisation of their fellow citizens (Caropreso, 2024b).

Kestenberg (1981a, 1988b, 1992; Kestenberg & Kestenberg, 1987) further argued that, besides the image of the tyrannical parent, Nazi ideology also embodied another parental trope: the sacrificial parent who renounces their own needs for their children. She suggested that, through the doubling of the image of the omnipotent and the powerless, saviour and aggressor, the Nazi regime could present itself as the injured party. Jewish people and other persecuted groups were viewed as the "bad children," providing both moral alibi and justification for violence. In this sense, Kestenberg (1981a, 1988b, 1992) argued that scapegoating was not only a political tactic but also an intrapsychic manoeuvre that allowed the denial and displacement of murderous impulses while preserving a self-image of righteousness (Caropreso, 2024b). Kestenberg's drive-theory-based formulations on superego development in authoritarian and oppressive conditions delivered a warning that, under certain cultural and familial conditions, the conscience of any community can be infantilised, fractured, and enlisted in the service of violence. She (1998a, 1998b) concluded that the antidote to an oppressive superego is not the imposition of new authority but reflective ownership of one's moral life.

Kestenberg's studies on the Nazi Holocaust were original in scope and methodology. Their defining feature was their kinaesthetic, developmental, and psychohistorical approach. Her studies were concerned with the developmental consequences of oppression and dehumanisation for the vulnerable – most specifically, children. As mentioned before, Judith and Milton Kestenberg devoted much of their lives to supporting the establishment of survivors' groups. They attended conferences worldwide on the topic of psychohistory and the victimisation of children (Kestenberg & Kestenberg, 1990). They participated in a meeting organised by the Freud Centre of the University of Jerusalem, focusing on the effects of war and militarisation on children in various places such as Cambodia, Mozambique, Palestine, Argentina, and Israel. They echoed concerns about the militarisation of children in Palestine and Israel and critiqued the State of Israel for not fostering good relationships. Kestenberg concluded that examining the effects of the Nazi Holocaust revealed profound insights about survivors' experience and human development, as well as the psychological and cultural consequences of oppressive (parental and governmental) authorities (Kestenberg & Kahn, 1998; Caropreso, 2024a, 2024b).

Between Tradition and Reform

Kestenberg grounded her psychodynamic theory of movement in classical psychoanalytic theory that linked bodily movement to pleasure seeking, drive-discharge, and ego defences (Breuer & Freud, 1895/1955; Freud, 1919, 1925, 1953, 1957a, 1957b, 1960, 1961, 1975; Ferenczi, 1952a, 1952b, 1955, 1994a, 1994b, 1994c; Abraham, 1913, 1949). Her focus was also closely aligned with several psychoanalytic movement researchers of the 1950s–1960s. She followed Deutsch's (1947, 1952) clinical observations on parallels between psychic states and postural change. Fries and Woolf's (1954) studies on congenital activity types and Mittelmann's (1957, 1958, 1960) studies also shaped her concepts. However, her main conceptual influences were Paul Schilder's (1942, 2013) work on body-image formation, Mahler's (1952, 1968; Mahler et al., 1975) and Erikson's (1950a, 1950b, 1959) developmental ego-psychology, Anna Freud's (1951, 1962, 1965; Freud et al., 1965) metapsychological framework and *Diagnostic Profile*, and Winnicott's (1958, 1960) object-relations perspective.

Although Kestenberg's work (1965a, 1965b, 1967a, 1967b) was conceptually closely aligned with these traditions, her developmental movement studies also differed significantly in both focus and the precision of her classificatory system. Rather than treating movement as a set of discrete behavioural units, she drew on Laban's dance and movement theory to classify it according to underlying qualitative dynamics. Kestenberg retained Laban's (1950, 1954, 2008; Laban & Lawrence, 1947) *Effort* categories and dimensional planes, but she extended this framework by developing the Labanian idea of *Flow* into separate categories of *Tension-Flow* and *Shape-Flow*, and by further elaborating *Shaping*. She also retained Laban's view of the moving body as animated by vibratory energies and tensions through which movement generates specific somatoaffective states in the mover and can influence others. In this sense, and in line with Laban, she understood movement as carrying therapeutic potential not only for individuals but also for society (as demonstrated by her Center for Parents and Children).

Kestenberg assigned qualities of *Tension-Flow* to component drives and traced the motor mechanisms of drive-discharge, distribution, and regulation. She emphasised the movement correlates of primary- and secondary-processes, early defences, and pre-ego functions. An Eriksonian epigenetic view of psychic development and the continuity between id and ego implicitly underpinned her developmental theory. These are reflected in her proposal of a cumulative sequence of movement patterns across distinct id- and ego-derivative categories, and in the assumption that congenital drive endowment shapes preferences for early defences, executive functions, coping mechanisms, and object-relations. In this view, drive-derivative *Tension-Flow* patterns come under the control of the ego-derived categories of *Pre-Efforts* and *Efforts*, while *Shape-Flow* becomes subordinated to complex *Shaping*.

Central notions of Kestenberg's framework included *Tension-Flow* attunement, *Shape-Flow* adjustment, and the principle of affinity as an indicator of intra- or interpersonal harmony or conflict. This principle implies a grammatical organisation to movement behaviour, proposing that clashes between affective *Tension-Flow* patterns and object-related *Shape-Flow* patterns signify intrapersonal conflicts between the drive aim and object. In her framework, clashes between ego-regulated *Efforts* and *Shaping* suggest tensions between adaptive aims and relational schemas; in gesture-posture sequences, such clashes may point to conflict between ego and superego structures. Drawing on her infant observations, she further argued that interpersonal clashes between mother and infant were critical in preventing developmental trauma. She proposed that such conflicts could be addressed through methods of *movement retraining* and creative arts-based interventions applied to parent–infant psychotherapy, family support, and child guidance (Kestenberg, 1965a, 1965b, 1967a; Kestenberg et al., 1971).

If we consider that Freud's work changed the paradigm of medical investigation from looking to listening, then Kestenberg further shifted it towards kinaesthetic listening. Freud developed the anatomy of narrative in his psychoanalytic technique; Kestenberg conceived of the psychodynamic vocabulary of movement. In the Freudian view, the psychic material underlying a symptom is revealed through language; for Kestenberg, it is revealed through the specific constellation of kinetic patterns within an individual's movement repertoire. Through her *Movement Profile*, she proposed that congenital preferences in drive-discharge and organisation, ego attitudes and functions, self–other schemas, and intra- or interpersonal conflicts could be visualised.

She used Labanotation as a symbolic system to represent various aspects of the observed movement sequence. However, she also developed her own inscription method that reached beyond what Laban's system captured. She documented the qualities of muscle tension through kinaesthetic free-hand tracing. Her method rendered the nuances of somatoaffective processes that would otherwise be imperceptible into readable waveforms. Freud (1964b, p. 160) noted the qualitative variations in tension between pleasure and unpleasure. Through her *Tension-Flow* concepts, Kestenberg formalised these qualities and developed a drawing practice to visualise them. Kestenberg's *Tension-Flow Curve*, as a distinct mode of visual inquiry, had an additional methodological particularity. It necessitated kinaesthetic attunement between bodies. This meant that she attuned to the mover's *Tension-Flow* and channelled its salient qualitative features into the movement of her hands and on to the paper. In this sense, the curves are the outcome of an embodied abstracting process that makes the multilayered complexity of movement readable while enabling the inquiry into how the *Tension-Flow* constellations participate in meaning-making about affective experience. Kestenberg's practice of movement-abstraction also employed the method of structuring. She quantified her qualitatively gathered kinaesthetic data and organised them into diagrams. The visually emerging patterns of the graphs, such as their relative widths, carried interpretive value. Structuring as a visual mode of inquiry in science is often aimed at making relations visible for comparison and classification. It is also a communicative practice that enables a community to share observations (Ambrosio, 2023). These were the considerations embedded in Kestenberg's movement profiling method. She translated embodied experience into graphs, aiming to make bodily movement not only thinkable but also communicable within psychoanalysis, child guidance, and therapeutic practice.

Kestenberg's body of work is marked by various internal ambivalences, reflected in her oscillation between reformist and conservative stances. Her traditionalist tendencies were most apparent in her continued commitment to

Freudian theory. Even though she critiqued classical psychoanalysis for neglecting the inner-genital organs in contrast to the clitoris and penis in psychosexual development, she joined the search for the 'essentially feminine', aligning with Freudian anatomical determinism. Following Bonaparte (2018), Deutsch (1925, 1930), and Greenacre (1950, 1948), she conceived of female sexuality as a developmental duality organised by contradiction (Birksted-Breen, 1993, p. 22). Kestenberg (1956b, 1956c) emphasised that children of both sexes pass through an *inner-genital* phase, characterised by feminine identifications and expressions, before entering the phallic phase, marked by paternal identification, penis envy in girls, and consolidation of the Oedipal situation. Although she proposed that the *inner-genital* phase is also present in boys, her developmental approach remained firmly situated within a Freudian, phallocentric framework (Kestenberg, 1973a). She described the girl's phallic phase as a "*misfortune*" that ends only when she overcomes penis envy and "*her hopelessness*" through the fantasy of growing a penis (Kestenberg, 1973a, p. 277). She further argued that the girl's turn away from the mother stems from a recognition that the mother lacks control over her own body and depends on the father's power. Kestenberg (1965a, 1965b, 1967a, 1967b, 1971a, 1985) proposed an adaptive, adult bisexual position grounded in the integration of *inner*- and *outer-genital* sensations as well as feminine and masculine tendencies. She identified this fusion as foundational to sex-specific identity, parental attitudes, and social adaptation. While this gestured towards a more nuanced perspective on the development of gender identity, Kestenberg also maintained strongly conservative assumptions, grounded in heteronormativity and gender stereotypes. She devised typologies of femininity, categorising women as mother, career woman, and wife, the integration of which she viewed as essential for the consolidation of feminine development. Furthermore, she critiqued movements towards women's equality and expressed concern about social practices that, in her view, delayed parenthood (Kestenberg, 1980b, p. 319, 1973a, 1980a, 1989; Kestenberg & Marcus, 1979; Kestenberg & Robbins, 1975).

On the other hand, Kestenberg's placing bodily movement at the centre of psychoanalytic inquiry was a pioneering effort. Her focus on internal bodily sensations, through which she reconsidered notions of activity and passivity, expanded libidinal theory to internal organs. Her emphasis on holding drives and ego processes to equal significance in psychoanalysis also demonstrated a progressive attitude. She addressed lesser-discussed topics such as fetal movements and proposed viewing parenthood as a developmental stage. In her later papers, she also emphasised mutual attunements between caregiver and infant and introduced the notion of *transsensus*, gesturing towards a bio-psycho-social view of development. Her work readily transgressed disciplinary boundaries between art and science, between body and mind. She integrated psychoanalytic developmental theory with dance studies and drew inspiration from Eastern medicine. When psychoanalysis was largely indifferent to the psychological consequences of the Nazi Holocaust, Kestenberg created new frameworks for understanding the developmental and intergenerational impact of persecution. Her concept of *transposition* enriched the psychoanalytic understanding of transgenerational trauma transmission with an embodied depth. Her somatically informed interviewing technique expanded the methodology of psychohistorical research.

Notes

1 Investing an object, person, or activity with libidinal energy.
2 In psychoanalysis, the term denotes the subject's mode of relating to the world, encompassing the complex outcomes of personality organisation, comprehension of objects and their phantasised aspects, as well as specific types of defence. The term is frequently used to refer to a particular subject's object-relations or to describe types of object-relationships, such as the oral object-relationship. In psychoanalytic terminology, the word 'object' is used to refer to subjects insofar as they are the objects of instinctual drives directed towards them. The concept of relationship here signifies the interconnection between the ways a subject constitutes their objects and the manner in which these objects influence the subject's actions (Laplanche & Pontalis, 1988, p. 277).
3 Curated Archive/Study notes & Literature/Study Notes/Notes on Spielrein/Notes on Jung/Notes on Hug-Hellmuth.
4 The oldest grandson of Sigmund Freud, the child playing the Fort/Da game in "Beyond the Pleasure Principle" (Freud, 1920/1975), who later trained and worked with his aunt, Anna Freud, at the Hempstead Clinic (Lupke, 2008).
5 "One of the two principles which, according to Freud, govern mental functioning: the whole of psychical activity is aimed at avoiding unpleasure and procuring pleasure. Inasmuch as unpleasure is related to the increase of quantities of excitation, and pleasure to their reduction, the principle in question may be said to be an economic one" (Laplanche & Pontalis, 1988, p. 322).
6 "Dynamic process consisting in a pressure (charge of energy, motricity factor) which directs the organism towards an aim. According to Freud, an instinct has its source in a bodily stimulus; its aim is to eliminate the state of tension obtaining at the instinctual source; and it is in the *object*, or thanks to it, that the instinct may achieve its aim" (Laplanche & Pontalis, 1988, p. 213).
7 Erotogenic or erogenous zone is a Freudian term for regions of the skin or mucous membrane that can become sites of sexual excitation. These areas function as primary sources of excitation and, in the Freudian framework, include oral, anal, and genital zones (Laplanche & Pontalis, 1988, p. 154).
8 For Freud, early sexuality is polymorphous and fragmented into component (partial) drives tied to varied erogenous zones; thus, a component instinct is specified by a somatic source (oral, anal, phallic erogenous zones), a tension-reducing aim, and an object. These partial drives operate independently in the early years of development yielding fragmented satisfactions and are later fused within successive libidinal arrangements and finally reorganised under genital primacy. Through developmental vicissitudes (learning, prohibition, frustration, identification, culture), originally diffuse pressures become attached to particular representations, producing highly individualised aims, objects, and modes of gratification. For example, an infant's diffuse oral tension is first relieved by sucking; as this drive attaches to particular representatives (the breast, bottle, caregiver), it crystallises

into recognisably oral aims and objects (food or kissing) (Laplanche & Pontalis, 1988, pp. 74–75, 127–129; Mitchell & Black, 2016, Chapter 1).

9 "Freud distinguishes three forms of masochism: erotogenic, feminine and moral. [...] By 'feminine masochism' one is naturally tempted to understand a 'masochism of women'. Freud certainly used such terms to mean the 'expression of the feminine essence', but in the context of the theory of bisexuality feminine masochism is an immanent possibility for any human being regardless of sex" (Laplanche & Pontalis, 1988, p. 245).

10 Cathexis is a psychoanalytic economic concept meaning "the fact that a certain amount of psychical energy is attached to an idea or to a group of ideas, to a part of the body, to an object" (Laplanche & Pontalis, 1988, p. 62).

11 "Process revealed by analytic investigation: in phantasy, the subject transposes objects and their inherent qualities from the 'outside' to the 'inside' of himself. Introjection is close in meaning to incorporation" (Laplanche & Pontalis, 1988, p. 228).

12 "The zones of the vagina and anus are confused into one representation. Cloacal theory is [...] sexual theory of children which ignores the distinction between vagina and anus. For Freud [...] [i]t is starting from this sort of undifferentiated state of affairs that 'the vagina, an organ derived from the cloaca, has to be raised into the dominant erotogenic zone'" (Freud, 1958, as cited in Laplanche & Pontalis, 1988, pp. 69–70).

13 Developed by F. M. Alexander, an alternative therapy technique that links poor posture to various health conditions.

14 A form of manual therapy in which a practitioner primarily uses finger and palm pressure to promote relaxation and well-being, drawing on concepts from traditional East Asian medicine.

15 John Newport Langley (1852–1925) was a British physiologist who made foundational discoveries about the nervous system.

16 Charles Bell (1774–1842) was a Scottish surgeon whose work gained widespread recognition from the mid-nineteenth century onward and laid the foundations for physiologically oriented psychology.

17 Carl Lange (1834–1900) was a Danish physician whose work made contributions to neurology, psychology, and psychiatry.

18 Freudian psychic development proceeds as drives differentiate along a phylogenetically programmed course (Yadlin-Gadot, 2022, p. 121). He argued that, owing to certain organs' dense innervation, they have enduring potential for sexual excitation and serve as erogenous zones. During development, different zones typically achieve temporary primacy and organise affect and phantasy. Based on this, he proposed the sequence of psychosexual stages – oral, anal, phallic – in which modes of gratification and relational themes shift as development proceeds. Childhood sexuality culminates around ages five to six in a genital organization that gathers earlier pregenital impulses (oral, anal, etc.) under genital primacy. This is achieved by the resolution of the Oedipus complex (Mitchell & Black, 2016, Chapter, 1).

19 In his topographic model of the mind, Freud posited three mental areas, the Unconscious (Ucs), Preconscious (Pcs), and Conscious (Cs), and two modes of mental functioning: primary- and secondary-processes. Primary-process thinking, located in the topos of the Unconscious, he viewed as characterised by unbound, impulsive free energy, absence of time, and logic driven by the pleasure-principle towards wish-fulfilment. In contrast, secondary-processes, related to the Preconscious-Conscious systems, he proposed to be linear and logical and to employ binding of energy to delay gratification according to the reality-principle. His model separated the Pcs-Cs from the Ucs by the repression barrier, which instated

the dynamic and conflictual nature of the psyche. Conflict between the aims of the pleasure and reality principles create excess energy that needs to be discharged or warded off by defences to maintain equilibrium within the organism (Aragno, 2022, pp. 204–205).

20 "One of the two principles which for Freud govern mental functioning. The reality principle is coupled with the pleasure principle, which it modifies: in so far as it succeeds in establishing its dominance as a regulatory principle, the search for satisfaction does not take the most direct routes but instead makes detours and postpones the attainment of its goal according to the conditions imposed by the outside world. Viewed from the economic standpoint, the reality principle corresponds to a transformation of free energy into bound energy; from the topographical standpoint, it is essentially characteristic of the preconscious-conscious system; and from the dynamic perspective, psycho-analysis seeks to base the intervention of the reality principle on a particular type of instinctual energy said to be more specifically in the service of the ego (Laplanche & Pontalis, 1988, p. 379).

21 In psychoanalysis, conflict means the clash of incompatible inner demands. It can be manifest (e.g., a wish versus a moral rule) or latent, surfacing indirectly in symptoms, behavioural or character disturbances. Mental life reflects shifting compromises between drives, agencies, and defences attempting to manage unpleasure and maintain psychic cohesion. Conflict is considered constitutive of psychic life and might arise on several planes: drive versus ego defence, agency versus agency, drive versus drive. From a structural viewpoint, conflict can form between agencies, id-ego-superego, and within an agency (e.g., rival paternal vs. maternal identifications in the superego). Conflict could also form between instincts, such as between binding/organizing and unbinding/destructive tendencies of the life versus death drives (Laplanche & Pontalis, 1988, pp. 359–360; Mitchell & Black, 2016, Chapter 1).

22 Urethral erotism, the mode of libidinal gratification linked to urination, including pleasure in discharge and in control (e.g., "letting it flow," "holding back"), was recognised by Freud as part of infantile sexuality (1953). He argued that, clinically and developmentally, it becomes salient in the second phase of infantile masturbation (around the fourth year), when the urinary apparatus can function as an agent for the still-immature genital apparatus, roughly coinciding with the phallic phase. Characterologically, several psychoanalysts (Abraham, 1954; Klein, 1932; Sadger, 1910) linked urethral eroticism and sadism to fantasies of omnipotence and "burning" ambition (Laplanche & Pontalis, 1988, pp. 478–480). However, as urethral erotism was thought to remain tightly interwoven with phallic erotism, no independent urethral phase was posited before Kestenberg.

23 Abraham (1949) proposed that the anal sadistic phase contains two levels within it, an earlier one with the tendency to expel and lose the object and a later one concerned with retaining and controlling the object. This drive towards retaining the object comes to the fore in Kestenberg's anal sadistic *Strain-Release Rhythm*.

24 Although Kestenberg does not state this explicitly, her categories of sadistic/fighting and libidinal/indulging motor patterns resonate with Jacobson's (1964) extension of the Freudian libidinal drive in which libido integrates split images of self and object (good/bad), while aggression promotes differentiation, sharpening boundaries and establishing distinct representations of self and other. Evoked by gratification, libido incorporates; evoked by frustration, aggression differentiates. Recurring cyclicality of these forces together supports the consolidation of a coherent, stable identity (Mitchell & Black, 2016, Chapter 2).

25 These kibbutzim were established between 1943 and 1949 on lands associated with Palestinian villages, namely: Khiyam al-Walid, Wadi'Ara, Qaytiyya, Yasur

and al-Muftakhira whose communities were displaced during the Nakba. For more information on the circumstances of settlements please visit the Interactive Encyclopedia of the Palestine Question - https://www.palquest.org/.

26 See Kestenberg's hand-drawn early *Tension-Flow* notations in Curated Archive/Movement Notation & Profiles/Flow Writing/1 & 2 Hand-drawn Tension-Flow Notation – 1964.

27 Curated Archive/Movement Notation & Profiles/Shape-Flow Design Curve.

28 Further examples of Kestenberg's Flow-Writing can be found in the Curated Archive/Movement Notation & Profiles/Flow Writing & Hand-drawn Tension-Flow Curve.

29 Examples of Labanotation symbols used by Kestenberg can be found in Curated Archive/Movement Notation & Profiles/Labeling with Symbols.

30 Examples of these labels can be seen in Figure 2.1, such as OS representing oral sadistic *Biting Rhythm*, O standing for oral libidinal *Sucking Rhythm*, P standing for phallic libidinal *Jumping Rhythm*, AS denoting anal sadistic *Twisting Rhythm*, and FSP representing a mix of feminine libidinal *Undulating Rhythm* and phallic sadistic *Leaping Rhythm*.

31 Example of a calculation sheet can be found at Curated Archive/Movement Notation & Profiles/Calculation Sheet Tension-Flow Attributes.

32 Curated Archive/Child Development Research/Charter & Certificate of Incorporation by University of the State of New York

33 Albert J. Solnit (1919–2002) was a child psychiatrist and psychoanalyst and director of the Yale Child Study Centre between 1966 and 1983.

34 Curated Archive/Child Development Research/An Ounce of Prevention Leaflet/ISOPC Leaflet.

35 Curated Archive/Child Development Research/Center for Parents and Children/Early Project Proposal 2.

36 Curated Archive/Child Development Research/Center for Parents and Children/Early Project Proposal 1.

37 Curated Archive/Child Development Research/Membership Letter.

38 CDR newsletters were published twice a year between 1978 and 1990. Curated Archive/Child Development Research/Center for Parents and Children/Newsletters.

39 Curated Archive/Child Development Research/Center for Parents and Children/Judith Kestenberg at the Center/Kestenberg at the Center with a camera 1 and 2.

40 Curated Archiver/Child Development Research/Center for Parents and Children/Infant Parent Assessment Scale.

41 Curated Archive/Unpublished Papers/Prevention or Infant Therapy, Kestenberg & Buelte, 1978.

42 See various movement and embodiment sessions for parents in Curated Archive/Child Development Research/Center for Parents and Children/Photos from the Center.

43 Curated Archive/Child Development Research/Center for Parents and Children/Educational Booklet.

44 Curated Archive/Child Development Research/Center for Parents and Children/Photos from the Center/The special doll.

45 Curated Archive/Unpublished Papers/Expressive Arts in Prevention, Judith Kestenberg.

46 Volkmar Glaser (1912–1997) was a German pioneer of psychosomatic breath and body therapy.

47 Curated Archive/Child Development Research/Mission Statement.

48 Curated Archive/Child Development Research/4R Policy.

49 Curated Archive/Child Development Research/ISOPC Leaflet.
50 Curated Archive/Unpublished Papers/Milton Kestenberg – Healing Power of Creativity 1987.
51 Curated Archive/Unpublished Papers/Pregenital Sources of the Moral and Corrupt Superego – Judith Kestenberg – 1988.
52 Freud proposed in *Totem and Taboo* that, in early human society, the primal father threatened his sons with castration. His sons united against him and killed him. This led to collective guilt and instated the first taboo of incest and murder. Working through this guilt, they started to worship the father and a totem. Freud related the development of superego and cultural consciousness to this process (Freud, 1912–1913, as cited in Laplanche & Pontalis, 1988, pp. 58–59).

References

Abraham, K. (1913). A constitutional basis of locomotor anxiety. In J. Strachey (Ed.), *Selected papers on psychoanalysis* (pp. 235–243). Hogarth.

Abraham, K. (1949). A short study of the development of the libido, viewed in the light of mental disorders. In *Selected papers of Karl Abraham, M.D.* (Trans. D. Bryan & A. Strachey, pp. 418–503). The Hogarth Press and the Institute of Psycho-Analysis. (Original work published in 1924)

Abraham, K. (1954). The narcissistic evaluation of excretory processes in dreams and neurosis. In *Selected papers on psycho-analysis* (Trans. D. Bryan & A. Strachey, pp. 318–322). Basic Books. (Original work published in 1920).

Ambrosio, C. (2023). Drawing as a pragmatist visual epistemology. In G. Anderson-Tempini & J. Dupré (Eds.), *Drawing processes of life: Molecules, cells, organisms* (pp. 52–82). Intellect. doi:10.1386/9781789387094_4.

American Psychoanalytic Association. (1976). Record of Milton E. Jucovy funding application, “Children of survivors of the Holocaust” (RG 16, Fund for Psychoanalytic Research, 1975–May 1977). American Psychoanalytic Association Collection. Oskar Diethelm Library, New York, NY, United States.

American Psychoanalytic Association. (1978a). Record of Judith Kestenberg funding application, “Siblings as objects” (RG 16, Fund for Psychoanalytic Research, May 1978–May 1979). American Psychoanalytic Association Collection. Oskar Diethelm Library, New York, NY, United States.

American Psychoanalytic Association. (1978b). Record of Milton Jucovy funding application, “Effects of the Holocaust” (RG 16, Fund for Psychoanalytic Research, December 1977–May 1978). American Psychoanalytic Association Collection. Oskar Diethelm Library, New York, NY, United States.

Anthony, E.J., & Koupernik, C. (Eds.). (1973). *The child in his family: The impact of disease and death*. John Wiley.

Aragno, A. (2022). A revised psychoanalytic model of mind and communication: Studies in body–mind continuity. In J. Mills (Ed.), *Psychoanalysis and the mind–body problem* (pp. 204–226). Routledge. doi:10.4324/9781003090755-10

Bartenieff, I., & Lewis, D. (2013). *Body movement: Coping with the environment* (1st ed.). Routledge. (Original work published in 1980). doi:10.4324/9781315025445

Behrens, N. (1997). Nekrolog Prof. Dr. med. Volkmar Glaser (1912–1997). *Physikalische Medizin, Rehabilitationsmedizin, Kurortmedizin*, 7, 291–292.

Bell, B. (1984). A new childcare concept takes root in Roslyn. *Roslyn News*, 23 February.
Benedek, T. (1952). *Psychosexual functions in women*. Ronald Press.
Benedek, T. (1959). Parenthood as a developmental phase: A contribution to the libido theory. *Journal of the American Psychoanalytic Association*, 7(3), 389–417. doi:10.1177/000306515900700301
Benedek, T. (1970). The family as a psychological field. In E.J. Anthony & T. Benedek (Eds.), *Parenthood: Its psychology and psychopathology* (pp. 109–136). Little, Brown.
Bergmann, M.S., & Jucovy, M.E. (Eds.). (1982). *Generations of the Holocaust*. Basic Books.
Berlowe, J.B., & Kestenberg, J.S. (1972). Movement profile scoring [Unpublished manuscript]. Box 55, Manuals, forms, and scoring sheets. Kestenberg papers (collection in process). Manuscript Division, Library of Congress, Washington, DC, United States. (Materials discovered by the author in Janet Kestenberg Amighi's private collection.)
Birklein, S.B. (2018). Contours of vitality in movement. In J. Kestenberg Amighi, S. Loman, & K.M. Sossin (Eds.), *The meaning of movement: Embodied developmental, clinical, and cultural perspectives of the Kestenberg Movement Profile* (2nd ed., pp. 243–265). Routledge. doi:10.4324/9781351038706
Birksted-Breen, D. (1993). General introduction. In D. Birksted-Breen (Ed.), *The gender conundrum. Contemporary psychoanalytic perspectives on femininity and masculinity* (pp. 1–39). Routledge.
Birnholz, J.C., Stephens, J.C., & Faria, M. (1978). Fetal movement patterns: A possible means of defining neurologic developmental milestones in utero. *American Journal of Roentgenology*, 130, 537–540.
Bonaparte, M. (2018). Passivity, masochism and femininity. In R. Grigg, D. Hecq, & C. Smith (Eds.), *Female sexuality: The early psychoanalytic controversies* (pp. 266–274). Routledge. (Original work published in 1935). doi:10.4324/9780429474675
Borgos, A. (2017). Pszichoanalitikus elméletek nőiségképe. Freudtól a feminista pszichoanalízisig [Image of women in psychoanalytic theory. From Freud to feminist psychoanalysis]. In M. Kovács (Ed.), *Társadalmi nemek. Elméleti megközelítések és kutatási eredmények* [Gender. Theoretical approaches and research outcomes] (pp. 21–37). ELTE Eötvös.
Borgos, A. (2019). Nőtörténeti dokumentumok a pszichoanalízis-történetben [Documents of women's history in the history of psychoanalysis]. In C. Pléh, *A pszichológiatörténet-írás módszerei és a magyar pszichológiatörténet* [Methodologies of the history of psychology and the history of Hungarian psychology] (pp. 76–90). Gondolat.
Borowitz, E. (1978a). Speaking to mothers on problems of separation. *Child Development Research News*, 1(2), 4.
Borowitz, E. (1978b). Attachment behaviour and contact functioning. *Modern Psychoanalysis*, 3(1), 85–109.
Brierley, M. (1936). Specific determinants in feminine development. *The International Journal of Psychoanalysis*, 17, 163–180.
Breuer, J., & Freud, S. (1955). *The standard edition of the complete psychological works of Sigmund Freud: Vol. 2 (1893–1895). Studies on hysteria* (Ed. & Trans. J. Strachey). Hogarth Press and the Institute of Psycho-Analysis. (Original work published 1895)
Buelte, A. (1978). Movement retraining. *Child Development Research News*, 1(2), 2.
Buelte, A. (1979). Movement retraining. *Child Development Research News*, 2(1), 1.

Bühler, C. (1930). *The first year of life* (Trans. P. Greenberg and R. Ripin). John Day.
Caropreso, F. (2024a). The research trajectory of Judith Kestenberg: From the study of movements to research with child victims of the Holocaust. *S:I.M.O.N. Shoah: Intervention. Methods. Documentation*, 11(1), 67–90. doi:10.23777/sn.0124/art_fcar01
Caropreso, F. (2024b). The psychological motivations of Nazism and its effect on the superego according to Judith Kestenberg. *Critical Hermeneutics*, 8(2), 259–282. doi:10.13125/CH/6106
Center for Parents and Children. (n.d.a). Consent forms [Unpublished archival materials]. Center for Parents and Children, Box 18–29, Kestenberg papers (collection in process). Manuscript Division, Library of Congress, Washington, DC, United States. Materials discovered by the author in Mark Sossin's private collection.
Center for Parents and Children. (n.d.b). Center books [Unpublished archival materials]. Center for Parents and Children, Boxes 15–17, Kestenberg papers (collection in process). Manuscript Division, Library of Congress, Washington, DC, United States. Materials discovered by the author in Mark Sossin's private collection.
Center for Parents and Children. (n.d.c). Staff notes [Unpublished archival materials]. Center for Parents and Children, Box 30, Staff Files, Kestenberg papers (collection in process). Manuscript Division, Library of Congress, Washington, DC, United States. Materials discovered by the author in Mark Sossin's private collection.
Center for Parents and Children. (n.d.d). Mother–Infant Interaction Scale [Unpublished archival materials]. Child Development Research, Box 34, Assessment Forms, Kestenberg papers (collection in process). Manuscript Division, Library of Congress, Washington, DC, United States. Materials discovered by the author in Mark Sossin's private collection.
Center for Parents and Children. (n.d.e). Weinberg father interviews [Unpublished archival materials]. Box 34, Staff Files, Kestenberg papers (collection in process). Manuscript Division, Library of Congress, Washington, DC, United States. Materials discovered by the author in Mark Sossin's private collection.
Child Development Research. (n.d.a). 4R policy [Unpublished document]. Materials located by the author in Janet Kestenberg Amighi's private collection.
Child Development Research. (n.d.b). Mission statement [Unpublished document]. Child Development Research, Box 34, Articles of incorporation, bylaws, and mission statement, Kestenberg papers (collection in process). Manuscript Division, Library of Congress, Washington, DC, United States. Materials discovered by the author in Janet Kestenberg Amighi's private collection.
Child Development Research. (n.d.c). An Ounce of Prevention CDR leaflet [Unpublished archival materials]. Child Development Research, Box 35, Brochures and membership forms, Kestenberg papers (collection in process). Manuscript Division, Library of Congress, Washington, DC, United States. Materials discovered by the author in Janet Kestenberg Amighi's private collection.
Child Development Research. (n.d.d). List of board members and interviewees [Unpublished archival materials]. Child Development Research, Box 35, Brochures and membership forms, Kestenberg papers (collection in process). Manuscript Division, Library of Congress, Washington, DC, United States. Materials discovered by the author in Janet Kestenberg Amighi's private collection.
Child Development Research. (1971–1987). Parent letters [Unpublished archival materials]. Child Development Research Center, Box 35–36, Correspondence,

General, Kestenberg papers (collection in process). Manuscript Division, Library of Congress, Washington, DC, Unites States. (Materials discovered by author in K. Mark Sossin's private collection.)

Child Development Research. (1974, November 30). Parent Letter [Unpublished archival materials]. Child Development Research Center, Correspondence, General, 1971–1974, Box 35, Kestenberg papers (collection in process). Manuscript division, Library of Congress, Washington, DC, United States. Materials discovered by author in K. Mark Sossin's private collection.

Child Development Research. (1978). *Child Development Research News* [Unpublished]. Child Development Research, Box 37, Newsletters, Kestenberg papers (collection in process). Manuscript Division, Library of Congress, Washington, DC, United States. (Materials discovered by the author in Janet Kestenberg Amighi's private collection.)

Child Development Research. (1985). *Child Development Research News*, 8(1). Materials discovered by the author in Janet Kestenberg Amighi's private collection.

Child Development Research. (1990). *Newsletter of the International Study of Organised Persecution of Children*, 7(2). Jerome Riker International Study of the Organized Persecution of Children, Box 48, Newsletters, Kestenberg papers (collection in process). Manuscript Division, Library of Congress, Washington, DC, United States. Materials discovered by the author in Janet Kestenberg Amighi's private collection.

Coates, S.W. (2004). John Bowlby and Margaret S. Mahler: Their lives and theories. *Journal of the American Psychoanalytic Association*, 52(2), 571–601. doi:10.1177/00030651040520020601

Comparetti, M.A. (1981). The neurophysiological and clinical implications of studies on fetal motor behavior. *Seminars in Perinatology*, 5, 183–189.

Csabai, M., & Erős, F. (2000). *Testhatárok és énhatárok. Az identitás változó keretei* [Body- and self-boundaries. Changing framework of identity]. Jószöveg.

Deutsch, F. (1947). Analysis of postural behavior. *Psychoanalytic Quarterly*, 16, 195–213.

Deutsch, F. (1952). Analytic posturology. *Psychoanalytic Quarterly*, 21, 196–214.

Deutsch, H. (1925). The psychology of women in relation to the functions of reproduction. *International Journal of Psychoanalysis*, 6, 405–418.

Deutsch, H. (1930). The significance of masochism in the mental life of women. *International Journal of Psychoanalysis*, 11, 48–60.

Deutsch, H. (1944). *The psychology of women: A psychoanalytic interpretation* (Vol. 1). Grune & Stratton.

Deutsch, H. (1945). *The psychology of women: A psychoanalytic interpretation: Vol. 2. Motherhood.* Grune & Stratton.

Eickhoff, F. (1989). On the borrowed unconscious sense of guilt and the palimpsestic structure of a symptom: Afterthoughts on the Hamburg Congress of the IPA. *International Review of Psycho-Analysis*, 16, 323–329.

Erikson, E.H. (1937). Configurations in play: Clinical notes. *Psychoanalytical Quarterly*, 6, 139–214.

Erikson, E.H. (1950a). *Childhood and society.* W.W. Norton.

Erikson, E. (1950b). Growth and crises of the healthy personality. Symposium on the Healthy Personality, Supp. 2, Problems of Infancy and Childhood. *Transactions of Fourth Conference*, March 1950. (Ed. M.J.E. Senn). Josiah Macy, Jr. Foundation.

Erikson, E.H. (1959). *Identity and the life cycle.* International Universities Press.

Ferenczi, S. (1952a). Thinking and muscle innervation. In J. Rickman (Ed.), *Further contributions to the theory and technique of psycho-analysis* (pp. 230–232). Basic Books. (Original work published in 1919)

Ferenczi, S. (1952b). Stages in the development of the sense of reality. In S. Ferenczi, *First contributions to psycho-analysis* (Trans. E. Jones, pp. 213–239). Hogarth Press and Institute of Psycho-Analysis. (Original work published in 1913)

Ferenczi, S. (1955). Laughter. In *Problems and methods of psychoanalysis* (Vol. 3, pp. 177–182). Basic Books.

Ferenczi, S. (1994a). Embarrassed hands. In J. Rickman (Ed.), *Further contributions to the theory and technique of psychoanalysis.* Karnac. (Original work published in 1914)

Ferenczi, S. (1994b). Rubbing the eyes as a substitute for onanism. In J. Rickman (Ed.), *Further contributions to the theory and technique of psychoanalysis.* Karnac. (Original work published in 1914)

Ferenczi, S. (1994c). Psychoanalytical observations on tic. In J. Rickman (Ed.), *Further contributions to the theory and technique of psychoanalysis.* Karnac. (Original work published in 1921)

Fogelman, E. (2017). The evolution of a second-generation Holocaust survivor identity. Available from: https://evafogelman.com/publications/the-evolution-of-a-second-generation-holocaust-survivor-identity/

Fogelman, E. (2019). Second generation identity. In I. Brenner (Ed.), *The handbook of psychoanalytic Holocaust studies: International perspectives* (pp. 83–89). Routledge. doi:10.4324/9780429292965-10

Freud, A. (1946). *The psycho-analytical treatment of children: Technical lectures and essays* (Trans. N. Procter-Gregg). Imago.

Freud, A. (1951). Observations on child development. *The Psychoanalytic Study of the Child*, 6, 18–30.

Freud, A. (1962). Assessment of childhood disturbances. *The Psychoanalytic Study of the Child*, 17(1), 149–158. doi:10.1080/00797308.1962.11822843

Freud, A. (1965, 17 November). Letter to J. S. Kestenberg [Unpublished archival material]. Box 3, Anna Freud, Kestenberg papers (collection in process). Manuscript Division, Library of Congress, Washington, DC, United States. Discovered by the author in Mark Sossin's private collection.

Freud, A., Nagera, H., & Freud, W.E. (1965). Metapsychological assessment of the adult personality: The Adult Profile. *The Psychoanalytic Study of the Child*, 20(1), 9–41. doi:10.1080/00797308.1965.11823225

Freud, W.E. (1967). Assessment of early infancy: Problems and considerations. *The Psychoanalytic Study of the Child*, 22(1), 216–238. https://doi.org/10.1080/00797308.1967.11822598

Freud, W.E., & Freud, I. (1976). The well-baby clinic. *Child Psychiatry and Human Development*, 7(2), Winter.

Freud, S. (1919). A child is being beaten: A contribution to the study of the origin of sexual perversions. In J. Strachey (Ed. & Trans.), *The standard edition of the complete psychological works of Sigmund Freud* (Vol. 17, pp. 175–204). Hogarth Press.

Freud, S. (1925). Inhibitions, symptoms and anxiety. In J. Strachey (Ed. & Trans.), *The standard edition of the complete psychological works of Sigmund Freud* (Vol. 20, pp. 75–173). Hogarth Press.

Freud, S. (1931). Female sexuality. In *The standard edition of the complete psychological works of Sigmund Freud* (Vol. 21, pp. 221–244). Norton.

Freud, S. (1932). New introductory lectures on psychoanalysis. In J. Strachey (Ed. & Trans.), *The standard edition of the complete psychological works of Sigmund Freud* (Vol. 22, pp. 1–183). Norton.

Freud, S. (1953). Three essays on the theory of sexuality. In J. Strachey (Ed. & Trans.), *The standard edition of the complete psychological works of Sigmund Freud* (Vol. 7, pp. 125–245). Hogarth Press. (Original work published in 1905)

Freud, S. (1957a). Instincts and their vicissitudes. In J. Strachey (Ed. & Trans.), *The standard edition of the complete psychological works of Sigmund Freud* (Vol. 14, pp. 111–140). Hogarth Press. (Original work published in 1915)

Freud, S. (1957b). The unconscious. In J. Strachey (Ed. & Trans.), *The standard edition of the complete psychological works of Sigmund Freud* (Vol. 14, pp. 159–215). Hogarth Press. (Original work published in 1915)

Freud, S. (1960). The psychopathology of everyday life. In J. Strachey (Ed. & Trans.), *The standard edition of the complete psychological works of Sigmund Freud* (Vol. 6, pp. 1–296). Hogarth Press. (Original work published in 1901)

Freud, S. (1961). The ego and the id. In J. Strachey (Ed. & Trans.), *The standard edition of the complete psychological works of Sigmund Freud* (Vol. 19, pp. 3–66). Hogarth Press and Institute of Psycho-Analysis. (Original work published in 1923)

Freud, S. (1964a). Femininity. In J. Strachey (Ed. & Trans.), *The standard edition of the complete psychological works of Sigmund Freud* (Vol. 22, pp. 112–135). Hogarth Press. (Original work published in 1933)

Freud, S. (1964b). The economic problem of masochism. In J. Strachey (Ed. & Trans.), *The standard edition of the complete psychological works of Sigmund Freud* (Vol. 19, pp. 155–170). Hogarth Press.

Freud, S. (1975). Beyond the pleasure principle. In J. Strachey (Ed. & Trans.), *The standard edition of the complete psychological works of Sigmund Freud* (Vol. 18, pp. 7–64). Hogarth Press. (Original work published in 1920)

Fries, M.E. (1944). Psychosomatic relationships between mother and infant. *Psychosomatic Medicine*, 6.

Fries, M.E., & Woolf, P.J. (1954). Some hypotheses on the role of the congenital activity type in personality development. *The Psychoanalytic Study of the Child*, 8, 48–64. doi:10.1080/00797308.1953.11822760

Fügedi, J. (2015). Lábán Rudolf – az európai színpadi táncnyelv megújítója [Rudolf Laban – the innovator of European stage dance]. Retrieved from: https://real.mtak.hu/80762/1/Fugedi_Janos_Laban%20Rudolf%20%E2%80%93%20az%20eurapai%20szinpadi%20tancnyelv%20megujitoja.pdf

Furman, E. (1973). The impact of the Nazi concentration camps on the children of survivors. In E.J. Anthony & C. Koupernik (Eds.), *The child in his family: The impact of disease and death* (Vol. 2, pp. 379–384). John Wiley.

Geissmann, C., & Geissmann, P. (1998a). Hermine Hug-Hellmuth: Pioneer and most obstinate of Freud's disciples. In *A history of child psychoanalysis* (pp. 33–61). Taylor & Francis e-Library.

Geissmann, C., & Geissmann, P. (1998b). Part III: Today: the spread of child psychoanalysis throughout the world from 1945: the United States of America. In *A History of Child Psychoanalysis* (pp. 210–230). Taylor & Francis e-Library.

Gober, S. (2014). The development of a measure of Margaret Mahler's theory integrating the infant, the mother, and their dyadic relationship during the infant's first five months of life [Doctoral dissertation, Rutgers, The State University of New

Jersey]. Rutgers University Community Repository (RUcore). https://rucore.libraries.rutgers.edu/rutgers-lib/42338/

Gonzalez-Dolginko, B. (1985). Creativity. *Child Development Research News*, 8(1) [Unpublished archival materials]. Kestenberg papers (collection in process). Library of Congress, Washington, DC, United States. Materials discovered by the author in Janet Kestenberg Amighi's private collection.

Gonzalez-Dolginko, B. (1988). Passing the torch. *Child Development Research News*, 10(1), 1–2 [Unpublished archival materials]. Kestenberg papers (collection in process). Library of Congress, Washington, DC, United States. Materials discovered by the author in Janet Kestenberg Amighi's private collection.

Gonzalez-Dolginko, B. (2021). *Applying developmental art theory in art therapy treatment and interventions: Illustrative examples through the life cycle.* Routledge.

Green, V., & Joyce, A. (2017). Revised diagnostic profile 2016: Revisions, rationale, and further thoughts. *Journal of Infant, Child, and Adolescent Psychotherapy*, 16(2), 138–148. doi:10.1080/15289168.2017.1309132

Greenacre, P. (1950). Special problems of early female sexual development. *The Psychoanalytic Study of the Child*, 5(1), 122–138. doi:10.1080/00797308.1950.11822888

Greenacre, P. (1948). Anatomical structure and superego development. *American Journal of Orthopsychiatry*, 18(4), 636–648. https://doi.org/10.1111/j.1939-0025.1948.tb05125.x

Hartmann, H. (1958). *Ego psychology and the problem of adaptation.* International Universities Press.

Hartmann, H., Kris, E., & Loewenstein, R.M. (1946). Comments on the formation of psychic structure. *The Psychoanalytic Study of the Child*, 2(1), 11–38. doi:10.1080/00797308.1946.11823535

Hartmann, H., Kris, E., & Loewenstein, R.M. (1949). Notes on the theory of aggression. *The Psychoanalytic Study of the Child*, 3, 9–36.

Herzog, D. (2016). The libido wars. In *Cold War Freud: Psychoanalysis in an age of catastrophes* (pp. 21–55). Cambridge University Press. doi:10.1017/9781139680455.002

Herzog, D. (2019, 6 June). Post-Holocaust trauma and the creation of PTSD [Weinmann Lecture]. United States Holocaust Memorial Museum, Washington, DC, United States. https://www.ushmm.org/m/pdfs/20190606-weinmann-dagmar-herzog.pdf

Horney, K. (1924). On the genesis of the castration complex in women. *International Journal of Psychoanalysis*, 5, 50–65.

Horney, K. (1926). The flight from womanhood: The masculinity-complex in women, as viewed by men and women. *International Journal of Psychoanalysis*, 7, 324–339.

Horney, K. (1928). The problem of the monogamous ideal. *International Journal of Psychoanalysis*, 9, 318–331.

Horney, K. (1933). The denial of the vagina: A contribution to the problem of the genital anxieties specific to women. *International Journal of Psychoanalysis*, 14, 57–70.

Horney, K. (1939). *New ways in psychoanalysis.* W.W. Norton.

Hug-Hellmuth, H.von. (1914). Kinderpsychologie, Pädagogik . *Jahrbuch für psychoanalytische und psychopathologische Forschungen*, 6, 393–404.

International Study of Organised Persecution of Children Files. (n.d.). Shadows of lost childhood exhibition invitation [Unpublished archival materials]. Jerome Riker International Study of the Organized Persecution of Children, Box 44, Brochures, Kestenberg papers (collection in process). Manuscript Division, Library of

Congress, Washington, DC, United States. Materials discovered by the author in Janet Kestenberg Amighi's private collection.

Jacobson, E. (1937). Development of the feminine superego. *International Zeitschrift für Psychoanalyse*, 23.

Jacobson, E. (1964). *The self and the object world.* International Universities Press.

Jucovy, M.E. (1985). Telling the Holocaust story: A link between the generations. *Psychoanalytic Inquiry: A Topical Journal for Mental Health Professionals*, 5(1), 31–49. doi:10.1080/07351698509533574

Kahn, C. (1998). Part I. Psychohistorical Perspectives. In J. Kestenberg & C. Kahn (Eds.), *Children surviving persecution: An international study of trauma and healing* (pp. 11–18). Praeger.

Kangisser Cohen, S., Fogelman, E., & Ofer, D. (2019). Introduction. In *Children in the Holocaust and its aftermath: Historical and psychological studies of the Kestenberg Archive* (pp. 1–12). Berghahn Books. doi:10.2307/j.ctvw04hks.4

Kaplan, S. (1978). Fellows in child psychiatry from the Long Island Jewish-Hillside Medical Center participate in center's program. *Child Development Research News*, 1(2), 2 [Unpublished archival materials]. Child Development Research, Box 37, Newsletters, Kestenberg papers (collection in process). Manuscript Division, Library of Congress, Washington, DC, United States. Materials discovered by the author in Janet Kestenberg Amighi's private collection.

Keilson, H.A., & Sarphatie, H.R. (1979). *Sequentielle Traumatisierung bei Kindern: Deskriptiv-klinische und quantifizierend-statistische Untersuchung zum Schicksal der jüdischen Kriegswaisen in den Niederlanden* [Sequential traumatisation in children: A clinical and statistical follow-up study on the fate of Jewish war orphans in the Netherlands]. Ferdinand Enke.

Kestenberg Amighi, J., & Loman, S. (1990). The past of the Kestenberg Movement Profile: A panel discussion with Kestenberg, J. S., Buelte, A., Marcus, H., Berlowe, J., & Lamb, W. In S. Loman & P. Lewis (Eds.), *The Kestenberg Movement Profile: Its past, present applications, and future directions* (pp. 9–32). Retrieved from https://aura.antioch.edu/facbooks/25

Kestenberg Amighi, J., Loman, S., & Sossin, K.M. (Eds.) (2018). *The meaning of movement, embodied developmental, clinical and cultural perspectives of the Kestenberg Movement Profile* (2nd ed.). Routledge.

Kestenberg J.S. (n.d.a). CV [Unpublished curriculum vitae]. Downstate Medical Health Center, Medical Research Library, Archives and Special Collections Department. New York, NY, United States.

Kestenberg, J.S. (n.d.b). CV [Unpublished curriculum vitae]. Documents of Judith S. Kestenberg (1937–1999). New York Psychoanalytic Association and Society A. A. Brill Library, Archives and Special Collections. New York, NY, United States.

Kestenberg, J.S. (n.d.c). Outline for a project for interdisciplinary center for child development. Discovered by the author in Mark Sossin's private collection.

Kestenberg, J.S. (n.d.d). Books and study notes [Unpublished archival materials]. Box 6, Notes, miscellaneous, Box 10, Books, Kestenberg papers (collection in process). Manuscript Division, Library of Congress, Washington, DC, United States. Discovered by the author in Mark Sossin's private collection.

Kestenberg, J.S. (1945). Early reactions to tensions. Presentation at the 283rd Meeting of the New York Psychoanalytic Society. Documents of Judith S. Kestenberg (1937–

1999). New York Psychoanalytic Association and Society A. A. Brill Library, Archives and Special Collections. New York, NY, United States.

Kestenberg, J.S. (1946). Early fears and early defenses. *The Nervous Child*, 4(1), 56–70.

Kestenberg, J.S. (1947). Review of The Psychoanalytic Treatment of Children by Anna Freud. *Psychoanalytic Quarterly*, 16, 553–556.

Kestenberg, J.S. (1950). Notes on early ego development [Paper presentation, Panel C: Problems of early ego development (M. S. Mahler, Chair; M. Friend, Reporter; participants: P. Greenacre, H. Hartmann, E. Sylvester). *The 1950 Mid-Winter Meeting Program. Bulletin of the American Psychoanalytic Association*, 6(4), 72–81.

Kestenberg, J.S. (1953). Notes on ego development. *International Journal of Psychoanalysis*, 34(2), 111–122.

Kestenberg, J.S. (1953–1978). Longitudinal study of infant observation [Unpublished archival materials]. Box 58, Kestenberg papers (collection in process). Manuscript Division, Library of Congress, Washington, DC, United States. Materials discovered by the author in Mark Sossin's private collection.

Kestenberg, J.S. (1954). A phase in the development of female sexuality. Presentation, Psychoanalytic Study Group, Seattle, United States.

Kestenberg, J.S. (1956a). Vicissitudes of female sexuality. *Journal of the American Psychoanalytic Association*, 4, 453–475.

Kestenberg, J.S. (1956b, 16 March). On the development of maternal feelings in early childhood: Observations and reflections [Presentation]. Meeting of the New York Psychoanalytic Society, Documents of Judith S. Kestenberg (1937–1999). New York Psychoanalytic Association and Society A. A. Brill Library, Archives and Special Collections. New York, NY, United States.

Kestenberg, J.S. (1956c). On the development of maternal feelings in early childhood: Observations and reflections. *The Psychoanalytic Study of the Child*, 11, 257–291. doi:10.1080/00797308.1956.11822936

Kestenberg, J.S. (1957, 26 August). Letter to Irmgard Bartenieff [Letter]. Irmgard Bartenieff papers (Collection 0390-SCPA), Correspondence, 1929–1981, Professional letters, 1929–1980. Michelle Smith Performing Arts Library, University of Maryland Archives, MD, United States.

Kestenberg, J.S. (1965a). The role of movement patterns in development. I. Rhythms of movement. *Psychoanalytic Quarterly*, 24(1), 1–36. doi:10.1080/21674086.1965.11926334

Kestenberg, J.S. (1965b). The role of movement patterns in development. II. Flow of tension and effort. *Psychoanalytic Quarterly*, 24(4), 517–563. doi:10.1080/21674086.1965.11926363

Kestenberg, J.S. (1966). Rhythm and organization in obsessive-compulsive development. *International Journal of Psychoanalysis*, 47(2), 151–159.

Kestenberg, J.S. (1967a). The role of movement patterns in development. III., Control of shape. *Psychoanalytic Quarterly*, 26(3), 356–409. doi:10.1080/21674086.1967.11926431

Kestenberg, J.S. (1967b). Phases of adolescence: With suggestions for a correlation of psychic and hormonal organizations. II. Prepuberty diffusion and reintegration. *Journal of the American Academy of Child Psychiatry*, 6(4), 577–614. doi:10.1016/s0002-7138(09)61691-5

Kestenberg, J.S. (1968). Outside and inside, male and female. *Journal of the American Psychoanalytic Association*, 16(3), 457–520. doi:10.1177/000306516801600307

Kestenberg, J.S. (1971a, 23 February). Development of the young child expressed through bodily movement. Presentation. 565th Meeting Proceedings, New York

Psychoanalytic Society and Institute, A. A. Brill Library & Archives. Documents Judith S. Kestenberg (1937–1999). New York Psychoanalytic Association and Society A. A. Brill Library, Archives and Special Collections. New York, NY, United States.

Kestenberg, J.S. (1971b). From organ-object imagery to self- and object representations. In J.B. McDevitt & C.F. Settlage (Eds.), *Separation-individuation: Essays in honor of Margaret S. Mahler* (pp. 75–99). New York International University Press.

Kestenberg, J.S. (1972a, 28 September). Letter to Irmgard Bartenieff [Letter]. Irmgard Bartenieff papers (Collection 0390-SCPA), Correspondence, 1929–1981, Professional letters, 1929–1980. Michelle Smith Performing Arts Library, University of Maryland, MD, United States.

Kestenberg, J.S. (1972b, 7 September). Letter to Mahler. Margaret Mahler Correspondences, Kestenberg, J. S. (1969–1975, n.d.). Margaret S. Mahler papers (MS 1138), Series I, Box 11, Folder 272. Beinecke Rare Book and Manuscript Library, Yale University, NH, United States.

Kestenberg, J.S. (1973a). Nagging, spreading excitement, arguing. *International Journal of Psychoanalytic Psychotherapy*, 2(3), 265–297.

Kestenberg, J.S. (1973b, 24 September). Letter to Marianne Kris. Ernst Kris and Marianne Kris Papers, Correspondences, Box 36, Kestenberg, Judith S., 1959–1975, Manuscript Division, Library of Congress, Washington, DC, United States.

Kestenberg, J.S. (1974a, 14 July). Letter to Marianne Kris. Ernst Kris and Marianne Kris Papers, Correspondences, Box 36, Kestenberg, Judith S., 1959–1975, Manuscript Division, Library of Congress, Washington, DC, United States.

Kestenberg, J.S. (1974b). Profiles. Laban/Bartenieff Institute of Movement Studies (LIMS) records (0339-SCPA), Student files, Certification projects. Michelle Smith Performing Arts Library, University of Maryland Archives, College Park, MD, United States.

Kestenberg, J.S. (1975a). Preface. In *Children and parents: Psychoanalytic studies in development* (pp. xv–xxvii). Jason Aronson.

Kestenberg, J.S. (1975b). Attunement and clashing in mother-child interaction. In *Children and parents: Psychoanalytic studies in development* (pp. 157–171). Jason Aronson.

Kestenberg, J.S. (1975c). Development of the young child from birth to latency as expressed through bodily movement II. In *Children and parents: Psychoanalytic studies in development* (pp. 235–267). Jason Aronson.

Kestenberg, J.S. (1976). Regression and reintegration in pregnancy. *Journal of the American Psychoanalytic Association, Supplement – Female Sexuality*, 24(5), 213–250.

Kestenberg, J.S. (1978). Transsensus-outgoingness and Winnicott's Intermediate Zone. In S.A. Grolnick & L.B. Barkin (Eds.), *Between reality and fantasy; Winnicott's concepts of transitional objects and phenomena* (pp. 61–75). Jason Aronson.

Kestenberg, J.S. (1980a). Pregnancy as a developmental phase. *Journal of Biological Experience: Studies in the Life of the Body*, 3, 58–66.

Kestenberg, J.S. (1980b). The three faces of femininity. *Psychoanalytic Review*, 67(3), 313–335.

Kestenberg, J.S. (1980c). Maternity and paternity in the developmental context. *Psychiatric Clinics of North America*, 3(1), 61–79.

Kestenberg, J.S. (1980d). Psychoanalysis of children of survivors from the Holocaust: Case presentations and assessment. *Journal of the American Psychoanalytic Association*, 28(4), 775–804.

Kestenberg, J.S. (1980e). Research news. *Child Development Research Newsletter*, 2(2).

Kestenberg, J.S. (1981a). The psychological consequences of punitive institutions. *Israel Journal of Psychiatry and Related Sciences*, 18(1), 15–30.

Kestenberg, J.S. (1981b). The Centre for Parents and Children. How do we do things in the Centre? *Child Development Research News*, 3(2).

Kestenberg, J.S. (1981c). Notes on parenthood as a developmental phase, with special consideration of the roots of fatherhood. In S. Orgel & B.D. Fine (Eds.), *Clinical psychoanalysis* (pp. 199–234). Downstate Psychoanalytic Institute Twenty-Fifth Anniversary Series, Vol. 3. Jason Aronson.

Kestenberg, J.S. (1982). A metapsychological assessment based on an analysis of a survivor's child. In M.S. Bergmann & M.E. Jucovy (Eds.), *Generations of the Holocaust* (pp. 137–158). Columbia University Press.

Kestenberg, J.S. (1985). The role of movement patterns in diagnosis and prevention. In D.A. Shaskan & W.I. Roller (Eds.), *Paul Schilder: Mind explorer* (pp. 97–161). Human Sciences Press.

Kestenberg, J.S. (1987). Empathy for the fetus. In T. Verny (Ed.), *Pre- and perinatal psychology: An introduction* (pp. 138–150). Human Sciences Press.

Kestenberg, J.S. (1988a). Memories from early childhood. *Psychoanalytic Review*, 75 (4), 562–571.

Kestenberg, J.S. (1988b). Pregenital sources of the moral and corrupt superego with some suggestions about the makeup of the Nazi superego [Unpublished document]. Presented at the National Psychological Association for Psychoanalysis. Materials discovered by the author in Mark Sossin's private collection.

Kestenberg, J.S. (1989). What are the ingredients of bonding postnatally? Paper presented at the International Congress on Pre and Perinatal Psychology and Medicine, Jerusalem.

Kestenberg, J.S. (1990) What are the ingredients of bonding prenatally? *International Journal for Prenatal and Perinatal Studies*, 119–124.

Kestenberg, J.S. (1992a). Children under the Nazi yoke. *British Journal of Psychotherapy*, 8(4), 374–390.

Kestenberg, J.S. (1992b). Kindheit und Wissenschaft. Eine biographische Skizze. In L. M. Hermanns (Ed.), *Psychoanalyse in Selbstdarstellungen* (Vol. 1, pp. 147–202). Edition Diskord.

Kestenberg, J.S. (1998a). Adult survivors, child survivors and children of survivors. In J. Kestenberg & C. Kahn (Eds.), *Children surviving persecution: An international study of trauma and healing* (pp. 56–66). Praeger.

Kestenberg, J.S. (1998b). Nazi fathers. In J. Kestenberg & C. Kahn (Eds.), *Children surviving persecution: An international study of trauma and healing* (pp. 124–138). Praeger.

Kestenberg, J.S., Berlowe, J., Buelte, A., Hershey, M., & Robbins, E. (1971). Development of the young child as expressed through bodily movement I. *Journal of the American Psychoanalytic Association*, 19(4), 746–764.

Kestenberg, J.S., & Borowitz, E. (1990). On narcissism and masochism in the fetus and the neonate. *Pre- and Perinatal Psychology Journal*, 5(1), 87. Retrieved from ProQuest Central.

Kestenberg, J.S., & Brenner, I. (1986). Children who survived the Holocaust – the role of rules and routines in the development of the superego. *The International Journal of Psychoanalysis*, 67(3), 309–316.

Kestenberg, J.S., & Brenner, I. (1996a). *The last witness: The child survivors of the Holocaust*. American Psychiatric Press.

Kestenberg, J.S., & Brenner, I. (1996b). Superego in young child survivors. In J.S. Kestenberg & I. Brenner, *The last witness: The child survivor of the Holocaust* (pp. 53–69). American Psychiatric Press.

Kestenberg, J., & Buelte, A (1977a). Prevention, infant therapy and the treatment of adults: 1. Towards understanding mutuality. *International Journal of Psychoanalytic Psychotherapy*, 6, 339–367.

Kestenberg, J., & Buelte, A. (1977b). Prevention, infant therapy and the treatment of adults: 2. Mutual holding and holding oneself up. *International Journal of Psychoanalytic Psychotherapy*, 6, 368–396.

Kestenberg, J.S., & Freud, A. (1955–1969). Correspondence with Kestenberg, Judith. Anna Freud Papers, 1895–1982, Box 54. Manuscript Division, Library of Congress, Washington, DC, United States.

Kestenberg, J.S., & Javaid, G.A. (1983). Entrancement of the mother with her young baby: Implications for the older sibling. *Dynamic Psychotherapy*, 1(1), 38–51.

Kestenberg, J.S., & Kahn, C. (Eds.). (1998). *Children surviving persecution: An international study of trauma and healing*. Praeger.

Kestenberg, J.S., & Kestenberg, M. (1982). The background of the study. In M.S. Bergmann & M.E. Jucovy (Eds.), *Generations of the Holocaust* (pp. 33–45). Basic Books.

Kestenberg, J.S., & Kestenberg, M. (1987). Child killing and child rescuing. In G.G. Neuman (Ed.), *Origins of human aggression: Dynamics and aetiology* (pp. 139–154). Human Sciences Press.

Kestenberg, J.S., & Kestenberg, M. (1990). Research news. *Newsletter of the International Study of Organised Persecution of Children*, 7(2), 12–13.

Kestenberg, J.S., & Marcus, H. (1979). Hypothetical monosex and bisexuality: A psychoanalytic interpretation of sex differences as they reveal themselves in movement patterns of men and women. In N.M. Coleman & J. Ikenberry (Eds.) *Psychosexual Imperatives* (pp. 146–181). Human Sciences Press.

Kestenberg, J.S., Marcus, H., Sossin, K.M., & Stevenson, R. (1994). The development of paternal attitudes. In S.H. Cath, A.R. Gurwitt, & J.M. Ross (Eds.), *Father and child: Developmental and clinical perspectives* (pp. 205–218). Routledge. doi:10.4324/9781315799056-15

Kestenberg, J.S., & Robbins, E. (1975). From early rhythms of socialization to the development of community spirit. In J.S. Kestenberg, *Children and parents: Psychoanalytic studies in development* (pp. 443–461). Jason Aronson.

Kestenberg, J.S., & Sossin, K.M. (1979). *The role of movement patterns in development (Vols. 1–2)*. Dance Notation Bureau Press.

Kestenberg, J.S., & Weinstein, J. (1978). Transitional objects and body-image formation. In S.A. Grolnick & L.B. Barkin (Eds.), *Between reality and fantasy; Winnicott's concepts of transitional objects and phenomena* (pp. 75–97). Jason Aronson.

Kestenberg, M. (1982). Discriminatory aspects of the German indemnification policy: A continuation of persecution. In M.S. Bergmann & M.E. Jucovy (Eds.), *Generations of the Holocaust* (pp. 62–79). Basic Books.

Kestenberg, M. (1985). Legal aspects of child persecution during the Holocaust. *Journal of the American Academy of Child Psychiatry*, 24(4), 381–384.

Kestenberg, M. (1987, 27 December). The healing power of creativity [Unpublished presentation]. University of California, Los Angeles. Box 10, Articles, co-authored by Judith and Milton Kestenberg, Kestenberg Papers (collection in process).

Manuscript Division, Library of Congress, Washington, DC, United States. Materials discovered by the author in Janet Kestenberg Amighi's private collection.

Kivnick, H.Q., & Wells, C.K. (2014). Untapped richness in Erik H. Erikson's rootstock. *The Gerontologist*, 54(1), 40–50. doi:10.1093/geront/gnt123

Klein, M. (1928). Early stages of the Oedipus conflict. *International Journal of Psychoanalysis*, 9, 167–180.

Klein, M. (1932). *The psycho-analysis of children*. Hogarth Press.

Krystal, H. (1968). *Massive psychic trauma*. International University Press. Retrieved from: https://archive.org/details/massivepsychictr0000unse/page/n5/mode/2up

Krystal, H. (1984). Review of the book *Generations of the Holocaust*, edited by M.S. Bergmann & M.E. Jucovy. *The Psychoanalytic Quarterly*, 53(3), 466–473.

Krystal, H., & Niederland, W.G. (Eds.). (1971). Psychic traumatization: Aftereffects in individuals and communities. *International Psychiatry Clinics*, 8(1).

Laban, R. (1950). *The mastery of movement on stage*. Macdonald & Evans.

Laban, R. (1954). *Principles of dance and movement notation*. Macdonald & Evans.

Laban, R. (2008). *Koreográfia* [Choreography]. (Trans. J. Fugedi). L'Harmattan. (Original work published in 1926)

Laban, R., & Lawrence, F.C. (1947). *Effort*. Macdonald & Evans.

Laemmli, W.E. (2016). The choreography of everyday life: Rudolf Laban and the making of modern movement. Doctoral dissertation, University of Pennsylvania. Retrieved from: https://repository.upenn.edu/entities/publication/8f9a810d-1d39-46f7-a40a-2f57f833f645

Laemmli, W.E. (2021). When words fail. Conference presentation. 25 June, Magdeburg University, Magdeburg, Germany.

Laemmli, W.E. (2022). Taylorism transfigured: Industrial rhythm and the British factory. *Grey Room*, 88, 102–126. doi:10.1162/grey_a_00351

Lamb, W. (1961). *Correspondence course in movement assessment*. Unpublished.

Lamb, W., & Watson, E. (1979). *Body code: The meaning in movement*. Routledge & Kegan.

Lambert, B. (1991). Milton Kestenberg, 79, lawyer who won Holocaust reparations. *The New York Times*, 21 November.

Lange, C.G., & James, W. (1922). The emotions (Vol. 1). In K. Dunlap (Ed.), *Psychology classics: A series of reprints and translations*. Williams & Wilkins. Retrieved from https://dn760004.eu.archive.org/0/items/emotions00lang/emotions00lang.pdf

Langley, J.N. (1921). *The autonomic nervous system, Part I*. W. Heffer.

Lanzkowsky, P. (2012). Philip Lanzkowsky interviewed by Howard A. Pearson [Oral history project]. American Academy of Pediatrics. Elk Grove Village, IL. Retrieved from https://www.aap.org/pediatrichistorycenter

Lampl-de Groot, A. (1928). The evolution of the Oedipus complex in women. *The International Journal of Psychoanalysis*, 9, 332–345.

Laplanche, J., & Pontalis, J.-B. (1988). *The language of psycho-analysis*. (Trans. D. Nicholson-Smith). Karnac. (Original work published in 1973)

Laufer, M. (1965). Assessment of adolescent disturbances: The application of Anna Freud's diagnostic profile. *The Psychoanalytic Study of the Child*, 20(1), 99–123. doi:10.1080/00797308.1965.11823227

Laufer, M. (1973). The analysis of a child of survivors. In E.J. Anthony & C. Koupernik (Eds.), *The child in his family: The impact of disease and death* (Vol. 2, pp. 363–373). John Wiley.

Loman, S. (1980). Dance therapy internship program: Attunement. *Child Development Research News*, 2(2).

Loman, S. (2016). Judith S. Kestenberg's Dance/Movement Therapy legacy: Approaches with pregnancy, young children, and caregivers. *American Journal of Dance Therapy*, 38(2), 225–244.

Lupke, H. (2008). Obituary for W. Ernest Freud. *International Journal of Prenatal and Perinatal Psychology and Medicine*, 20(1/2), 77–78.

Mahler, M.S. (1952). On child psychosis and schizophrenia: Autistic and symbiotic infantile psychoses. *The Psychoanalytic Study of the Child*, 7(1), 286–305. doi:10.1080/00797308.1952.11823164

Mahler, M.S. (1968). *On human symbiosis and the vicissitudes of individuation*. International University Press.

Mahler, M.S., & Furer, M. (1966). Development of symbiosis, symbiotic psychosis, and the nature of separation anxiety: Remarks on Weiland's paper. *International Journal of Psycho-Analysis*, 47(4), 559–560.

Mahler, M.S., & McDevitt, J.B. (1982). Thoughts on the emergence of the sense of self, with particular emphasis on the body self. *Journal of the American Psychoanalytic Association*, 30(4), 827–848. doi:10.1177/000306518203000401

Mahler, M.S., Pine, F., & Bergman, A. (1975). *The psychological birth of the human infant: Symbiosis and individuation*. Basic Books.

Marcus, H. (1981). The father's project. *Child Development Research News*, 3(2).

Meehan, B. (1979). Child development class. *Child Development Research News*, 2(1).

Midgley, N. (2013). *Reading Anna Freud*. Routledge. doi:10.4324/9780203078876

Mitchell, S.A., & Black, M.J. (2016). *Freud and beyond: A history of modern psychoanalytic thought*. Basic Books.

Mittelmann, B. (1957). Motility in the therapy of children and adults. *The Psychoanalytic Study of the Child*, 12, 284–319.

Mittelmann, B. (1958). Psychodynamics of motility. *International Journal of Psychoanalysis*, 39, 196–199.

Mittelmann, B. (1960). Intrauterine and early infantile motility. *The Psychoanalytic Study of the Child*, 15, 104–127. doi:10.1080/00797308.1960.11822571

Müller, J. (1932). A contribution to the problem of libidinal development of the genital phase in girls. *International Journal of Psychoanalysis*, 13, 361–368.

Naszkowska, K. (2023). Give me permission to remember: Judith S. Kestenberg and the memory of the Holocaust. In L. Henik & L. Aron (Eds.), *Contemporary psychoanalysis and Jewish thought: Answering a question with more questions* (pp. 197–217). Routledge.

Naszkowska, K. (2024a). Introduction: History is the fruit of power. *American Imago*, 81(4), 461–476. doi:10.1353/aim.2024.a951890

Naszkowska, K. (2024b). Language is mother. *American Imago*, 81(4), 571–597. doi:10.1353/aim.2024.a951896

New York Psychoanalytic Society & Institute. (1937–1945). 283rd Meeting of the New York Psychoanalytic Society, Scientific Session Program, Training Documents, Judith S. Kestenberg (1937–1999). New York Psychoanalytic Association and Society A. A. Brill Library, Archives and Special Collections. New York, USA.

Noth, I. (2015). Beyond Freud and Jung: Sabina Spielrein's contribution to child psychoanalysis and developmental psychology. *Pastoral Psychology*, 64(3), 279–286. doi:10.1007/s11089-014-0621-5

Passos-Ferreira, C. (2022). Freud's views on mental causation. In J. Mills (Ed.), *Psychoanalysis and the mind–body problem* (pp. 69–87). Routledge. doi:10.4324/9781003090755-4

Polat, B. (2021). Mental hygiene, psychoanalysis, and interwar psychology: The making of the maternal deprivation hypothesis. *Isis*, 112(2), 266–290. doi:10.1086/714599

Porter, J.N. (1979). Social psychological aspects of the Holocaust. In B.L. Sherwin & S.G. Ament (Eds.), *Encountering the Holocaust: An interdisciplinary survey* (pp. 189–222). Impact Press.

Rapaport, D. (1959). A historical survey of psychoanalytic ego psychology. In E.H. Erikson (Ed.), *Identity and the life cycle: Selected papers* (Vol. 1, No. 1). International Universities Press.

Reich, W. (1945). *Character-analysis: Principles and technique for psychoanalysts in practice and in training*. (Trans., T.P. Wolfe). Orgone Institute Press.

Reubens, M. (1978). Center's role in a psychiatrist's training. *Child Development Research News*, 1(2), 3 [Unpublished archival materials]. Child Development Research, Box 37, Newsletters, Kestenberg papers (collection in process). Manuscript Division, Library of Congress, Washington, DC, United States. Materials discovered by the author in Janet Kestenberg Amighi's private collection.

Rosenberger, L. (1973). Children of survivors. In E.J. Anthony & C. Koupernik (Eds.), *The child in his family: The impact of disease and death* (Vol. 2, pp. 375–377). John Wiley.

Ruprecht, L. (2015). Gesture, interruption, vibration: Rethinking early twentieth-century gestural theory and practice in Walter Benjamin, Rudolf von Laban, and Mary Wigman. *Dance Research Journal*, 47(2), 23–41. doi:10.1017/S0149767715000200

Sadger, I. (1910). Über Urethralerotik [On urethral eroticism]. *Jahrbuch für psychoanalytische und psychopathologische Forschungen*, 2, 409–450.

Schenk-Danzinger, L. (1963). Fundamental ideas and theories in Charlotte Bühler's lifework. *Journal of Humanistic Psychology*, 3(2). doi:10.1177/002216786300300202

Schilder, P. (1942). *Mind: Perception and thought in their constructive aspects.* Columbia University Press.

Schilder, P. (2013). *The image and appearance of the human body* [E-book]. Routledge. (Original work published in 1950)

Schmincke, C. (2012). Die Psychotonik Volkmar Glasers (1912–1997) [Glaser's psychotonics]. *Deutsche Zeitschrift für Akupunktur*, 55(2), 19. doi:10.1016/j.dza.2012.06.005

Schur, M. (1960). Bela Mittelmann 1899–1959. *The Psychoanalytic Quarterly*, 29(2), 240–240. doi:10.1080/21674086.1960.11926173

Sigal, J.J., & Rakoff, V. (1971). Concentration camp survival: A pilot study of effects on the second generation. *Canadian Psychiatric Association Journal*, 16(5), 393–397. doi:10.1177/070674377101600503

Sossin, K.M. (1978). Studying the self. *Child Development Research News*, 1(2), 7 [Unpublished archival materials]. Child Development Research, Box 37, Newsletters, Kestenberg papers (collection in process). Manuscript Division, Library of Congress, Washington, DC, United States. Materials discovered by the author in Janet Kestenberg Amighi's private collection.

Sossin, K.M. (1987). Reliability of the Kestenberg Movement Profile. *Movement Studies*, 2, 23–28.

Sossin, K.M. (2007). The history and future of the Kestenberg Movement Profile. In S. Koch & S. Bender (Eds.), *Movement analysis – Bewegungsanalyse* (pp. 103–119). Logos.

Sossin, K.M. (2018). Musings on theoretical and research contributions of the KMP within the context of nonverbal studies. In J. Kestenberg Amighi, S. Loman, & M.K. Sossin (Eds.), *The meaning of movement, embodied developmental, clinical and cultural perspectives of the Kestenberg Movement Profile* (2nd ed., pp. 287–316). Routledge.

Sossin, K.M., & Birklein, S. (2006). Nonverbal indices of stress in parent–child dyads: Implications for individual and interpersonal affect regulation and intergenerational transmission. In S. Koch & I. Bräuninger (Eds.), *Advances in Dance/Movement Therapy: Theoretical perspectives and empirical findings* (pp. 128–141). Logos.

Spielrein, S. (2015). The origin of the child's words papa and mama: Some observations on the different stages in language development. (Trans., B. Wharton). In C. Covington & B. Wharton (Eds.), *Sabina Spielrein: Forgotten pioneer of psychoanalysis* (2nd ed., pp. 233–248). Brunner-Routledge. (Original work published in 1922)

Stein, A. (2009). Feminism, therapeutic culture, and the Holocaust in the United States: The second-generation phenomenon. *Jewish Social Studies*, 16(1), 27–53. doi:10.2979/jss.2009.16.1.27

Thelen, E., & Adolph, K.E. (1994). Arnold L. Gesell: The paradox of nature and nurture. In R.D. Parke, P.A. Ornstein, J.J. Rieser, & C. Zahn-Waxler (Eds.), *A century of developmental psychology* (pp. 357–387). American Psychological Association. doi:10.1037/10155-027

Thompson, N.L. (2003). Marie Bonaparte's theory of female sexuality: Fantasy and biology. *American Imago*, 60(3), 343–378.

Trossman, B. (1968). Adolescent children of concentration camp survivors. *Canadian Psychiatric Association Journal*, 13(2), 121–123. doi:10.1177/070674376801300205

University of the State of New York. (1970, 26 June). Official incorporation of the Child Development Research [Unpublished document]. Child Development Research, Box 34, Articles of incorporation, bylaws, and mission statement, Kestenberg Papers (collection in process). Manuscript Division, Library of Congress, Washington, DC, United States. (Materials discovered by the author in Janet Kestenberg Amighi's private collection.)

Verny, T. (1981). *Secret life of the unborn child.* Summit.

Wahl, C. (1984). *Laban/Bartenieff movement studies: Contemporary applications.* Human Kinetics.

Weinberg, R. (1981). Some aims and purposes: Table play, gross motor activities & snack time. *Child Development Research News*, 3(2), 5–9.

Weinstein, J. (1978). Notes on the changing image of women's bodies. *Child Development Research News*, 1(2), 6 [Unpublished archival materials]. Child Development Research, Box 37, Newsletters, Kestenberg papers (collection in process). Manuscript Division, Library of Congress, Washington, DC, United States. Materials discovered by the author in Janet Kestenberg Amighi's private collection.

Winnicott, D.W. (1958). Transitional objects and transitional phenomena. In *Collected papers: Through paediatrics to psycho-analysis* (pp. 229–242). Basic Books. (Original work published 1951)

Winnicott, D.W. (1960). The theory of the parent–infant relationship. *The International Journal of Psychoanalysis*, 41, 585–595.

Winnik, H.Z. (1968). Contribution to symposium on psychic traumatization through social catastrophe. *The International Journal of Psychoanalysis*, 49(2), 298–301.
Wolfs, B. (2022). The psychoanalytic milieu of Margaret Mahler: Historical and contemporary perspectives on the separation-individuation process. *WUPJ*, 10.
Yadlin-Gadot, S. (2022). Lacan on mind and body. In J. Mills (Ed.), *Psychoanalysis and the mind–body problem* (pp. 119–136). Routledge. doi:10.4324/9781003090755-6

Chapter 3

An Ambivalent Reception

Movement Studies

> I think she always felt that she did not get recognition for the movement work in her own field. It was the dance/movement therapists who welcomed her, not the psychoanalysts.
>
> (Kestenberg Amighi, personal communication, 13 November 2021)

In Psychoanalysis

Kestenberg's work was discussed at two plenary meetings of the New York Psychoanalytic Society, once on 13 March 1956 and again on 23 February 1971. The first discussion concerned her paper "On the Development of Maternal Feelings in Early Childhood" (Kestenberg, 1956). As discussed in Chapter 2, Kestenberg identified *inner-genital* tensions in girls as the root of maternality, proposing that the externalisation of these diffuse, unlocalisable tensions gives rise to doll play, nurturing behaviour, and the wish for a child. Four discussants addressed Kestenberg's paper. The first discussant, Dr Abbott (1956, pp. 2–5), concurred with Kestenberg about vaginal tensions coinciding with the development of maternal behaviour in girls while also challenging her tension externalisation hypothesis. Dr Abbott presented a case involving an 8-year-old girl who exhibited precocious sexual development, a lack of interest in doll play, pronounced vaginal masturbation, and early onset of menstruation. By working through the tensions in analysis and a shift in the mother's attitude, the patient discontinued masturbatory behaviour, began engaging in doll play, and demonstrated maternal behaviours. Dr Abbott contended that it was, in fact, the altered mother–daughter relationship that facilitated the girl's identification with her mother, which contributed to the emergence of maternal behaviour through imitation (Abbott, 1956). Kestenberg (1956) further argued that this case supports her view that doll play and maternal behaviour are initiated or associated with the suppression of vaginal excitations.

Rudolf Loewenstein (1898–1976), the next commentator, critiqued Kestenberg's overemphasis on instinctual drives and argued that circumstances inhibit or reinforce instinctual development. He clarified that all

DOI: 10.4324/9781003559955-4

aspects of the complex maturational process may contribute to the development of maternality, not only the biologically determined vaginal tensions. He further elaborated, drawing on his work with Hartman and Kris, that ego aspects, such as congenital preferences for certain types of defence mechanisms, interfere with drive development; thus, ego development may play a crucial role in the development of maternal attitudes (Loewenstein, 1956, pp. 6–11). Loewenstein emphasised that identification with the mother as an ego-ideal may be an essentially decisive factor. He further problematised that, even though, according to Kestenberg, girls lack pronounced genital tensions compared with boys' genital sensations, she still maintained that their maternality originates from the projections of such fleeting, almost "non-existent" sensory experiences (Loewenstein, 1956, p. 10). Kestenberg (1956) clarified that she did not suggest these tensions were absent, but rather that they possess a diffuse and undefined quality, making them difficult to localise or confirm through visual or tactile means, in contrast to boys' genital sensations. This indirect relationship to knowledge about their genitals subsequently shapes girls' overall relationship to knowledge, predisposing them to favour more indirect and intuitively constructed ideas as opposed to the deductive and scientific methods typically preferred by boys. Edith Jacobson (1897–1978), the final discussant, endorsed Kestenberg's findings. She observed the significance of early vaginal tensions in her clinical work; however, she had not previously considered focusing on the methods of externalisation of these tensions, which she identified as a significant contribution of Kestenberg's (Jacobson, 1956, pp. 11–16).

In 1971, three discussants, Margaret Mahler, Albert Solnit, and Eleanor Galenson (1916/1917–2011) commented on Kestenberg's paper entitled "Development of the Young Child Expressed Through Bodily Movement" (Kestenberg, 1971). Mahler highlighted the importance of observational data as empirical support for psychoanalytic metapsychology. She called Kestenberg's movement categorisation framework an "ingenious method, a kind of alphabet" that "placed psychoanalytic infant observation in a truly new key" (Mahler, 1971, p. 1). She particularly praised the epigenetic sequence of zonal development and corresponding changes in body-image/body-ego organisation in Kestenberg's developmental movement theory. Through her observational research, Mahler confirmed the aptness of Kestenberg's interpretation of the correlation between the onset of teething, oral sadistic (Snapping-Biting) *Tension-Flow Rhythms*, and the infant's distancing tendencies, exemplified by pulling away or practising standing up in the mother's lap. Mahler (1971, p. 7) further emphasised the precision of Kestenberg's concepts concerning the achievement of vertical bodily alignment in conjunction with the development of representational intelligence. She also endorsed Kestenberg's designation of a separate urethral phase, which she believed to be easily verifiable from the libidinal investment in various kinds of water play of 3-year-olds.

The next discussant, Solnit (1971), praised Kestenberg's comprehensive developmental assessment and considered her categorisation of *Tension-Flow Rhythms* by erogenous zones and their association with phase-specific needs particularly valuable. He added that her emphasis on pre-ego manifestations could fill important gaps in psychoanalytic theory. However, Solnit critiqued Kestenberg for her use of "psychosomorphic" language, especially in relation to her concepts of *Shape-Flow*, which he found ambiguous. He added that, owing to its metaphorical character, Kestenberg's terminology did not lend itself easily to the advancement of psychoanalytic theory (Solnit, 1971, p. 4).

Galenson (1971), the final commentator, also critiqued Kestenberg (1971) for her systematic sequentialisation of phase-specific aspects of the development of drives, ego, and object-relations. She argued that Kestenberg's heightened focus on maturational processes that determine phase development disregarded the effects of external factors and inner bodily changes. Galenson further elaborated that, to adequately appreciate the complex interplay of many events within a single phase of development, psychodynamic assessment must resist the pull of an overly clear-cut systematisation. Galenson's example concerned Kestenberg's concept of the urethral phase, suggesting that the reorganisation of the child's body-ego into a more fluid, mobile, and overflowing state results not only from dominant urethral drives but also from the emergence of independent walking and running, and from the growing physical distance between mother and child. She further elaborated that Kestenberg demonstrated well how specific modes of patterning originating in given erogenous zones generalise to dominate the given phase's mode of functioning; however, she argued that, in the oral phase, not only are libidinal oral *Sucking* patterns frequent, but visual fixation and scanning with the eyes also dominate. Here, Galenson (1971) aimed to highlight the range of behaviours that characterise a developmental phase, emphasising that not only the motor but also the visual-perceptual apparatus contributes to the expression of drives and the emergence of object-relatedness.

In 1975, an anthology of Kestenberg's papers was published, accompanied by a foreword written by Phyllis Greenacre. Greenacre characterised Kestenberg's work as a significant advancement in psychoanalysis, highlighting its holistic perspective on the individual and its essential technical and methodological innovations (Greenacre, 1975, p. xiv). Subsequently, Goldings (1978) reviewed the publication and described Kestenberg as a pioneer at the intersection of bodily processes and mental activity. Goldings noted that Kestenberg's methods challenged conventional scientific standards, yet were valuable for generating hypotheses and broadening psychoanalytic understanding (Goldings, 1978). However, he also observed that Kestenberg's work faced scepticism within the psychoanalytic community, reportedly owing to a perceived neglect of ego-psychology.

Estelle Borowitz (1985), a collaborator of Kestenberg's at the Center for Parents and Children, sought to integrate Heinz Kohut's (1913–1981) self-psychology and concepts of narcissism with Kestenberg's *Shape-Flow* category, emphasising their relevance to the development of object-relations. Borowitz noted that, for Kestenberg, psychic patterns are reflected in motor patterns, and the self develops through the child's embodied interactions with the environment. Instead of distinguishing the self from other psychic structures, she argued that it is rooted in the body and inseparable from affective and drive processes. Borowitz further explained that, while Kohut emphasised maintaining self-cohesion through empathic mirroring between the infant and caregiver, Kestenberg focused on integration achieved through the coordination of bodily tension and shape patterns. She asserted that Kestenberg's perspective locates the emergence of self- and object-constancy in the lived experience of movement, ultimately leading to the perception of oneself as a unified whole. Borowitz (1985) also emphasised that both theorists view narcissism not as pathological but as a necessary and enduring aspect of psychic life. La Barre (in Kestenberg, 1990b), another collaborator of Kestenberg's, argued that Kestenberg's adaptation of drive-theory had the potential to revolutionise psychoanalytic theory and practice; its implications have yet to be fully explored. She further asserted that Kestenberg's *Movement Profile* provided new avenues for exploring long-standing questions in psychoanalysis, offering fresh insights into the complexities of human experience.

Apart from these commentaries, Kestenberg's psychodynamic vocabulary, developmental movement theory, and *Movement Profile* did not generate sustained interest in the field of psychoanalysis. With the exception of those of her trainees and collaborators, no focused studies have revisited or examined her movement concepts. A recollection from Susan Loman (dance/movement therapist) underscored a disconnect between Kestenberg and psychoanalysts at the time:

> During a conference where she presented a case, she tried to explain her findings by pointing to the poster of her patient's Movement Profile that she had constructed. She pointed to sections of the profile to illustrate specific movement patterns, but it was clear to me that the audience did not understand what these movements were. This disconnect made me realise how hard it was to clearly present movement concepts to non-movers. (Loman, personal communication, 15 November 2022)

During my archival research, I encountered traces of Kestenberg's disappointment at the neglect of her movement-centred work in her annotated copies of books on infant research in psychoanalysis. In the margins, she disputed contemporaneous findings and commented on the absence of references to her own studies (Kestenberg, n.d.). Her frustration is also underscored in a letter from Bartenieff to Lamb in which she reported that Kestenberg was so disheartened by her colleagues' hesitancy towards her movement studies that she considered abandoning the line of inquiry altogether (Bartenieff, 1963, p. 2).

In Creative Arts Therapies

Kestenberg's movement studies found particularly receptive ground among the emerging action-focused therapies (Levy, 1988), where her *Movement Profile* was both implemented and further developed. Her movement-focused developmental framework, together with her psychiatric background, made her work especially relevant to the professionalisation of creative arts therapies, particularly dance/movement therapy. The efforts of Penny Lewis, Susan Loman, Carol Fishman, Beth Gonzalez-Dolginko, Janet Kestenberg Amighi, and Mark Sossin facilitated the dissemination of Kestenberg's ideas beyond psychoanalytic circles, introducing them to a broader community of creative arts therapy practitioners.

During the 1970s, several first-generation American dance/movement therapists incorporated the Kestenberg Movement Profile (KMP) into their clinical practices (Loman & Merman, 1996; Lewis, 1972, 1990; Lewis & Loman, 1992). Lewis (1990) found Kestenberg's *Shape-Flow* category to be a particularly sensitive indicator of post-traumatic difficulties. She identified frequent occurrences of *Unipolar Shrinking, Bipolar Narrowing*, and *Neutral Flow* as the distinctive motor constellation among people with traumatic histories. Susan Loman played a pivotal role in advancing Kestenberg's work and facilitating its integration into American dance/movement therapy. Loman taught the KMP at the Laban Institute for Movement Studies to a diverse group of mental health professionals, dancers, and movement researchers. From the late 1980s, Loman directed the master's programme in Dance/Movement Therapy at Antioch University New England, where she implemented a practicum programme modelled after the Center for Parents and Children (Loman, personal communication, 15 November 2022).

Loman and Fishman, alongside Kestenberg (Kestenberg et al., 1979), presented their formulations on the relevance of arts-based methods in psychotherapy at the Conference of the New England Council of Creative Therapies and later, in 1983, at the Creative Arts Therapy Department of the Pratt Institute. Their presentations drew on their clinical experience of applying the KMP in dance/movement therapy and in child guidance at the Center for Parents and Children. They argued that infants localise and identify objects based on their physical properties, motion, shape, and location. They disputed the classical psychoanalytic idea that the pleasurable aspect of play derives from its relation to the discharge of excess energy and contended that it is, in fact, related to the pleasure derived from the recognition of the ability to make an impact on the external environment through physical movement. They argued that the body-image formation is based on the creative exchange of kinaesthetic experiences between bodies. They proposed a view of expressive movements as creative, transitional phenomena appearing at the frontiers of the internal and external world; at the merger and separation of self and other. They further maintained that *Tension-Flow Rhythms* and *Shape-Flow* patterns can be observed in any medium of art as fundamental expressions of vitality. Therefore, not only dance/movement therapy but also other creative arts therapies could use the KMP as an assessment framework (Kestenberg et al., 1979).

Loman and Merman (1996; Loman, 1998) argued that the KMP is an appropriate tool for evaluating therapeutic efficacy. They highlighted the importance of a clearly articulated theoretical framework in dance/movement therapy that integrates developmental and movement theories, supports both qualitative and quantitative data collection for treatment planning, and facilitates effective communication of clinical information within multidisciplinary teams. Furthermore, they maintained that the KMP can support the development of therapeutic skills. They argued that Kestenberg's concept of attunement enables therapists-in-training to cultivate the embodied skills needed to establish good rapport with clients. They also proposed that dance/movement therapists' awareness of their own movement repertoires enhances therapeutic competence (Loman & Merman, 1996). As a result of these initiatives, in the 1990s, 12 dance/movement therapy trainees dedicated their master's theses to exploring the application of the KMP in various settings (Atley, 1991; Berger, 1994; Binette, 1993; Bridges, 1989; Daigle, 1993; Korn, 1990; Lemon, 1990; Merman, 1990; Ojala, 1995; Stupka-Malloy, 1992; Watkins, 1995; Williams, 1994).

In 1989, the first conference on the Kestenberg Movement Profile was organised by the Dance/Movement-Therapy graduate programme at Antioch University New England (Loman & Lewis, 1990). Presenters reported on the application of the KMP in dance/movement therapy practice (Lewis, 1990) and in cross-cultural research (Kestenberg Amighi, 1990). A panel discussion addressed the future applications of the KMP; it featured Frances La Barre, a psychoanalyst; Penny Lewis and Hillary Merman, dance/movement therapists; and Ellen Goldman, a Laban Movement Analyst. In her review of the conference publication, Martha Davis (1992), a key figure in movement behaviour research at the time, acknowledged the conceptual rigour and complexity of the KMP but questioned whether the drive towards systematisation did justice to the dynamic, open-ended nature of human behaviour. She also noted the scarcity of publications that translated the KMP's psychoanalytic terminology into more accessible language for those unfamiliar with its conceptual framework. Davis's (1992) observations were addressed through the popularisation efforts of Kestenberg Amighi, Loman, Lewis, and Sossin, culminating in the publication of *The Meaning of Movement: Developmental and Clinical Perspectives of the Kestenberg Movement Profile* (1999). This volume presented the KMP theory in its entirety, with clinical case studies and revised terminology to aid accessibility for a broader audience, including creative arts therapists, professionals in child development, and lay readers interested in embodiment perspectives.

In Nonverbal Communication Research

Kestenberg became peripherally associated with the transdisciplinary field of nonverbal communication research, which developed in the 1950s and culminated in the establishment of the Institute for Nonverbal Communication Research (INCR) by Martha Davis in 1978. Kestenberg served on the advisory board of the institute alongside pioneering nonverbal behaviour researchers in the psy-sciences and affiliated humanities, such as Margaret Mead (1901–1978), anthropologist; Albert Scheflen (1920–1980), psychiatrist; Norbert Freedman (1922–2011), psychoanalyst; Israel Zwerling (1917–1993), psychiatrist; and William S. Condon (1896–1968), psychologist (*Kinesis*, 1978, p. 2). The INCR sponsored various seminars on pioneering methods in nonverbal communication research, such as a 12-week course in developmental movement patterns, including the KMP (*Kinesis*, 1978, p. 4). The INCR provided funding for the publication of the *Kinesis* Report journal and several scientific conferences. Although Kestenberg served on the institute's advisory board, she did not publish in *Kinesis* and, according to Davis's recollections, even though she attended INCR-sponsored conferences, she did not present her own research (Davis, personal communication, 31 January 2023). Davis was nonetheless an enthusiastic advocate of Kestenberg's work and initiated her nomination for the Marconi Prize in 1980. The Marconi Fellowship Award recognised individuals who made significant contributions to communication science and technology, especially those whose work promoted the well-being of children through nonverbal means (Davis, 1980). Representing the INCR, Davis wrote to Albert Solnit to request a letter of recommendation supporting Kestenberg's nomination. According to Davis's letter, Kestenberg welcomed the prospect of being nominated. However, no documentation has been found to confirm whether the nomination was ultimately submitted or pursued.

Holocaust Studies

Kestenberg's psychohistorical studies on the Nazi Holocaust encountered a quite dissimilar reception to her movement-focused work within psychoanalysis. Her concepts on transgenerational trauma transmission embedded themselves into the canon of the psychoanalytic approach to trauma, and the unique scope of her Holocaust studies was praised by many of her contemporaries.

Coleman (1974), in a review of a psychoanalytic study of child survivors, noted that the new case material reinforced Kestenberg's hypothesis that Holocaust survivors bear deep psychological wounds which may negatively impact their children's emotional development. Coleman also highlighted that some of the described symptoms resemble schizophrenia, echoing Kestenberg's caution about the importance of distinguishing trauma-related manifestations from psychotic disorders, both for diagnostic clarity and to avoid jeopardising survivors' access to indemnification. Auerhahn and Prelinger

(1983) used Kestenberg's formulations about children of survivors living in their parents' past in their case study on first- and second-generation survivors. Blum (1983) demonstrated that trauma is transmitted across generations through the child's profound identification with a Holocaust survivor parent. Drawing on Kestenberg's (1980) concept of *transposition*, Blum argued that the mother's unresolved mourning and emotional withdrawal establish a psychic environment in which the child internalises her trauma. According to Blum, this process gives rise to the child's ambivalent wish to "*kill or cure*" the parent, reflecting both the inherited, unprocessed trauma and the child's struggle for individuation. Auerhahn and Laub (1984) described the emotional dynamic between survivors of the Nazi Holocaust and their children as grounded in the survivors' unresolved longing to reclaim a lost past. Following Kestenberg's (1980) insights, they suggest that survivors' intense emotional investment in their children and the children's reciprocal efforts to revive or embody their parents' experiences together express an unconscious wish to restore what was destroyed, using the next generation as a means to continue an interrupted life.

Eickhoff (1986, 1989) applied Kestenberg's notion of transposition in his case study on a daughter of a Nazi sympathiser. In Freedman's (1988) opening speech at the Institute for Psychoanalytic Training and Research in May 1986, he reflected on Kestenberg's (1982) important distinction between the psychological legacies of children of Holocaust survivors and those of Nazi descendants. He recounted Kestenberg's formulation that, while children of survivors must resist intrusions of ambivalent trauma into their superegos via the internalised images of both persecutor and victim, children of Nazis persecutors need to confront their own conscience without the shared experience of the Holocaust trauma – a proposition Freedman found deeply illuminating.

Abramovitch (1992) emphasised Kestenberg's substantial contributions to the understanding of the psychological experiences of children of survivors. He noted her precise observations that survivors frequently do not conform to standard diagnostic categories, at times appearing emotionally detached or showing signs of psychosis, while simultaneously exhibiting unexpected ego strength. Abramovitch (1992) found Kestenberg's term "*transmitted traumatic neurosis*" exceptionally useful to describe the condition in which children become preoccupied with traumatic events that they did not personally experience. Fonagy (1999) mentioned the innovative nature of Kestenberg's Holocaust studies for their emphasis on the bodily aspect of trauma transmission and for differentiating *transposition* from the process of identification. Kafka (1999) offered a nuanced appraisal of Kestenberg's studies. He praised the psychoanalytic developmental approach employed to identify and interpret discernible patterns of psychological response to extreme trauma. He found the emphasis on continuity in both therapy and research interviews particularly valuable. However, Kafka also critiqued some of Kestenberg's interpretations, which he viewed as speculative, such as her hypothesis that

Nazi infanticidal violence represented a projection of their own wish to destroy their children, and her invocation of the death instinct to explain survivors' wish to die. He cautioned that such interpretations risked oversimplifying the horrors of the Nazi Holocaust (Kafka, 1999). Berger (1994) also critiqued Kestenberg and her collaborators for psychologising the Nazi Holocaust. As he proposed, one cannot be cured of being a Holocaust survivor. He argued that it is not a psychological but rather an ontological condition for which therapy is not the answer, and that the Nazi Holocaust transcends the clinical realm. MacLennan (1999), reviewing Kestenberg and Kahn (1998), regarded the volume as an invaluable resource for mental health professionals working with traumatised children and adults, and as a valuable contribution to trauma studies overall.

Judith Kestenberg became well known for her Holocaust studies within the international psychoanalytic community and in the American Jewish community. Her daughter, Janet Kestenberg Amighi, recalled that, a year before her mother's death, she accompanied her to a conference of the New York Psychoanalytic Society. As Judith was wheeled into the room by her nurse, the audience rose and applauded her. Kestenberg Amighi attributed this warm reception to her mother's Holocaust work, yet expressed surprise, as she had believed her mother never felt fully appreciated by the New York psychoanalytic community (Kestenberg Amighi, personal communication, 13 November 2021). Similarly, Silvia Birklein (KMP-trained psychoanalyst) observed that many psychoanalysts were familiar with Kestenberg primarily through her Holocaust studies (Birklein, personal communication, 11 November 2022). Thus, Judith Kestenberg's body of work has been divided between her two principal projects. While her psychohistorical studies of the Nazi Holocaust were widely recognised, her movement-focused work received limited attention in American psychoanalysis and psychiatry.

References

Abbott (1956, March 16). Discussion of Judith S. Kestenberg: On the development of maternal feelings in early childhood. Meeting Proceedings, New York Psychoanalytic Society Documents of Judith S. Kestenberg (1937–1999). New York Psychoanalytic Association and Society A. A. Brill Library, Archives and Special Collections. New York, NY, United States.

Abramovitch, H. (1992). Review of the book *Generations of the Holocaust*, edited by M. S. Bergmann & M. E. Jucovy. *Journal of Analytical Psychology*, 37(2), 245–246.

Atley, S.H. (1991). In search of a standard form of assessment: The Kestenberg Movement Profile as a diagnostic tool and treatment guide integrated into the practice of dance therapy. Unpublished master's thesis, Antioch New England Graduate School, NH, United States.

Auerhahn, N., & Laub, D. (1984). Annihilation and restoration: Post-traumatic memory as pathway and obstacle to recovery. *International Review of Psycho-Analysis*, 11, 327–344.

Auerhahn, N., & Prelinger, E. (1983). Repetition in the concentration camp survivor and her child. *International Review of Psycho-Analysis*, 10, 31–46.
Bartenieff, I. (1963, 16 January). Letter to Warren Lamb. Irmgard Bartenieff Papers (0390-SCPA), Correspondence, 1929–1981, Professional letters, 1929–1980. Michelle Smith Performing Arts Library, University of Maryland, United States.
Berger, K.J. (1994). Language of motion: An introduction to the Kestenberg Movement Profile. Unpublished master's thesis, Antioch New England Graduate School, NH, United States.
Binette, L. (1993). A KMP analysis of moshing: The study of a communal ritual dance amongst adolescent males of the 1990s. Unpublished master's thesis, Antioch New England Graduate School, NH, United States.
Blum, H. (1983). The psychoanalytic process and analytic inference: A clinical study of a lie and loss. *International Journal of Psychoanalysis*, 64, 17–33.
Borowitz, E. (1985). Origins of the self as viewed in the self-psychology of Heinz Kohut and the movement analysis of Judith Kestenberg. Doctoral dissertation, Union Graduate School for the Union of Experimenting Colleges and Universities, Cincinnati, OH, United States.
Bridges, L. (1989). Measuring the effect of dance/movement therapy on the body image of institutionalized elderly using the Kestenberg Movement Profile and projective drawings. Unpublished master's thesis, Antioch New England Graduate School, NH, United States.
Coleman, M. (1974). Review of the book *The child of two survivors: A report of an unsuccessful therapy* by M. Lipkowitz. *Psychoanalytic Quarterly*, 43, 334–335.
Daigle, R. (1993). Application of the Kestenberg Movement Profile to the clinical assessment of the mother–autistic child dyad. Unpublished master's thesis, Antioch New England Graduate School, NH, United States.
Davis, M. (1980, September 26). Letter to Albert Solnit [Unpublished archival material]. Box 35, Correspondences, Kestenberg papers (collection in process). Manuscript Division, Library of Congress, Washington, DC, United States. Discovered by the author in Kestenberg Amighi's private collection.
Davis, M. (1992). Flowing into the mainstream isn't free. *American Journal of Dance Therapy*, 14(1), Spring/Summer.
Eickhoff, F. (1986). Identification and its vicissitudes in the context of the Nazi phenomenon. *International Journal of Psychoanalysis*, 67, 33–44.
Eickhoff, F. (1989). On the "borrowed unconscious sense of guilt" and the palimpsestic structure of a symptom: Afterthoughts on the Hamburg Congress of the IPA. *International Review of Psycho-Analysis*, 16, 323–329.
Fonagy, P. (1999). The transgenerational transmission of holocaust trauma. *Attachment & Human Development*, 1(1), 92–114. doi:10.1080/14616739900134041
Freedman, N. (1988). The setting and the issues. *Psychoanalysis and Contemporary Thought*, 11(2), 197–212.
Galenson, E. (1971, February 23). Discussion of Judith S. Kestenberg: Development of the young child expressed through bodily movement I. 565th Meeting Proceedings, New York Psychoanalytic Association and Society Meeting Notes, A. A. Brill Library, Archives and Special Collections.
Goldings, H.J. (1978). Review of the book *Children and parents: Psychoanalytic studies in development*, by J. S. Kestenberg. *The Psychoanalytic Quarterly*, 47, 124–127.

Greenacre, P. (1975). Foreword. In J.S. Kestenberg, *Children and parents: Psychoanalytic studies in development* (pp. xiii–xiv). Jason Aronson.

Jacobson, E. (1956, March 16). Discussion of Judith S. Kestenberg: On the development of maternal feelings in early childhood. Meeting Proceedings, New York Psychoanalytic Society Documents of Judith S. Kestenberg (1937–1999). New York Psychoanalytic Association and Society A. A. Brill Library, Archives and Special Collections. New York, USA.

Kafka, J.S. (1999). Book review and commentary: *The Last Witness: The Child Survivor of the Holocaust* (J. S. Kestenberg & I. Brenner, 1996). *Journal of Applied Psychoanalytic Studies*, 1(3), 277–279.

Kestenberg Amighi, J. (1990). The application of the KMP cross-culturally. In S. Loman & P. Lewis (Eds.), *The Kestenberg Movement Profile: Its past, present applications, and future directions* (pp. 114–125). Retrieved from https://aura.antioch.edu/facbooks/25

Kestenberg-Amighi, J., Loman, S., Lewis, P., & Sossin, K.M. (Eds.). (1999). *The meaning of movement: Developmental and clinical perspectives of the Kestenberg Movement Profile.* Gordon & Breach.

Kestenberg, J.S. (n.d.). Books and study notes [Unpublished archival materials]. Box 6, Notes, miscellaneous, Box 10, Books. Kestenberg papers (collection in process). Manuscript Division, Library of Congress, Washington, DC, United States. Discovered by the author in Mark Sossin's private collection.

Kestenberg, J.S. (1956, March 16). On the development of maternal feelings in early childhood: Observations and reflections [Presentation]. Meeting of the New York Psychoanalytic Society, Documents of Judith S. Kestenberg (1937–1999). New York Psychoanalytic Association and Society A. A. Brill Library, Archives and Special Collections. New York, NY, United States.

Kestenberg, J.S. (1971, February 23). Development of the young child expressed through bodily movement. Presentation. 565th Meeting Proceedings, New York Psychoanalytic Society and Institute, A. A. Brill Library & Archives. Documents Judith S. Kestenberg (1937–1999). New York Psychoanalytic Association and Society A. A. Brill Library, Archives and Special Collections. New York, NY, United States.

Kestenberg, J.S. (1980). Psychoanalysis of children of survivors from the Holocaust: Case presentations and assessment. *Journal of the American Psychoanalytic Association*, 28(4), 775–804.

Kestenberg, J.S. (1982). Introduction to persecutor's children. In M.S. Bergmann & M. E. Jucovy (Eds.), *Generations of the Holocaust* (pp. 161–167). Basic Books.

Kestenberg, J.S. (1990). Future directions of the KMP. Panel discussion with Goldman, E., LaBarre, F., Lewis, P., Merman, H., & Sossin, K. M. In S. Loman & P. Lewis (Eds.), *The Kestenberg Movement Profile: Its past, present applications, and future directions* (pp. 155–173). Retrieved from https://aura.antioch.edu/facbooks/25

Kestenberg, J.S., & Kahn, C. (Eds.). (1998). *Children surviving persecution: An international study of trauma and healing*. Praeger.

Kestenberg, J.S., Loman, S., & Fishman, C. (1979). A multicreative approach to prevention with infants, toddlers, and their parents. Conference presentation, unpublished. Presented at the New England Council of Creative Therapies Conference, Brown University, United States.

Kinesis. (1978). A news journal for nonverbal communication research, 1(1).

Korn, S. (1990). Rhythms of life: The Kestenberg Movement Profile and dance therapy. Video master's thesis, Lesley College, Cambridge, MA, United States.

Lemon, J. (1990). The use of dance/movement therapy in professional sport: A Kestenberg Movement Profile of Joe Montana. Unpublished master's thesis, Antioch New England Graduate School, NH, United States.

Levy, F. (1988). *Dance/movement therapy: A healing art.* The American Alliance for Health, Physical Education, Recreation and Dance.

Lewis, P. (1972). *Theory and methods in dance/movement therapy.* Kendall/Hunt.

Lewis, P. (1990). The Kestenberg Movement Profile in the psychotherapeutic process with borderline disorders. In S. Loman & P. Lewis (Eds.), *The Kestenberg Movement Profile: Its past, present applications, and future directions.* Retrieved from https://aura.antioch.edu/facbooks/25

Lewis, P., & Loman, S. (1992). Movement components of affect: Tension-flow attributes within the Kestenberg Movement Profile (KMP). In American Dance Therapy Association 27th Annual Conference Proceedings. American Dance Therapy Association.

Loman, S. (1998). Employing a developmental model of movement patterns in dance/movement therapy with young children and their families. *American Journal of Dance Therapy*, 20(2), 101–115. doi:10.1023/A:1022100511657

Loman, S., & Lewis, P. (1990). *The Kestenberg Movement Profile: Its past, present applications, and future directions.* Retrieved from https://aura.antioch.edu/facbooks/25

Loman, S., & Merman, H. (1996). The KMP: A tool for dance/movement therapy. *American Journal of Dance Therapy*, 18(1), 29–52. doi:10.1007/BF02360220

Loewenstein, R. (1956, March 16). Discussion of Judith S. Kestenberg: On the development of maternal feelings in early childhood. Meeting Proceedings, New York Psychoanalytic Society Documents of Judith S. Kestenberg (1937–1999). New York Psychoanalytic Association and Society A. A. Brill Library, Archives and Special Collections. New York, USA.

Mahler, M.S. (1971, February 23). Discussion of Judith S. Kestenberg: Development of the young child expressed through bodily movement I. 565th Meeting Proceedings, New York Psychoanalytic Association and Society Meeting Notes A. A. Brill Library, Archives and Special Collections.

MacLennan, B.W. (1999). Review of the book *Children surviving persecution: An international study of trauma and healing*, edited by J. S. Kestenberg & C. Kahn. *Journal of Child and Adolescent Group Therapy*, 9(2), 253–255.

Merman, H. (1990). The use of precursors of effort in dance/movement therapy. In S. Loman & P. Lewis (Eds.), *The Kestenberg Movement Profile: Its past, present applications, and future directions.* Antioch New England Graduate School.

Ojala, E. (1995). Dance/movement therapy with a developmentally disabled adolescent utilizing the Kestenberg Movement Profile. Unpublished master's thesis, Antioch New England Graduate School, NH, United States.

Solnit, A. (1971, February 23). Discussion of Judith S. Kestenberg: Development of the Young Child Expressed through Bodily Movement I. 565th Meeting Proceedings, New York Psychoanalytic Association and Society Meeting Notes, A. A. Brill Library, Archives and Special Collections.

Stupka-Malloy, A. (1992). The KMP explored: An illustrated presentation of the Tension-Flow Rhythms. Unpublished master's thesis, Antioch New England Graduate School, NH, United States.

Watkins, A. (1995). An application of the Kestenberg Movement Profile and ritual: A case study. Unpublished master's thesis, Antioch New England Graduate School, NH, United States.

Williams, A. (1994). Dance/movement therapy and drama therapy as co-modalities with an adolescent population. Unpublished master's thesis, Antioch New England Graduate School, NH, United States.

Chapter 4

Issues of Belonging in the Psychological Sciences

In what follows, I'm seeking to illuminate the processes in the disciplinary history of the mid- to late-twentieth-century American psy-sciences that contributed to the uneven and selective reception of Kestenberg's work. Rather than treating this ambivalent reception as reflecting the value and coherence of her theories, this chapter approaches it as contingent upon shifting institutional, methodological, and theoretical considerations in mental health research and practice. The discussion will provide a focused account of changes in the landscape of American psychological sciences, with particular attention to the disciplines and fields within which Kestenberg worked. These changes include the rise and subsequent decline of psychoanalysis within American psychiatry; the emergence of ego-psychology, infant observation studies, and child guidance; and the shift toward community mental health, interactional frameworks, nonverbal communication, and the proliferation of new psychotherapeutic modalities. These developments, spanning the 1940s to the 1980s, unfolded within the broader context of the Cold War and were shaped by changing political demands, institutional priorities, and funding structures. As the psy-sciences became increasingly differentiated, shifting scientific priorities redefined central research questions, the criteria for legitimate knowledge, and the standing of particular methodologies. These proved consequential for the reception of Kestenberg's work.

Evolving Landscapes

At the turn of the century, mental health care in the United States was characterised by an extensive network of state mental hospitals that provided inpatient care, supported by significant statutory budgets. Psychiatry was a predominantly institutionalised profession with most clinicians working in state hospitals (Grob, 1991, pp. 5–24). The traditional approach in psychiatry was an assumed sharp distinction between illness and health expressed in drastic somatic and behavioural symptoms. This paradigm began to shift gradually at the turn of the century, driven by the contributions of Sigmund Freud (1856–1939), Adolf Meyer (1866–1950), and William Alanson White

DOI: 10.4324/9781003559955-5

(1870–1937). They challenged the strict separation between mental health and disease and emphasised the importance of life history in the aetiology of mental disorders (Grob, 1991, p. 6). Mental illness increasingly became recognised as a preventable public health issue. Polat (2021, p. 272) noted that many contended that psychiatry historically prioritised the treatment of severe mental illness while overlooking the role of environmental factors in the development of psychological disturbances. In 1909, the National Committee for Mental Hygiene was established in New York City to prevent mental illness by promoting emotional well-being. This led to the establishment of child guidance clinics in the 1920s across the United States (and in Britain), and psychiatry expanded its scope to provide mental health guidance to the general population. Polat (2021, pp. 272–278) explained that, during the first decades of the twentieth century, American psychiatry struggled to separate from medicine and establish its disciplinary identity. Through the reframing of itself as a discipline that can prevent social issues by identifying pathogenic environmental factors through methods such as mental testing, direct observation, and psychoanalytic investigation, it could leave the walls of the asylum and offer itself as a psycho-social technology with a wider scope (Polat, 2021; Grob, 1991).

Polat (2021, pp. 269–270) demonstrated that psychiatric and psychoanalytic investigations, such as the life-history method and personality assessment, dominated the first epoch of child guidance. In the 1930s, the focus shifted towards mixed-methods approaches combining direct observation and psychometric assessments. In the 1940s, attention to normal and abnormal development grew in child guidance. Under pressure from funding agencies and to keep up with academic publishing standards, psychoanalytic psychiatrists set out to develop norm-based instruments to validate psychoanalytic developmental notions. This introduced a shift towards larger-scale, experimental assessments of children, away from the individual case-study format (Polat, 2021, p. 285). Psychiatry's expanding engagement with prevention, development, and environmental causation altered its clinical remit while also generating new methods for observing and measuring psychological development. Psychoanalytic theory provided a theoretical hinge for early child guidance practitioners in establishing the link between psychological and developmental disturbance in children and pathogenic environmental factors. Practitioners applied analytic developmental interpretations to the emotional states they observed in children (Polat, 2021, p. 290). Aligned with the ethos of child guidance and psychiatry's increasing focus on prevention and environmental causation, Kestenberg developed a psychoanalytic assessment framework specifically designed to support diagnosis and prevention in developmental psychiatry. She sought a systematic framework for observing development through movement, positioning motor specificities as indicators of psychological organisation and potential developmental disturbance.

Kestenberg began to formulate these ideas during her internship in the Child Psychiatry Department of Bellevue Hospital, during a period marked by the economic downturn of the 1930s, which severely affected most public psychiatric institutions in the United States. Staff ratios had to be curtailed, and developments were halted. During the war years, overcrowding in mental health hospitals and deteriorating environmental conditions posed further problems (Grob, 1991, p. 3). State mental hospitals provided long-term care for a growing population of patients with chronic behavioural and underlying somatic disorders. The Second World War marked a turning point, as the conditions of inpatient care worsened and new ideas about non-institutional care started to emerge. Grob (1991, p. 8) explained that clinicians' wartime experiences reinforced evidence for the effectiveness of outpatient treatment, underscored the impact of environmental and combat-related factors on mental health, and strengthened confidence in preventive psychiatry. These developments fostered the emergence of a new generation of psychiatrists who emphasised the socio-environmental determinants of mental illness and promoted psychodynamic, community-based approaches to care. In 1946, the landmark Mental Health Act was passed, establishing the National Institute of Mental Health (NIMH) in 1949, under the leadership of Robert Felix (1904–1990) (Hale, 1995, p. 252). Felix advocated for community psychiatry, and the NIMH funded a diverse range of projects in biological, psychodynamic, and social sciences (Hale, 1995). The NIMH also played a significant role in supporting training in psychiatry and psychoanalysis, allocating funding for psychoanalytically oriented research in psychiatry as well as in affiliated fields such as social sciences, social work, and family support. Hale (1995, p. 222) reported that psychoanalytic institutes "between 1948 and 1961 received $1,121,030" from the NIMH (Herzog, 2016a, p. 46).

During the war years, psychoanalysis exerted an increasingly significant influence on American psychiatry, a trend that persisted until the mid-1960s. A younger cohort of psychoanalytically oriented psychiatrists who came to dominate the field in the postwar period shaped this development. These practitioners were sceptical of organic treatment methods and favoured non-directive approaches (Hale, 1995, pp. 245–247). Their preference for psychoanalysis was informed by their wartime experiences that highlighted the inadequacy of existing psychiatric approaches. Psychoanalysis seemed to provide this generation with new insights and frameworks to understand the underlying aspects of psychological disturbances (Hale, 1995; Aron & Starr, 2013). Between 1947 and 1965, psychoanalysis maintained a substantial presence in medical school education in the United States. Psychoanalytic training schools were established at Columbia University, Downstate Medical Centre in Brooklyn, and New York University (Hale, 1995, p. 253; Herzog, 2016b). The influence of psychoanalysis on psychiatry training was supported by generous governmental funding. "The two largest recipients of NIMH funding were Yale and the University of California, Los Angeles, where psychoanalysts headed the psychiatry departments"

(Herzog, 2016a, p. 46). These developments were exemplified in Kestenberg's career as she held a faculty position at the Department of Psychiatry at Downstate Medical Centre and served as a training analyst at the State University of New York.

The postwar expansion of psychiatry into community-based and preventive domains created both an opportunity and challenges for psychoanalysis. Although psychoanalytic concepts became increasingly influential in psychiatric training and practice, ongoing questions remained regarding the extent to which psychoanalysis could contribute to a general psychology of the mind and human behaviour (Hale, 1995). This highlighted the need to support psychoanalytic concepts with empirical evidence. It was within this context that mid-century American psychoanalysis began to reformulate itself in closer alignment with empirical inquiry. This medical and scientific orientation was profoundly influenced by the emigration of European analysts during the 1930s, a movement driven by escalating anti-Semitism in Europe and the rise of the Third Reich. Many of the émigrés came from medical backgrounds and had extensive clinical experience. Their ambitions aligned well with the interests of American psychiatric psychoanalysts (Hale, 1995, p. 231).

It was ego-psychology, heralded by European émigrés, that addressed this challenge of making psychoanalysis more scientific. It was developed into a prominent movement of American psychoanalysis by Heinz Hartmann, Rudolph Loewenstein, Marianne and Ernst Kris (1900–1957), David Rapaport (1911–1960), Phyllis Greenacre, Edith Jacobson, Margaret Mahler, and Anna Freud (who was based in England but exerted significant influence on American psychoanalysis) (Hartmann, 1958; Hartmann et al., 1949; Hale, 1995; Midgley, 2013; Herzog, 2016b). They addressed questions traditionally associated with academic psychology, such as perception, intelligence, and learning. They also had an interest in systematically embedding the role of the environment in psychoanalytic theory (Hale, 1995, p. 233). Ego-psychologists, such as Anna Freud, frequently pursued preventive objectives, aiming to reduce the incidence of neurosis in children. Achieving this goal required a comprehensive examination of normal developmental processes (Hale, 1995; Polat, 2021; Midgley, 2013). These theorists re-examined the mechanisms underlying aggressive drives, emphasising the ego's regulatory and autonomous functions. They reconsidered the Freudian postulate (Freud, 1923/1961) and argued that the ego does not develop from the id but rather emerges from an undifferentiated phase of innate givens. Hartmann's key contributions were to posit a conflict-free sphere of the ego and the mechanism of drive naturalisation in the service of adaptation. He theorised that aggressive drives could also be decoupled from their instinctual aims, just as the libido can be through sublimation; this was the process of neutralisation for Hartmann. The ability to neutralise had significance for the development of object-relationships; that is, one had to be able to sublimate aggressive instincts to form enduring relationships. This neutralised energy was also thought to contribute significantly to reality testing and mastery, as it supplies the ego and superego with the power for action (Hartmann, 1958; Hartmann et al., 1949; Hale, 1995, p. 236). The maturational processes that could develop outside of conflict included motor development, thinking, perception, intention, and language. He argued that many defences served adaptive ends, such as denial and avoidance, which could help escape from danger. Both concepts became increasingly influential in orienting analysts' attention to the study of the total personality. Eissler (1953) defined the core clinical parameters of ego-psychology, establishing an austere framework characterised by the analyst's objectivity, neutrality, and detachment, and the focus on intrapsychic conflict and a balance between aggressive and libidinal drives (Wallerstein, 2002). Within this framework, treatment objectives shifted to enhancing productivity, improving overall functioning, and facilitating adaptation to the environment (Hale, 1995, pp. 233–235). Hale (1995) added, "the strength of ego-psychology lay in its attempts at orderly propositions, more comprehensive systemic theory and the reappraisal of drives" (p. 244).

Hartmann identified potential in psychoanalytically informed infant observation to address gaps in developmental theory. He argued that psychoanalytic theory should guide observation and generate hypotheses for empirical testing. By reframing psychoanalytic theory around normal development, adaptive functioning, and ego capacities, ego-psychology helped legitimise new, empirical forms of inquiry within psychoanalysis. These shifts supported the incorporation of direct observation, longitudinal study, and normative developmental assessments into psychoanalytic research, specifically within child guidance and preventive psychiatric contexts (Polat, 2021; Hale, 1995). This integration of direct observational methods into psychoanalytic developmental inquiry within the framework of child guidance was the focal point of the work at Anna Freud and Mahler's research nurseries (Polat, 2021, p. 284). Freud's studies at Hampstead responded to topical questions of the time regarding the effectiveness of psychoanalysis in prophylactic psychiatry. Mahler's study of the separation-individuation process was also among the first in psychoanalysis to systematically integrate clinically derived concepts of early development with empirical evidence from infant observation (Gergely, 2000). Kestenberg's work resonated strongly with the developmental and adaptive orientation of ego-psychology, as evidenced by her efforts to conceptualise movement patterns associated with the development of ego functions and regulatory mechanisms (Kestenberg, 1946, 1953, 1965b, 1967).

In 1950, at a meeting of the American Psychoanalytic Association in Detroit, René Spitz presented a paper on the relevance of direct observation of infants. His lecture clearly demonstrated the focus of psychoanalytic psychiatry at the time. He argued for observational studies of development to identify developmental norms and deviations in service of a preventive approach in psychiatry. He stressed the need for experimental studies and scientific measures integrated with psychoanalytic theory. Spitz (1950) reported having drawn upon Gesell's (Gesell & Amatruda, 1947) and Bühler's (1930) developmental observational studies and applied the Baby Tests; however, he critiqued that neither of these studies accounted sufficiently for the understanding of the personality of the child. Spitz called for a method to evaluate the relationships between different sectors of the personality, which he considered a new approach in infant psychiatry. He contended that, to understand infant development, psychoanalytic theory alone was insufficient; psychological and experiential methods of observation and testing were necessary. He stressed the relevance of an integrative approach and criticised the discriminatory use of observation and testing alone. He added that developmental observations enhanced understanding of environmental factors and, thus, could also inform preventive psychiatry (Spitz, 1950, pp. 72–73). As Polat explained (2021, p. 285), key disciplinary debates in mid-century American psychoanalysis centred on whether psychoanalysis could effectively support the early detection and management of psychopathology, and whether its emphasis on the individual psyche, combined with the limited use of diagnostic classifications, allowed the generation of scientifically valid claims regarding developmental issues (cf. Hale, 1995; Polat, 2021). Kestenberg's developmental movement studies were designed to address these theoretical and methodological concerns. Her developmental assessment framework, the *Movement Profile*, evaluated data from direct observation through a psychoanalytic lens, with particular attention to relational, affective, and developmental organisation in early life for the purposes of primary prevention (Kestenberg, 1974, 1985).

The popularity of psychoanalysis among the postwar generation of psychiatrists, the scientification efforts of ego-psychologists, and, as Herzog (2016a, 2016b) demonstrated, the discipline's changed relationship to theories of sexuality and its response to religious critiques contributed to the significant postwar expansion of psychoanalysis, which reached its highest point of prestige in the 1960s (Hale, 1995, p. 232). Herzog (2016b, p. 67) situated this ascent in the postwar climate in the United States characterised by a confluence of increased religiosity, psychologisation of religion, self-improvement ideals, and growing religious pluralism. Her study demonstrated (Herzog, 2016a, pp. 50–52) that in the late 1940s, across the United States, Canada, and Western Europe, various members of the clergy took a special interest in psychoanalysis, advocating their right to receive analytic training and even publishing works on the potential compatibility between Freudian theory and Catholicism. In 1952, it was Pope Pius XII[1] himself who commented on the issue of psychoanalysis. He emphasised that, while some of Freud's methods and theories were eccentric and clearly incompatible with the Catholic faith, such as the heightened focus on sex, the talking cure, if it veered away from the "sex talk," was acceptable and valuable (Herzog, 2016a, p. 51). At the same time, there were various feuds within American psychoanalysis itself about basic tenets of Freudian libido and psychosexual development theory. Modifications in the theory and practice by Karen Horney, Eric Fromm, Harry Stack Sullivan, and Franz Alexander all loosened the centrality of libido in relation to psychic life, shifting the emphasis on to feelings of anxiety, cultural factors, and interpersonal relationships (Herzog, 2016a, p. 23). These internal debates and external church critiques intensified the ambivalence of American analysts towards the topic of sex, contributing to the setting aside of libido theory and fixing their focus on adaptation, autonomy, and ego-strength as expressed in the influential paradigm of ego-psychology. Simultaneously, as Herzog (2016b, pp. 56–57) underscored, contemporaneous sexology research directly challenged psychoanalytic assertions regarding differences in sexual behaviours and capacities between women and men, which energised rivalry and competitiveness between psychoanalysts. These dynamics contributed to American psychoanalysis adopting a conformist position in the Cold War era, maintaining public legitimacy, advancing normative propositions about femininity, and pathologising homosexuality (Herzog, 2016a, p. 36). As Herzog (2016b, p. 67) explained:

> Psychoanalysis ascended in the decades of the Cold War precisely by offering a mixed, at once secular and religious, "moral sensibility" that reinforced conservative family values under the sign of "health," one that was expressly contemptuous of homosexuality and of any expression of female sexuality outside of marriage.

It is within this process of transformation of American psychoanalysis towards conformity and normativity that Kestenberg (1980a, 1980b, 1981; Kestenberg & Marcus, 1979) developed her formulations on sex-specific identity and parental attitudes, which were heavily saturated with hetero-normative, gender-stereotypical, and patriarchal assumptions.

By the mid-1960s, the momentum of social reform movements led to psychoanalysis being criticised as an authoritarian, patriarchal, and pathologising enterprise (Hale, 1995, p. 302). Women's rights activists directly attacked psychoanalysis for portraying women as intellectually subordinate to men and lacking sexual agency (Herzog, 2016b, p. 69). Additionally, the rise of self-help and popular psychology, to which psychoanalysts had contributed by popularising their concepts in the 1950s, began to challenge the authority of experts, driven by an anti-authoritarian impulse (Herzog, 2016b, pp. 70–72). Gradually, psychoanalysis appeared increasingly disconnected from the prevailing concerns of the public, contributing to the end of its "golden age" and to its subsequent marginalisation within American psychological sciences and mental health (Herzog, 2016b, p. 56).

The waning influence of psychoanalysis was also reinforced by the introduction of psychotropic drugs, which demonstrated the feasibility of community-based care through the pharmacological management of mental illness outside institutional settings (Grob, 1991, p. 124). This led to significant shifts in mental health policy, culminating in the enactment of the Community Mental Health Act in 1963 (Grob, 1991, p. 4). Psychiatrists' attention was drawn to the limitations of psychodynamic therapeutic approaches, and experimental methods, quantification, and repeatability were increasingly favoured (Hale, 1995, p. 301). As Herzog (2016b, p. 72) remarked: "psychiatry in the USA would rescue its own reputation and cultural esteem by dumping psychoanalysis overboard, and binding its professional future to a biomedical research agenda."

Between 1965 and 1985, all the favourable aspects that had contributed to the rise of psychoanalysis in American psychiatry before were on the decline. State and private funding for psychoanalytic research was depleted. Doubts about its validity and effectiveness spread widely. The testability of behavioural approaches and short-term therapies largely shifted public opinion in their favour (Hale, 1995, p. 312). Psychotherapeutic effectiveness was expected to be evaluated through standardised outcome assessments. Operationalising the core elements of psychoanalytic therapy for empirical testing proved difficult, raising fundamental questions about how therapeutic success should be defined and measured. The psychoanalytic case study tradition came to be dismissed as anecdotal rather than as scientific evidence informing practice. Eventually, psychoanalysis became the focal point of attacks within the psy-sciences led by behaviourists, and psychoanalysis detached from psychiatric reform (Hale, 1995, p. 301). It was within this shifting terrain, where the influence of psychoanalysis declined, and empirical demands intensified, that Kestenberg's work would come to occupy an increasingly ambiguous position. It fell out of sight in psychoanalysis but gained attention among emergent approaches of psychotherapy.

The postwar economic boom in the United States, combined with increased governmental funding for mental health and a shift towards community-based models, expanded opportunities in psychological services leading to the emergence of new psychotherapeutic modalities, including family therapy and action-oriented approaches such as dance, drama, music, and art therapy, many of them employing some adapted forms of psychoanalysis (Grob, 1991; Levy, 1988; Weinstein, 2013).

Amid the social rehabilitation efforts of the 1940s, American modern dancers carried their studio practices into clinical settings (Levy, 1988; Laemmli, 2016; Kormos, 2023a). Pioneering figures such as Marian Chace (1896–1970), Blanche Evan (1909–1982), Liljan Espenak (1905–1988), Mary Whitehouse (1911–1979), and Irmgard Bartenieff (Kestenberg's collaborator) began volunteering with veterans and treatment-resistant psychiatric populations, bringing creative movement improvisation into state mental hospitals. They initially drew on their autodidactic knowledge of psychoanalysis, psychology, and anthropology to theorise the healing potential of dance. They believed that the lived experience of the mentally ill could be understood through the language of bodily expression (Levy, 1988; Laemmli, 2016; Kormos, 2023a). Their volunteer efforts attracted the attention of leading figures in psychiatry, including Frieda Fromm-Reichmann (1889–1957) at Chestnut Lodge, Paul Schilder at Bellevue Hospital, and Israel Zwerling at Albert Einstein College of Medicine at Yeshiva University. Israel Zwerling (1917–1993) was a pioneer in community and social psychiatry and a major proponent of creative arts as therapies. He directed the social and community psychiatry division at Albert Einstein College of Medicine and the affiliated Jacobi Psychiatric Clinic at the Bronx State Hospital in the 1960s (Zwerling, 1989). He was the first psychiatrist to employ art, music, and dance therapists at a public hospital (Beels, 1989, pp. 3–8). This support from psychiatrists facilitated the professionalisation of the emerging discipline. In 1966, the American Dance Therapy Association was established, and, during the 1970s, the first formal training programmes in dance/movement therapy were introduced across the United States (Levy, 1988; Kormos, 2023a).

The transition to community mental health in the 1960s led to an influx of non-medical professionals into the mental health field, facilitating the formation of multidisciplinary teams and giving rise to new intra-disciplinary conflicts (Grob, 1991, pp. 293–294; Aron & Starr, 2013, pp. 107–109; Pickren, 2007). The increasing involvement of non-medical practitioners in psychiatric contexts raised significant questions regarding professional boundaries and authority. The introduction of alternative training pathways for these professionals challenged the traditional dominance of psychiatrists. Practitioners in social psychiatry, including dance/movement therapists, advanced alternative models of expertise and therapeutic intervention, culminating in pronounced disputes over professional competence (Grob, 1991, p. 122). Psychoanalytic psychiatrists attempting to reinforce disciplinary lines were not particularly welcoming to dance/movement therapists employing classical psychoanalytic frameworks. Examples of such disputes are the two commentaries by psychoanalytic psychiatrists, Kestenberg and Albert Solnit, on the paper by dance/movement therapist Elaine V. Siegel. Kestenberg (1973) praised Siegel's effort to synthesise analytic theory with a movement methodology but warned against offering psychoanalytic interpretations without rigorous analytic training. Solnit (1973) shared these concerns, urging caution about intuitive speculation and insisting that observational and analytic data should support, rather than alter, psychoanalytic technique. While acknowledging the value of collaboration with dance specialists, he stressed boundaries between areas of competence.

Bodies, Bonds, and Signals

Historical studies by Weinstein (2013) and Laemmli (2016) showed that the Cold War period in the United States brought interpersonal relations, somatic experience, and nonverbal expression into the centre of cultural and scientific attention. Concerns about the fragility of Western democracy made mental health a matter of social and political urgency. Studies on personality diagnostics linking developmental trauma, psychological predispositions, and prejudice intensified fears that individual beliefs could destabilise the social order. This orientation was already evident in Henry A. Murray's (1893–1988) psychoanalytically oriented profile of Adolf Hitler, commissioned by the U.S. Office of Strategic Services in 1943. The report aimed to provide psychologists and psychiatrists with a comprehensive personality assessment that could support predictions about Hitler's likely behaviour in the event of confrontation or forced surrender. Murray also argued that the profile had strategic value for US geopolitical planning, since it could serve as a template for understanding what he described as the psychology of the "typical Nazi," which he suggested was prevalent among many Germans. In his view, such insights were essential to postwar efforts to help transform Germany into a "peace-loving nation" (Murray, 1943, p. 2). Murray's analysis addressed developmental aspects, libidinal and sadistic drive patterns, and defence mechanisms, linking these dynamics to ensuing personality characteristics. It also included observations of bodily behaviour, such as jerky gestures, restlessness, and what he described as "effeminate" gestures and gait. As Laemmli (2016, p. 138) demonstrated, another example of postwar scientific and cultural attention to the potential social threat posed by individual attitudes was the widespread influence of *The Authoritarian Personality* study, first published in 1950 (Adorno et al., 1950/1993). The book promoted the idea of a distinct fascistic personality type, framing prejudice and anti-democratic attitudes as outcomes of identifiable psychological dispositions. Within this broader discourse, the body was increasingly conceptualised as a locus for trauma and repressed aggression, which were regarded as influential in shaping personality development and social attitudes. Irmgard Bartenieff and Judith Kestenberg, for example, emphasised the safe expression and regulation of aggression through bodily movement, framing this work as serving not only individual adjustment but also collective and societal well-being by helping to mitigate aggressive drives (Laemmli, 2016, pp. 45–47; Bartenieff & Lewis, 1980/2013, p. 145; Kestenberg, 1981). In turn, the prevention of delinquency, discrimination, and prejudice was increasingly understood as a psychological project, with particular attention given to adverse childhood experiences and pathological family dynamics (Weinstein, 2013). Significant theoretical and methodological shifts occurred in the psy-sciences, and pathology was relocated from the intrapersonal interior of the individual to the intersubjective space of groups and families. The focus moved from what happens within the individual to what happens between people (Weinstein, 2013, p. 6). Behavioural therapies increasingly focused on group dynamics and family systems as potential sources of illness (Hale, 1995; Grob, 1991). The family unit became a site of social governance and an object of scientific observation. It was viewed as a self-regulating, potentially pathology-maintaining system (Weinstein, 2013, Chapter 1). Invited by Israel Zwerling to work at the Jacobi Clinic at the Bronx State Hospital, Irmgard Bartenieff highlighted the growing emphasis on family observation and interpersonal dynamics in letters to her movement-notation teacher, Warren Lamb:

> The psychiatrists in the Clinic are interested in two aspects of notations: 1) making a full assessment of the patient under varying observation situations and at different times of their stay; 2) conducting family assessments of the patient's family together. (Bartenieff, 1963)
>
> The material I gathered up until this spring aroused so much interest, just as a description of movement dynamics, that my department. of Social Psychiatry at Yeshiva University wants to start training. (Bartenieff, 1964)

Psychopathology was no longer linked to a pathogenic agent but understood as a compromised relationship between the self and other or maladjustment to environmental factors (Weinstein, 2013, p. 5). This new orientation towards dynamics and interactive processes brought action and behaviour to the centre of clinical attention, replacing the emphasis on verbal language in clients' self-reports and on the therapist's verbal interpretation. The methodological approach shifted from diagnostic to descriptive. Weinstein (2013) explained that an "optic orientation" (p. 13) and naturalistic observation methods prevailed, with frequent use of uncut video recordings and one-way mirrors (pp. 142–145).

This tendency towards movement in Cold War American psy-sciences was demonstrated not only by pioneers of dance/movement therapy in emerging social-psychiatry settings developing new movement-analysis methods but also by various groups of researchers in the psy-sciences and affiliated humanities who turned to the study of nonverbal behaviour (Davis, 1982, 2001). While working at the Jacobi Clinic, Bartenieff devised her *Effort/Shape* analysis and a set of corrective motor principles later termed the *Fundamentals* (Bartenieff & Davis, 1965, 1972; Bartenieff, 1964). Bartenieff's assistant, Martha Davis (b. 1942), a clinical psychologist, began to develop her *Movement Signature Analysis* and the *Movement Psychodiagnostic Inventory* (Davis, 1997). Davis hypothesised that bodily movement serves as a sensitive indicator of shifts in mental and psychological states, and that observation of movement carries differential diagnostic value (Davis, 1981; Lausberg, 2014). She later devised the *Nonverbal Interaction and States Analysis* for psychotherapy process research, focusing on the postural shifts and gesticulation of interactants (Davis & Hadiks, 1990). Psychotherapists explored the concepts of therapeutic alliance, containment, and therapeutic change through notions of synchrony, mirroring, and echoing expressed in the bodily movements of client and therapist (Scheflen, 1965, 1970, pp. 457–472; Davis, 2001, p. 8; Kestenberg, 1978). Freedman and Bucci (1981) examined motor activity embedded in speech and thought, linking gesture and posture with characteristic cognitive attitudes.

In this Cold War milieu, as Martin-Nielsen (2010) demonstrated, studies of language and communication also came to the fore. In an era hyperaware of spies and propagandists, language came to be viewed as both a weapon and a tool to ensure democratic stability in the West and to cement the position of the United States in the new world order (Martin-Nielsen, 2010, p. 138). Generous federal funding was channelled into language programmes, which turned linguistics into a professional and technocratic enterprise. The various projects on machine translation and cryptography support the view that engineered, rule-based systems rooted in structural analysis could serve as a national security infrastructure (Martin-Nielsen, 2010, p. 142). This technocratic ethos expanded language programmes at the Foreign Service Institute and across universities and schools. Linguists aligned themselves with the 'hard sciences' and articulated mathematical rules of language, demonstrated in formal descriptions of structuralist linguistics. As Martin-Nielsen (2010) argued, these efforts reinforced Cold War confidence that human behaviour could be modelled, optimised, and technologically managed. This orientation, which treated linguistics and communication as tools tied to the geopolitical demands of the Cold War, also extended to the 'hidden' sphere of bodily communication. Numerous research projects attempted to formalise and operationalise the seemingly unruly nature of nonverbal communication, applying the same technocratic and structural logics to gesture, bodily expressions, and signals.

In the late 1940s, Elliot Chapple (1909–2000), an anthropologist, developed the interaction chronograph, a device intended to map the flow of interactional activity between conversational partners, revealing rhythmic patterns reflecting cultural norms and temperament (Saslow et al., 1955). Ray Birdwhistell (1918–1994), another anthropologist, coined the term kinesics to describe his approach to the study of nonverbal communication, drawing on structural linguistics. He worked on several projects for the Foreign Service Institute and the U.S. Department of State. His first book, *Kinesics*, was an internal publication for these agencies (Birdwhistell, 1952, 1955, 1970). In the 1950s and 1960s, several nonverbal communication labs were established across the United States. At the Eastern Pennsylvania Psychiatric Institute, Birdwhistell and Albert Scheflen (1920–1980) filmed psychotherapy and family-therapy sessions. They proposed the natural history approach, using uncut video footage capturing the whole body to preserve the behavioural stream in context (Scheflen, 1965, 1970; Davis, 2001). On the West Coast, at the Center for Advanced Study in the Behavioral Sciences at Stanford University, several psychiatrists, anthropologists, linguists, and kinesicists analysed social interaction through interviews (McQuown, 1971; Leeds-Hurwitz & Kendon, 2021). Gregory Bateson (1904–1980) and his collaborators (Bateson Project) studied family sessions with people diagnosed with schizophrenia to analyse meta-messages (largely nonverbal signals) (Weinstein, 2013, p. 50). In the 1970s, Kestenberg and her collaborators at the Center for Parents and Children examined clashes and matches in caregiver–infant nonverbal interaction. They offered embodied interventions to parents with the explicit aim of mitigating risks of developmental trauma and fostering healthy family bonds. In the 1980s, Davis et al. (1992; Davis & Dulicai, 1992) conducted studies on the body language profiles of world leaders, namely George W. Bush, Mikhail Gorbachev, Saddam Hussein, and Hitler, focusing on deception patterns, signs of stress, and changes in nonverbal behaviour in relation to political and personal crises.

In 1978, Davis founded the Institute for Nonverbal Communication Research (INCR). This scientific organisation brought together researchers and practitioners across the humanities and psy-sciences interested in the study of nonverbal behaviour (Davis, 1982, p. 23). The first congress of nonverbal behaviour research, "Interaction Rhythms," was held at Teachers College, Columbia University, 21–22 March 1979. Presenters examined the rhythms of movement behaviour from various perspectives. William S. Condon (psychologist) dealt with cultural micro rhythms and inter- and intrapersonal asynchrony in specific psychiatric pathologies; Daniel Stern (developmental psychiatrist and psychoanalyst) examined the rhythmic structure of somatic interactions in mother–infant dyads; Beatrice Beebe (clinical psychologist) presented a detailed frame-by-frame analysis of mother–infant communication including kinetic measures of interactive games, transitions, and maternal hand pauses, alongside coding of the infant's gaze, orientation, and facial expressions (Condon, 1982; Stern, 1982; Davis, 1982; Beebe et al., 1982). Davis remembered the emerging years of nonverbal communication research:

> The Institute for Nonverbal Communication Research (INCR) lasted only three and a half years due to financial pressures, but it played a formative role in shaping interdisciplinary dialogue about movement and interaction. I remember how exciting it was in the 1970s when developmental researchers, anthropologists, linguists, and psychologists were conferring together. They differed in focus across child development, conversation patterns, psychotherapy transactions, and social behaviour, but shared a common interest in synchrony, pacing, and energy concepts. [...] Daniel Stern referred to synchrony as the "atom of human bonding," and described pacing in mother–infant interactions. Beebe examined relational spacing, facial expression mirroring, and the timing of mother–infant interactions to advance the study of attachment behaviour. Researchers like William Condon and Paul Byers pushed interaction microanalysis even further, analysing aspects of body movement occurring in 1/40th of a second. (Davis, personal communication, 31 January 2023)

Building on Leammli (2016) and Weinstein (2013), in the Cold War context, research on bodily movement and nonverbal communication became part of broader efforts to clarify the connections between upbringing, mental health, and the stability of democratic society (Weinstein, 2013; Laemmli, 2016; Kormos, 2023b). Bodily movement was viewed as an indicator of disrupted personal and group dynamics. The evaluation and therapeutic retraining of movement (Kestenberg, 1975a; Kestenberg & Buelte, 1977a, 1977b) were considered promising for psycho-technological prevention of social problems, while movement interpretation within the field of communication research became connected to diplomatic and national-security concerns (Martin-Nielsen, 2010; Davis, 1982; Birdwhistell, 1952).

Mutual Regulations

In the early 1970s, "cracks had begun to appear in the ego-psychology monolith" (Wallerstein, 2002, p. 145), opening the field to object-relations-focused, social-constructivist, and two-person psychology perspectives. This intersubjective turn – with a pronounced interest in communication and the nonverbal – also fostered new methods and interests in infant observation research. Mahler's separation-individuation model, while foundational to developmental ego-psychology in the 1950s, received considerable criticism, and, by the late 1970s, many of its core claims had fallen out of favour (Wolff, 1959; Fantz, 1963; Meltzoff & Moore, 1977; Watson, 1972; Gergely, 2000). These critiques concerned the rejection of her normal autistic and symbiotic phases. Mahler based her developmental model on Freud's (2001, p. 220) view of the newborn who, like a chick in the egg, is closed off from the external environment. She argued that postnatal life starts with normal autistic and symbiotic phases in which the infant is viewed as functioning in an undifferentiated state of self-and-object. She claimed that, with the emergence of bodily awareness, the infant "hatches" from the merged state at between 5 and 9 months of age (Mahler et al., 1975, p. 44; Gober, 2014, p. 8). However, new infant observation data showed that infants possess sophisticated, innate capacities to process aspects of the external world from birth (Gergely, 2000). Fantz (1963) demonstrated an innate sensitivity to the contours and shapes of the human face. Meltzoff and Moore's (1977, 1989) studies showed an inborn capacity to imitate facial expressions, such as tongue protrusion. Stern (1998a) and Bower (1982; Kaye & Bower, 1994) exposed innate abilities for cross-modal information transfer. These newly found early perceptual mechanisms of self-and-other differentiation were incompatible with Mahler's concepts (Gergely, 2000; Mahler et al., 1975, pp. 41–44). Beebe (2014) noted that the 1960s marked a shift in developmental research towards an interactive systems approach, a bidirectional model, and the view of the competent infant, which prepared the stage for the microanalytic studies of infant–mother interactions that emerged in the early 1970s (Stern, 1971; Trevarthen, 1979). For the next two decades, vehement arguments rippled across the field of infant research over whether a bidirectional or mutual regulation model was correct. Eventually, it was Tronick and his collaborators' landmark studies, using time-series analysis, that shifted the disciplinary discourse towards viewing early mother–infant interactions as bidirectional (Beebe, 2014, p. 5; Tronick, 1989; Tronick & Cohn, 1989). Cohn and Tronick conducted several microanalytic studies investigating how mothers and infants coordinated their emotional expressions and behaviours, such as smiling, gaze direction, and vocalisations, in real time. To examine their interactional behaviours, they employed frame-by-frame time-series analysis, a method that can reveal patterns and trends in how variables change over time (Cohn & Tronick, 1987, 1988; Tronick & Cohn, 1989). They found evidence that both partners, parent and infant, were responsive to each other's moment-to-moment changes, which they understood to have a non-periodic organisation rather than resulting from mutual entrainment of rhythmic cycles. Their results challenged linear models of interaction and contributed fundamentally to the mutual regulation perspective in infant development research.

Kestenberg's Problematic Alliances

The ambitions, focus, and methods that Kestenberg applied in her developmental movement studies aligned with significant trends in American psy-sciences. She was a psychoanalytic psychiatrist, first working with children in various psychiatric hospitals, then shifting her focus to infant observation in a natural setting. She began her developmental observation studies amid the mid-century drive to gather empirical data to underscore psychoanalytic developmental concepts. She was a proponent of child guidance and community psychiatry, as reflected in the establishment of her child guidance centre. Her work formed close ties with the emerging psychotherapeutic modalities of the 1960s and supported the development of creative arts therapies. On the other hand, Kestenberg also countered various currents in the psy-sciences at the time.

Trends in scientific attention influence the adoption of theories and methodologies through what Peterson termed "intra-field boundary work" (Peterson, 2017, p. 71). These rhetorical strategies extend beyond the conventional distinction between science and 'pseudoscience' by regulating disciplinary focus and differentiating approaches from those of adjacent domains and subfields. Peterson argued that, in "densely populated epistemic environments," such as the mind sciences, boundary work constructs disciplinary identities and prevents prolonged theoretical disputes by establishing a "conceptually clear workspace" (Peterson, 2017, pp. 54–56). Scientific communities maintain coherence by cultivating a shared frame of focus that highlights particular objects, questions, and methods while marginalising others. These focus-management practices not only organise research problems but also shape normative images of the "good scientist," establish methodological hierarchies, and define the field's obligations to the public. Decisions regarding what remains in focus are based on value judgements about rigour and relevance. This management of disciplinary attention often intertwines with institutional power. Actors with greater authority are typically better positioned to determine what is considered central, credible, or worth pursuing. In the postwar era, internal pressures in American psychoanalysis, such as factionalism and endorsed paradigms, compounded with external pressures towards standardisation in the psychological sciences, contributed to some approaches gaining authority by aligning with ideals of scientific formalism and experimental design, while others, such as Kestenberg's movement studies, risked marginalisation by appealing to traditional alliances and unorthodox methods.

Beyond Freud and Mahler

In developing a framework for developmental assessment, Kestenberg reflected the mid-twentieth-century emphasis of American psychoanalysis on collecting empirical evidence for developmental concepts through direct observation of infants (Spitz, 1950; Midgley, 2013; Hale, 1995). Applying the positivist orientation of American ego-psychology, she anatomised movement into well-defined categories and elements and proposed a syntactic structure of movement comparable with that of symbolic language. However, at a time when American psychoanalysis became engrossed in ego-psychology rather than drive-theory, Kestenberg stressed the equal importance of instinctual and ego processes in psychic development. She asserted that instincts and ego do not form a dichotomy but, rather, a drive–defence continuum (Kestenberg, 1975a). Davis expressed that "Kestenberg was, in some ways, like Freud, a purist. I used to say that she was going to be the first researcher to empirically confirm Freud's psychosexual stages of development" (personal communication, 31 January 2023). Kestenberg's allegiance to Freudian drive-theory limited her alignment with the rising currents of ego-psychology; her opposition to Hartmann's autonomous sphere of the ego further complicated her position in psychoanalytic discourse at the time. La Barre (in Kestenberg, 1990b) noted that Kestenberg's psychodynamic framework reinterpreted drive-theory within a relational framework, rejecting the idea of drives as the sole motivational system. It integrated drive-theory with broader perspectives on affect, object-seeking, and mastery. However, the wider implications of this remained largely unexplored owing to the marginalisation of drive-theory amid the disciplinary shifts towards relational paradigms in the 1970s. La Barre further noted that resistance to Kestenberg's movement-focused work was influenced by the principle of analytic neutrality maintained by orthodox Freudians (in Kestenberg, 1990b). Kestenberg's recognition of the analyst's bodily presence in the analytic setting represented a departure from the classical expectation of analyst neutrality, thereby complicating her acceptance within the Freudian tradition as well.

Despite Kestenberg's pioneering infant research in the 1960s, her papers (Kestenberg, 1965a, 1965b, 1967; Kestenberg et al., 1971) were largely uncited by infant researchers of the 1970s and 1980s. This dismissal was likely influenced by Kestenberg's continued reliance on Mahler's symbiotic phase, which clashed with emerging trends in infant research that increasingly embraced the notion of a competent infant endowed with innate capacities for interaction. Mahler herself later softened her position on the normal autistic and symbiotic phases to align her framework more closely with contemporaneous infant studies (Coates, 2004, p. 595). Kestenberg's later publications also reflected this shift. She addressed emergent object-relatedness in her concept of *transsensus* (Kestenberg, 1978), elaborated the significance of mutuality in *Tension-Flow* and *Shape-Flow* attunement between caregiver and infant (Kestenberg & Buelte, 1977a, 1977b), and explored fetal movement patterns (Kestenberg, 1987, 1989, 1990a; Kestenberg & Borowitz, 1990). However, these considerations were never fully integrated into her overall developmental model, nor did they lead to a comprehensive revision. Moreover, while her developmental approach gradually moved towards mutuality, her *Movement Profile* method remained primarily individual-focused. As discussed earlier, it gathers qualitative, movement-based data to produce an individual personality profile. As part of child guidance, individual profiles of parents and their children were compared to identify areas of mismatch. This approach offered limited means for observing and documenting the simultaneous, mutually shaping processes between caregiver and infant that contemporaneous bidirectional models sought to capture. Kestenberg's close ties to Mahlerian concepts and her method's individualised lens did not substantially anchor her work within the field's emerging interaction-centred paradigms and contributed to its broader dismissal within the new trends of infant research.

The Body Problem: Somatic Languages at the Margin

Bodily processes occupy a central role in psychoanalytic theory and practice. Freud's concept of the unconscious, along with his topographic and structural models, elucidates the intricate ways in which the physical dimension (bodily drives, primary-processes) influences the mental realm (Jurist, 2022, p. 186). Despite Freud's emphasis on the somatic foundations of psychic life, the systematic study of bodily processes remained peripheral in classical psychoanalysis. Yadlin-Gadot (2022, p. 120) noted that: "For Freud, then, everything begins with the body. The drives are innate, as is their programmed development. The mind is formed in lieu of the drive's demands, and throughout life, they remain its driving force." However, she went on to elucidate that the bodily drives in the Freudian model are subordinated to the mind, through the proposition that optimal development strives towards a hierarchical dominance of the ego over the id's demands, thereby essentially marginalising the somatic. As discussed before, in the Freudian structural model, the id, the topos of the unconscious, is the structural element of the psyche understood as a reservoir of somatically generated energy. The ego is a formation born out of the external world's direct influence on the id through bodily perceptual and motor experiences. The ego is understood to gradually gain dominance over and come to regulate the id's internal strivings in accordance with external reality (Freud, 1923/1961; Yadlin-Gadot, 2022). The superego is viewed as embodying social norms, and the ego is oriented towards managing bodily drives, demands of reality, and the prohibitions of the superego. In Freud's account (more or less), uncomplicated functioning is associated with the dominance of the reality principle and the ego's taming of bodily drives (Yadlin-Gadot, 2022, pp. 120–121).

Thus, Freudian theory both resists and reinstates a dualist separation of mind and body. On the one hand, drive-theory brought the body into psychology (a non-dualist orientation). On the other hand, it preserved a hierarchical mind–body distinction through the ego and superego's mastery of the drives (a dualist tendency). Fonagy (2007, p. 40) added that, even when the Freudian unconscious incorporates the bodily, it tends to function as a detached container of abstractions, divorced from the body and the social environment. This left the specificities of somatic processes conceptually and methodologically secondary in Freudian theory (such as in the case of the psychoanalytic study of bodily movement). Bálint (1959) noted the same blind spot, remarking on how little Freud wrote about the psychology of movement and its relation to object-relations and the environment (pp. 117–118). Within the classical frame, bodily movement was largely understood as drive-discharge, an 'undeveloped' counterpart to the mind that requires containment rather than being a source of meaning in its own right (Knoblauch, 2017, p. 287).

Kestenberg's movement studies addressed this enduring problem in psychoanalysis. Employing the Freudian structural model, she aligned categories of movement with the id, ego, and superego. She also retained his developmental hierarchy by which drive-derived patterns progressively come under the regulation of ego-controlled movements. At the same time, she positioned bodily movement as the central object of metapsychology. She gestured towards a concept of the psyche in which the body has the mind within, and vice versa. She regarded movement experience as intrinsic to symbolic process and understood gestural movement as integral to ideation. She developed a grammar of movement that rendered somatic processes as complex and structured as symbolic language. By examining the vocabulary and modes of meaning-making through bodily movement, she framed somatisation not as regression but as an alternative mode of working-through. In this respect, her work challenged the dualist contention of a mind that thinks and a body that acts (Sheets-Johnstone, 2011). These considerations were viewed as at least unorthodox and at most problematic in psychoanalytic thought at the time.

Kestenberg's kinaesthetic terminology, rooted in Laban's dance studies, further deepened her disconnection from analysts at the time. Interdisciplinary work requires creating a simplified shared language through which concepts can travel across fields (Galison, 1996; Collins et al., 2007). Although Kestenberg (1965b; Kestenberg & Sossin, 1979) repeatedly published glossaries with her articles, analysts showed palpable reluctance to engage with the technical terms of her psychodynamic vocabulary of movement, compounded by their limited familiarity with kinaesthetic experience (Sossin, personal communication, 1 November 2022).

This reluctance was evident in the commentaries by Solnit and Galenson at the 1971 meeting of the New York Psychoanalytic Society. Galenson (1971) challenged Kestenberg's emphasis on the primacy of motor development and argued that a wide variety of functions, such as visual perception (fixation and scanning), mature simultaneously throughout development. This critique, however, reflects a limited grasp of Kestenberg's psychodynamic movement framework, which categorised underlying qualitative features of movement phenomena rather than discrete behavioural units. This means that eye movements such as scanning and fixation, as mentioned by Galenson, count as 'movement' in her system and would be classified by their qualitative properties. Solnit (1971) directly criticised Kestenberg for describing psychic and symbolic processes from a somatic perspective, calling her terminology ambiguous and her language "psychosomorphic." KMP-trained psychoanalyst Silvia Birklein's following statement (personal communication, 11 November 2022) further illuminates the issue of a somatic language in psychoanalysis:

> I am not sure the turning point in psychoanalysis towards a full recognition of embodiment has truly arrived. The difficulty, I believe, lies primarily at the level of theory. Theorising movement is inherently complex, and it remains challenging to move the body out of the realm of the primary-process, or what is often regarded as more primitive in comparison to the mind. Even today, the language of the Kestenberg Movement Profile (KMP), and, more broadly, any movement-focused terminology, remains largely unfamiliar to those without a background in dance or movement research. The challenge lies in the fact that the KMP cannot truly be learned without embodying its various patterns and understanding the framework through movement itself. Too often, people shy away from this embodied aspect of learning the system. When I conducted training within my psychoanalytic community, I noticed that participants often felt overwhelmed by the language of the KMP. It is so unfamiliar and unconventional that, even when I wrote articles specifically focused on the KMP and its concepts, I was frequently asked to modify the movement-focused terminology, though doing so inevitably diminished the embodied dimension of these ideas. I believe this challenge begins as an issue of language, but it extends further into the difficulty of translating between bodily experience, psychological understanding, and psychoanalytic theory. There seems to be a kind of dissociation at play, rooted, of course, in the enduring Cartesian dualism that continues to shape much of academic discourse.

The difficulty many analysts faced with Kestenberg's *Movement Profile* was not simply a matter of unfamiliar vocabulary but, perhaps, a broader problem of translation between very distinct epistemic cultures (Galison & Stump, 1996; Hacking, 1996; Knorr Cetina, 1999; Peterson, 2017). Disciplinary communities operating in the same broader scientific field are often separated by different methods, theories, and research practices. Thus, cross-field interaction necessitates bridging tools such as shared language, standardised practices, and specialised communication skills (Galison, 1996; Collins et al., 2007; Peterson, 2017). Kestenberg's project demanded precisely this kind of bridging between psychoanalytic developmental study and embodied practices. Despite her deliberate efforts, this divide persisted within a psychoanalytic context marked by limited embodied literacy and a persistent reluctance to recognise bodily movement as a valid medium for meaning-making.

Transgressing Boundaries

As discussed earlier, American psychoanalysis in the 1950s–1960s sought to build an empirical evidence base for its developmental concepts, expand into academic psychology, and maintain its close connection to psychiatry amid growing trends towards scientification and the proliferation of new psychotherapeutic modalities (Pickren, 2007; Hale, 1995). In this context, Kestenberg's work, largely influenced by dance studies, may have appeared potentially detrimental to the field's mid-century drive to scientifically stabilise its theory and practice. A quote from Sossin captures both the strength and the liability of Kestenberg's transdisciplinarity:

> Kestenberg was a bit different. She branched out and was always willing to train and learn from non-psychoanalytic psychotherapists, art therapists, music therapists, occupational and physical therapists, and movement specialists. At the time, very few psychoanalysts stepped out of their more constricted domains. (Sossin, personal communication, 1 November 2022)

Kestenberg's project, which integrated Labanian concepts with psychoanalytic theory and combined meridian concepts with Western neurology, resisted clear theoretical and methodological classification, which likely limited its uptake among clinicians of her time. She not only transgressed disciplinary boundaries but also collaborated extensively with non-clinicians, including Susan Loman, a dance/movement therapist; Arnhilt Buelte, an early years teacher; and Joan Weinstein, a social worker (Kestenberg & Buelte, 1977a, 1977b; Buelte, 1978, 1979; Kestenberg & Weinstein, 1978). This blurring of hierarchies between those holding specialised professional knowledge and those contributing experiential, practice-based knowledge may have further complicated analysts' engagement with her work at the time.

"Abandon Freud in Favour of Laban"

In the late 1960s, the emergent field of American dance/movement therapy needed a theoretical framework to legitimise its practices within the discourse of psy-sciences. Significant interest in Kestenberg's *Movement Profile* sprouted. By collating qualitative features of movement with psychoanalytic developmental concepts, it provided a vocabulary and an assessment framework for dance/movement therapy to legitimise itself as a psychotherapeutic modality. American dance/movement therapists critiqued the dominance of verbal approaches in traditional psychotherapy and sought to place embodied experience at the centre of their practices. They were sceptical of Freud's focus on verbal language and instead drew upon ideas from his dissident heirs, Jung, Reich, and Adler. Humanistic psychology and transpersonal/transcendental frameworks also shaped distinct approaches in the emerging field (Bernstein, 1979; Kormos, 2023a). Kestenberg's framework, rooted in Freudian drive theory, provoked concern within the field of dance/movement therapy. Loman explained that "terms such as phallic and sadistic were off-putting to dance/movement therapists at the time" (Loman, personal communication, 15 November 2022). Statements from Irmgard Bartenieff and Warren Lamb (Lamb was Kestenberg's teacher and collaborator) in their letter correspondence underscore this apprehension. In 1963, Bartenieff wrote to Lamb that Kestenberg's Freudian interpretations tended to "go overboard." She was specifically concerned that Lamb appeared to endorse Kestenberg's use of Freudian terms such as oral and anal. Bartenieff urged Lamb to "tactfully set her straight" (Bartenieff, 1963, p. 3). In his reply, Lamb stated: "I can certainly confirm what you say about Dr Kestenberg. She is a problem." Lamb credited Kestenberg as an exceptionally skilled observer and suggested that Freud was "at the root" of the problem. He further expressed scepticism that Kestenberg would completely "abandon Freud in favour of Laban" (Lamb, 1965, p. 1).

Amid the intradisciplinary tensions in the psy-sciences, particularly around the question of non-medical practitioners conducting psychotherapy, Kestenberg initially joined in on drawing clear jurisdictional boundaries, potentially to ensure the relevance and significance of her method as a movement-based metapsychological assessment framework. Her commentary on Siegel's (1973) psychoanalytically framed movement therapy with a child argued that Siegel risked misdiagnosing a child's symptoms. Kestenberg (1973) contended that only a comprehensive developmental understanding enables systematic interpretation of motor and verbal communications; therefore, rigorous psychoanalytic training should be considered a prerequisite for practitioners of psychoanalytic movement psychotherapy.

Even though Kestenberg championed creative arts therapies, such critiques potentially reinforced American dance/movement therapy's distancing itself from psychoanalysis. Consequently, the Kestenberg Movement Profile (KMP) was adapted to the disciplinary ambitions of dance/movement therapy, and its

Freudian terminology was revised to more descriptive, phenomenological language to avoid any association with a specific school of thought. 'Libidinal' and 'sadistic' (classifying drive-derivative movement patterns) were replaced by the terms '*indulging*' and '*fighting*', and the phallic-sadistic phase became the *outer-genital* fighting phase (Kestenberg Amighi et al., 1999, p. 56). This intervention to strengthen the theoretical connection between the KMP and creative arts therapies through these changes in terminology not only advanced the development of the KMP itself but also supported the professionalisation of American dance/movement therapy. At the same time, it detached Kestenberg's psychodynamic theory of movement and her *Movement Profile* from the field of psychoanalysis.

Evidence Norms and the Fate of Movement-Psychodynamics: The Case of Stern and Kestenberg

As discussed earlier, by the mid-1960s, pressures from funding agencies prompted psychoanalytic psychiatrists to abandon the case-study format in favour of empirical, experimental methods involving larger groups of subjects. As confidence in psychoanalytic theory declined, the traditional case study was increasingly dismissed as anecdotal rather than scientifically valid evidence informing practice (Hale, 1995, pp. 322–345). Methodological trends in infant and nonverbal behaviour research, driven by systems theory and a focus on interaction patterns (rather than psychoanalytic developmental concepts), energised the shift towards experimental designs (Davis, 2001, 1982, personal communication, 31 January 2023). Kestenberg's methodology did not follow these shifts. She derived her theory from clinical material and direct observation in small samples and presented most of her findings in a traditional psychoanalytic case-study form. In the mid-1980s, psychoanalytic infant observation rose to prominence through the works of Stern (1998a), Freedman and Bucci (1981), and others (Gilani et al., 1985), yet continuities with Kestenberg's earlier developmental movement studies were not drawn.

A striking example of disciplinary recognition and dismissal shaped by contemporaneous methodological paradigms can be seen in the differing receptions of Daniel N. Stern's (1934–2012) and Kestenberg's infant observation studies. While Stern's work occupies a central position in the historical canon of the psy-sciences, with his concepts of *affect-attunement* and *vitality affects* considered foundational to infant mental health research, Kestenberg's closely related concepts remained comparatively marginalised. Stern developed detailed formulations on the nonverbal interactional dynamics of the infant–mother dyad. His research emphasised the motor dimensions of attunement between mother and infant, as well as the rhythmic and sensorimotor qualities of the infant's perceptual world. He conceptualised *affect-attunement* between caregiver and infant as the qualitative matching of the underlying feeling tone of the behaviour, creating a shared affective experience (Stern,

1998b, pp. 141–142). This definition closely echoes Kestenberg's earlier concept of *kinaesthetic attunement*, the notion of shared affective states achieved through the matching of *Tension-Flow* and *Shape-Flow* qualities (Kestenberg, 1965b, 1967; Kestenberg et al., 1971). Stern (1998b) identified the underlying dimensions in which affect-attunement occurs. These were absolute intensity, intensity contour, temporal beat, rhythm, duration, and shape. He called these *vitality affects* and argued that they arise from internal biological rhythms within the body. Stern's *vitality affects* closely correspond to Kestenberg's *Tension-Flow* and *Shape-Flow* categories (Kestenberg, 1965a, 1965b, 1967, 1975b). Precisely, his absolute intensity equates to Kestenberg's degree of intensity conceptualised in *Low* or *High Intensity Tension-Flow Attribute*. Stern's intensity contour aligns with Kestenberg's rate of change, such as *Gradual* or *Abrupt Tension-Flow*. His dimension of rhythm is reflected in Kestenberg's *Tension-Flow Rhythms*, and his notion of shape corresponds to Kestenberg's *Shape-Flow* qualities.

Despite these strong conceptual parallels and the fact that Kestenberg's work in the 1960s preceded Stern's publications by nearly two decades, he made no substantive reference to her theoretical contributions. This is particularly notable given that Stern also used cursive line drawings in his studies to represent mother–infant rhythmicity, which closely resemble Kestenberg's *Tension-Flow Curves*. His only citation is in a footnote and refers to Kestenberg and Sossin (1979), which presents their work as movement notation rather than developmental theory (Stern, 1998a, p. 159). Later, Stern (2010) discussed Laban's and Warren Lamb's methods of movement analysis yet omitted any reference to Kestenberg, despite her substantial integration of Lamb's work with psychoanalytic developmental theory.

The divergent reception of Kestenberg's and Stern's work can be primarily attributed to the theoretical and methodological trends of the 1970s and 1980s. Stern's studies were well aligned with the rising focus on intersubjectivity and empiricism in infant research. He described simple actions that readers could easily imagine (Davis, 1992, p. 53). He presented the outcomes of his infant observations more in line with the traditions of empirical research. He described the research setting and observational categories and employed statistical methods (Stern, 1971, 1982, 1998a). His empirical approach to developmental observation aligned with the experimental drive of psychoanalysis at the time. Within the growing trend of scientification in psychoanalysis in the 1970s (Hale, 1995), disciplinary preference for larger experimental studies and the use of statistical methods problematised the relevance of Kestenberg's developmental movement studies. However, Birklein (personal communication, 11 November 2022) sharply noted the lack of precise terminology that influences the depth of research:

> While there is a growing interest in bodily processes within psychoanalytic research, the conceptualisation of movement itself often feels superficial. Discussions of somatic experience frequently stop at the level

of sensation, without extending into the interpretation of movement. In this regard, KMP-trained analysts have much to contribute, offering a sophisticated language and a systematic framework grounded in Kestenberg's original vision. Daniel Stern's infant observation studies, for example, displayed remarkable attention to the details of movement, how a child grasped a chair or looked up, but even they lacked a sufficiently precise vocabulary for categorising movement in clinical or developmental terms.

Kestenberg's developmental movement studies also remained peripheral within the broader field of nonverbal communication research owing to difficulties adapting to prevailing methodological trends. Davis noted that, despite the shared focus on infant development, there remained a noticeable disconnect between Kestenberg and other scholars associated with the INCR:

> Kestenberg's approach was strongly influenced by psychoanalysis and the work of Anna Freud. She and her group emphasised movement dynamics and flow qualities that were largely neglected in mainstream nonverbal behaviour research. Many researchers resisted studying movement dynamics in depth, preferring to focus on variables that are easier to describe and code, like direction, space, or proximity. There was a certain 'blindness to dynamics' within psychology, where the qualitative and expressive aspects of movement were marginalised. That blindness posed a particular challenge for Kestenberg, because her work focused on dynamics and flow at an extremely subtle, microanalytic level. It was complex and multilayered, and many researchers in nonverbal communication simply did not understand what she was describing. Perhaps concepts like shape flow and effort or tension flow seemed esoteric and less scientific to them. (Davis, personal communication, 31 January 2023)

As trends in scientification within psychoanalysis, the interpersonal turn, and the advancement of bidirectional interaction models in infant research favoured experimental designs and easily observable, readily representable behaviours, Kestenberg's developmental movement studies, with her kinaesthetic vocabulary and dance-derived methodology, were sidelined. Her peripheral position within the field of nonverbal communication research stemmed from the technical specificity and microanalytic focus of her approach.

Trauma Narratives and Postwar Identities

As previously discussed, the postwar history of the psychological sciences in the United States was marked by a shift towards community psychiatry and the proliferation of new psychotherapeutic modalities, such as dance/movement therapy and family therapy (Levy, 1988; Hale, 1995; Weinstein, 2013;

Laemmli, 2016). Interest in interpersonal dynamics and nonverbal behaviour grew, exemplified by infant mental health research in the 1970s and 1980s that focused on nonverbal infant–caregiver interactions. Community mental health placed strong emphasis on the prevention of trauma and adverse childhood experiences in relation to individual and societal well-being. Psy-sciences entered the privacy of family homes, provided guidance to children, and analysed family dynamics to identify pathogenic interactional patterns (Weinstein, 2013; Laemmli, 2016). The study of traumatic experience, its embeddedness in somatic processes, and its influence on transgenerational well-being were focal points of Kestenberg's later, psychohistorical studies on the effects of the Nazi Holocaust. Well received by contemporaries, it shaped psychoanalytic theory and practice relating to transgenerational trauma. The following section outlines the trends that facilitated the uncomplicated reception and broader dissemination of Kestenberg's Holocaust studies.

Arlene Stein (2009, p. 27) highlighted that, in the 1970s, about a quarter of a million children of Holocaust survivors became young adults in the United States. The cultural discourse of the decade was marked by widespread interest in ethnic heritage, migrant experiences, and community (Fogelman, 1988, p. 619). A confluence of therapeutic ethos and emancipatory trends fuelled by second-wave feminism and ethnic politics engendered social movements conducive to developing second-generation identities of Holocaust survivors. Psychotherapists who were themselves children of survivors (such as Judith Kestenberg, Eva Fogelman, and many of their collaborators) believed it was necessary to address the psychological health of the second generation. They organised survivor and consciousness-raising groups and collected testimonies from survivors. Fogelman reported hundreds of Holocaust survivor groups across the United States (Mason & Fogelman, 1984; Fogelman, 1988; Fogelman & Savran, 1979, 1980). As therapeutic notions such as trauma and recovery permeated the growing Holocaust memorial culture, storytelling, public disclosures, and community development came to be viewed as vehicles of personal healing and political activism (Stein, 2009, p. 36). Prevailing concepts of community mental health and the emphasis of second-wave feminism on personal reflection as a form of political action encouraged individuals to reinterpret past experiences of victimisation as narratives of survival. Broadening concepts of trauma became a "central cultural resource for narrating the self" (Stein, 2009, p. 29), and cultural heritage emerged as a significant element in the pursuit of identity (Stein, 2009, p. 34).

Within this cultural context, both Holocaust survivors and their children began to examine the impact of wartime experiences on subsequent generations. The participation of second-generation survivors in the emergent movement of "therapeutic politics of identity," as Stein (2009, p. 30) termed it, played a central role in shaping Holocaust consciousness in the United States (Stein, 2009, p. 30). These currents crystallised in interventions at the intersections of therapeutic practice and community development. In 1976,

Fogelman and Savran (Fogelman, 1988; Fogelman & Savran, 1979, 1980) established short-term therapeutic support groups for second-generation survivors of the Nazi Holocaust in the Boston area. One group consisted of children of survivors in their 20s and 30s, while another group included an older cohort who had been children during the Holocaust. According to Fogelman (1988), participants were motivated to join these groups to share Holocaust experiences in a safe, supportive environment. These short-term survivor groups integrated elements of psychological support, self-help, and community development. The group process was divided into four themes. The creation of group ethos was followed by a focus on intergenerational communication and the search for identity (Fogelman, 1988, p. 622). Later, they explored issues of mourning and loss and then worked towards the safe termination of the process. The leaders directly addressed guilt and self-destructive behaviours by facilitating social connections, fostering self- and group-acceptance. Verbalising feelings linked to family histories of persecution and hearing others' accounts of resilience were viewed as protective against self-destruction and as ways to generate new perspectives on identity (Fogelman, 1988, p. 639).

As Fogelman (2017) noted, with the growing involvement of psychological professionals in Holocaust memorial culture, numerous oral-history projects that collected personal survival testimonies adopted a life-history approach during the 1980s. Kestenberg's Holocaust studies followed this trend. Her ISOPC project emphasised a holistic view of the participants, whose experiences of persecution were understood within the broader fabric of their life histories. Kestenberg's studies aimed not only to uncover survivors' narratives and insert them into collective memory but also to inform mental-health professionals about the distinctive struggles of different groups of survivors (child survivors, children of survivors, first-generation and war children). The ultimate goal of the interviews was to help survivors integrate traumatic experiences (Fogelman, 2017). Kestenberg's efforts to create space for the narratives of second-generation survivors and her commitment to community-building were firmly situated within the main currents of the growing Holocaust awareness in the United States in the 1980s.

Insides and Outsides: Kestenberg's Work in Context

Looking at Kestenberg's work within the broader currents of American psysciences between the 1940s and 1980s reveals that her oeuvre both followed and resisted key intellectual and disciplinary trends of the period. Her *Movement Profile*, grounded in direct infant observation, incorporated the focus of the early twentieth-century child guidance movements, which were closely aligned with psychoanalytic psychiatry, which often employed personality assessment methods and infant observation with an interest in distinctions between normal and abnormal development (Polat, 2021). Kestenberg's developmental movement studies likewise focused explicitly on identifying congenital differences and examining the predictive and diagnostic significance of motor behaviour in relation to later psychopathology (Kestenberg, 1965a, 1965b, 1967; Kestenberg & Sossin, 1979). Her Center for Parents and Children collaborated with several psychiatric colleges and welcomed trainee psychiatrists, providing them with access to data on normal development.

Kestenberg joined the New York psychoanalytic community at a tumultuous time in the late 1930s, when battles over theoretical and methodological orthodoxy divided the field (Kestenberg, 1992; Hale, 1995; Herzog, 2016a; Aron & Starr, 2013). Waves of emigration from Europe, and the divergent intellectual and cultural orientations of American- and European-trained analysts, further intensified these tensions. European émigrés were more often politically left-leaning, and their analytic work frequently engaged with social work, psychosomatic medicine, and developments in theory and technique (Hale, 1995, p. 118). Kestenberg's professional profile reflected the European orientation. She brought a sustained commitment to community welfare and preventive, developmentally oriented work. This was demonstrated through her community-facing projects and collaborations with non-clinical professionals, including social workers, educators, and dance/movement therapists. She also pursued a distinctive somatic line of inquiry.

During the primary period of Kestenberg's developmental movement studies, from 1953 to 1977, psychoanalysis in the United States was primarily shaped by the dominant paradigm of ego-psychology. The ambitions of Kestenberg's movement studies, grounded in systematic infant observation, resonated with the mid-century scientific drive of ego-psychology. By prioritising longitudinal observation and the collection of normative developmental data, she joined broader efforts to anchor psychoanalytic concepts in empirical evidence, aiming to underscore their relevance in psychiatry amid disciplinary tensions within the psy-sciences (Grob, 1991; Hale, 1995; Pickren, 2007).

Kestenberg's efforts to develop an assessment framework for prophylactic psychiatry and child guidance also reflected the emergence of community psychiatry in the late 1960s. Midgley (2013, pp. 137–138) argued that, through the concept of developmental lines, Anna Freud intended to provide a practical framework for application across various areas of child guidance, opening up the discourse to those outside psychoanalysis. Similarly, Kestenberg contended that the knowledge gathered and presented in a *Movement Profile* could aid intervention and treatment planning across interdisciplinary contexts in developmental psychiatry and family support (Kestenberg, 1985). When applied in dance/movement therapy and child guidance settings, her *Movement Profile* similarly extended psychoanalytic assessment into broader community-based practices. The establishment of the Center for Parents and Children also aligned with mid-1960s funding trends, when most funding for psychoanalytic projects was granted to those embedded in affiliated fields such as family support or social work (Hale, 1995).

Kestenberg (1980a, 1980b, 1981; Kestenberg & Marcus, 1979) also concordantly aligned herself with the Cold War normativity and competitiveness of American psychoanalysis in relation to external pressures from church criticism and new sex research, demonstrated by Herzog (2016b). She engaged in passionate critiques of new sex research, tendentiously underscoring the relevance and authority of psychoanalysis in relation to the topic of sex. In her formulations on sex-specific identity and parental attitudes, she devised normative typologies of women based on traditional gender roles, problematising the postponement of parenthood and the pursuit of women's equality (Kestenberg, 1980a, p. 319, 1980c; Kestenberg & Marcus, 1979).

While Kestenberg shared many of the field's broader ambitions, she also challenged several key concepts in American psychoanalysis at the time. Her (1945, 1956a, 1956b) formulations on the development of female sexuality in the early 1950s reflected the centrality of reconsidering libido theory and basic Freudian tenets on female sexual development prevalent in American psychoanalysis at the time (Herzog, 2016a). While many shifted their focus away from sexuality on to adaptation and ego development, she revised the psychosexual stage theory, introduced the *inner-genital* phase, and emphasised the psychosexual significance of vaginal tensions. Amid the internal tensions within American psychoanalysis centring around the topic of sex, somewhat contrastingly, Kestenberg intended to reaffirm the relevance of the Freudian libido theory. Even though she explicitly aligned her work with that of Anna Freud, Kestenberg's *inner-genital* psychosexual phase did not find support from Freud (Kestenberg, 1991). Kestenberg also rejected the notion of the autonomous ego sphere in the 1950s and did not readily embrace the transition from drive-theory to object-relations and interpersonal approaches in the 1970s.

Factionalism and intellectual ruptures are woven through the history of psychoanalysis (Bálint, 1954; Bibring, 1954; Thompson, 1958; Greenacre, 1966; Eisold, 1994; Bergmann, 1993, 1997; Kirsner, 2009; Berman, 1995; Herzog, 2016a, 2016b; Aron & Starr, 2013; see also Makari, 2008). A pervasive intolerance of intellectual diversity marked mid-century American psychoanalysis, a tendency reported as especially pronounced within the New York Psychoanalytic Society (Eisold, 1994; Hale, 1995; Kirsner, 2009, p. 62). In the pursuit of "protecting psychoanalysis from marginalisation and dilution" among the emerging psychotherapeutic approaches, proponents of ego-psychology adopted heightened protective measures, emphasising established clinical parameters and a scientific orientation. It was not uncommon to dismiss or characterise alternative approaches as unanalytic when they departed from the prevailing adaptation-focus, dominant theoretical formulations, or preferred evidentiary frameworks (Wallerstein, 2002, p. 145). The consequences of deviating from accepted paradigms ranged from intellectual intimidation to dismissal to, at times, complete marginalisation of dissenting figures (Eisold, 1994). In this context, partial conceptual misalignments with the prevailing analytic paradigms led to Kestenberg's developmental movement studies being viewed as 'unanalytic' and subsequently dismissed within psychoanalytic circles. According to Kestenberg's (1992, p. 183) recollection, her disagreement with Hartmann over the origins of the ego even led to Hartmann "diagnosing" her with unresolved neurotic conflicts.

Kestenberg's methods of developmental study, likewise, sat uneasily with the growing experimentalism in infant research of the late 1970s, which increasingly embraced bidirectional interaction models and focused on readily observable, easily codified behaviours. By contrast, Kestenberg produced microanalytic studies that she presented in a case-study format using a technically demanding kinaesthetic lexicon. Stern's empirically framed account of attunement became canonical, while Kestenberg's approach was overlooked. This difference in reception highlights how evidence hierarchies and trends in scientific representation govern judgements of knowledge and validity.

Furthermore, Kestenberg's movement-focused work transcended disciplinary boundaries between dance studies, psy-sciences, and Western and Eastern medicine. Her methodology remained anchored in dance practice, resisting the pull of contemporaneous scientification trends in movement research and within the psy-sciences. Her eclectic reach fostered fertile innovations and won allies among American creative arts therapists but it also blurred the disciplinary home of her work and fuelled doubts about the scientific validity of her movement studies within psychoanalysis and psychiatry. Psychoanalytic traditionalists could dismiss it as insufficiently orthodox, and experimentalists could find it too technical.

Kestenberg examined bodily movement through the lens of Freudian metapsychology, developing the psychodynamic theory and vocabulary of movement. However, her work also retained explicit ties to the field of dance. Her observation method was grounded in kinaesthetic attunement. Her terminology was derived from movement experience and somatic sensations. Her muscle-tension inscription technique and the Laban-derived notation system required an embodied grasp of movement as a language. She foregrounded kinaesthetic attunement between bodies as a scientific instrument for qualitative psychological assessment and proposed her freehand tracing of muscle-tension flow as scientific documentation of bodily movement. She diagrammatically structured and visualised these embodied qualities in graphs. Kestenberg's in-depth focus on bodily movement was unique, and her vocabulary was largely unfamiliar to psychoanalysts and psychiatrists at the time, leading to the marginalisation of her movement psychodynamics. However, their hesitation cannot be attributed to terminology or the primacy of movement alone. Kestenberg's work conveyed a palpable "confusion of tongues" generated by the tension between her diagrammatic orientation, the systematising drive of mid-century American psychoanalysis, and the exploratory, phenomenological language borrowed from dance. A dynamic integration of the epistemic orientations of dance and psychoanalysis was not achieved, dividing her audience into psychoanalysts, who took some interest in her developmental assessment but were held at a distance by the language, and dance/movement therapists, who embraced its Labanian concepts but rejected its Freudian foundation.

The emerging field of American dance/movement therapy, in need of a psychologically grounded framework for movement assessment, proved more receptive to Kestenberg's *Movement Profile.* Through the dance/movement therapists' interventions, the *Movement Profile*'s Freudian foundations were loosened and reoriented to reflect the disciplinary alliances of the emerging profession. At the same time, psychoanalysts (including Kestenberg) responded to the proliferation of new psychotherapeutic modalities by asserting their authority over dance/movement therapists who used psychoanalytic interpretations. These gestures of boundary-making could also have accelerated dance/movement therapy's separation from psychoanalysis. As the new discipline of dance/movement therapy consolidated, it selectively retained Kestenberg's *Movement Profile,* which potentially contributed to its distancing from the psychoanalytic landscape. These intricacies of selective attention across the psy-sciences show that disciplinary boundaries and theoretical and methodological alliances were tension-filled areas in the postwar period. A drive towards disciplinary purity in psychoanalysis and psychiatry paralleled the emergence of new, more eclectic psychotherapy modalities, such as the creative arts therapies (Levy, 1988; Grob, 1991; Hale, 1995).

Cold War American psy-sciences, invested in the stability of the democratic project in the West, were marked by heightened interest in interpersonal processes and in preventing social and psychological ills through community mental health frameworks. Kestenberg believed that the study of bodily movement has the potential to enhance individual and societal well-being. This notion strongly echoed Laban's vitalist concepts, but it was also intimately tied to Cold War discourse (Laban, 1950, 1954, 2008; Laemmli, 2016; Weinstein, 2013). Kestenberg's child guidance centre positioned itself as a primary prevention project arising from concerns about the breakdown of family relationships, which may impede child development and, in turn, contribute to later psychological distress. Participation was framed as an investment in children and future generations and, therefore, in society as a whole (Bell, 1984). This preventive orientation was grounded in embodiment and movement. Staff at the centre developed movement-based parenting assessment scales, used observational films for movement notation, and constructed movement profiles to support child guidance interventions. These practices demonstrate that the study of movement behaviour was central to the center's efforts to prevent both individual and social ills. The postwar years saw a broadening of psychological discourse marked by the extension of psychiatric practice into communities and family homes (Grob, 1991; Weinstein, 2013). The centre also exemplified this domestic expansion and focus on family dynamics. Staff offered specialised knowledge classes for parents, aiming to enhance caregiving skills and foster personal growth. Parents were also encouraged to observe and journal about their children's development. Staff employed embodied, pedagogical methods, such as *movement retraining*, to synchronise the nonverbal interactions of parents and children, supporting their emotional attachment. The centre intended to foster a sense of community among parents through initiatives such as a newsletter that encouraged parents to share their parenting challenges. The dedicated fathers' group, which combined elements of a peer support group, also exemplifies the community-oriented approach.

Kestenberg's work also reflects the broader preoccupation in the Cold War period with decoding/deciphering foreign communications (Martin-Nielsen, 2010), as well as the growing interest in psychotechnological mediation of behaviour in the service of democratic stability (Laemmli, 2016). Grounded in postwar assumptions that linked individual adjustment to social well-being, Kestenberg treated the body as a messenger and movement as a language. In her view, the body is a repository of past experience, and habitual movement patterns reveal the psychosocial organisation of personality. She suggested that repressed aggression (which could lead to racial prejudice) is stored in the body and indicated in movement behaviour. Reorganising kinetic features of movement behaviour becomes therapeutic, and 'movement retraining' of parent–child interactions becomes preventive of both potential individual and social ills.

Central to her movement assessment framework was the idea of balance. She conceptualised 'healthy functioning' in motor terms as the balance between oppositional qualities of movement, avoiding extremes. As Laemmli (2016, p. 147) noted, this emphasis on balance echoes Cold War ideals invested in Western democratic stability, standing against the perceived extremes of authoritarianism. The Cold War era's focus on information-gathering, language, and communication, combined with technocratic and operational tendencies, is reflected in the diagrammatic orientation of Kestenberg's *Movement Profile*. This is particularly apparent in her muscle-tension inscription method. The hand-drawn curves, which trace variations in muscular tension and are linked to detailed somatoaffective nuances, convert the movement process into a stable, readable waveform, resembling EEG lines rendering brain activity into a visual, readable record. Kestenberg's *Tension-Flow Curves* were developed to register somatoaffective patterns, employing the examiner's kinaesthetic attunement as a route into otherwise inaccessible internal states. Through her profiling system, Kestenberg conceptualised embodied experience as a patterned signal that, when organised into diagrams and categories, becomes thinkable and manageable within the psy-sciences.

Kestenberg's Holocaust studies, also unique in their scope and embodied focus, were received with far less ambivalence than her developmental movement studies. This difference in reception likely stemmed from her Holocaust work's aligning with the main cultural currents of the growing Holocaust awareness of the 1980s.

Note

1 Also see Pius XII (1952).

References

Adorno, T.W., Frenkel-Brunswik, E., Levinson, D.J., & Sanford, R.N. (1993). *The authoritarian personality* (Studies in Prejudice series, Vol. 1). W. W. Norton. (Original work published in 1950)

Aron, L., & Starr, K. (2013). Psychoanalysis as war hero. In *A psychotherapy for the people: Toward a progressive psychoanalysis* (pp. 99–110). Routledge.

Bálint, M. (1954). Analytic training and training analysis. *The International Journal of Psychoanalysis*, 35(2), 157–162.

Bálint, M. (1959). Notes on some psychology of motility. In *Thrills and regressions* (pp. 117–118). International Universities Press.

Bartenieff, I. (1963, 16 January). Letter to Warren Lamb. Irmgard Bartenieff Papers (0390-SCPA), Correspondence, 1929–1981, Professional letters, 1929–1980. Michelle Smith Performing Arts Library, University of Maryland, MD, United States.

Bartenieff, I. (1964, 15 June). Letter to Warren Lamb. Irmgard Bartenieff Papers (0390-SCPA), Correspondence, 1929–1981, Professional letters, 1929–1980. Michelle Smith Performing Arts Library, University of Maryland, MD, United States.

Bartenieff, I., & Davis, M. (1965). Effort-shape analysis of movement: The unity of expression and function. New York: Albert Einstein College of Medicine, Yeshiva University, 1965. Box 6. Item 5. Martha Davis papers (0373-SCPA), Bartenieff and Lewis items, 1933–1994, undated. Michelle Smith Performing Arts Library, University of Maryland, MD, USA.

Bartenieff, I., & Davis, M. (1972). Effort-shape analysis of movement: The unity of expression and function. In *Research Approaches to Movement and Personality*. Arno Press.

Bartenieff, I., & Lewis, D. (2013). *Body movement: Coping with the environment* (1st ed.). Routledge. (Original work published in 1980.) doi:10.4324/9781315025445

Beebe, B. (2014). My journey in infant research and psychoanalysis: Microanalysis, a social microscope. *Psychoanalytic Psychology*, 31(1), 4–25. doi:10.1037/a0035566

Beebe, B., Gerstman, L., Carson, B., Dolins, M., Zigman, A., Rosesweig, H., Faughey, K., & Korman, M. (1982). Rhythmic communication in the mother–infant dyad. In M. Davis (Ed.), *Interaction rhythms: Periodicity in communicative behavior* (pp. 79–100). Human Sciences Press.

Beels, C.C. (1989). Israel Zwerling: Lessons from a career. *New Directions for Mental Health Services*, 42, 3–8. doi:10.1002/yd.23319894203

Bell, B. (1984). A new childcare concept takes root in Roslyn. *Roslyn News*, 23 February.

Bergmann, M.S. (1993). Reflections on the history of psychoanalysis. *Journal of the American Psychoanalytic Association*, 41(4), 929–955. doi:10.1177/000306519304100402

Bergmann, M.S. (1997). The historical roots of psychoanalytic orthodoxy. *International Journal of Psychoanalysis*, 78, 69–86.

Berman, E. (1995). On analyzing colleagues. *Contemporary Psychoanalysis*, 31(4), 521–539. doi:10.1080/00107530.1995.10746922

Bernstein, L.P. (Ed.). (1979). *Eight theoretical approaches in dance-movement therapy*. Kendall/Hunt.

Bibring, G.L. (1954). The training analysis and its place in psycho-analytic training. *The International Journal of Psychoanalysis*, 35(2), 169–173.
Birdwhistell, R. (1955). Background to kinesics. *ETC: A Review of General Semantics*, 13(1), 10–18.
Birdwhistell, R. (1970). *Kinesics and context: Essays on body motion communication.* University of Pennsylvania Press.
Birdwhistell, R.L. (1952). *Introduction to kinesics: An annotation system for analysis of body motion and gesture.* Washington, DC, Department of State, Foreign Service Institute.
Bower, T.G.R. (1982). *Development in infancy.* W.H. Freeman.
Buelte, A. (1978). Movement retraining. *Child Development Research News*, 1(2), 2.
Buelte, A. (1979). Movement retraining. *Child Development Research News*, 2(1), 1.
Bühler, C. (1930). *The first year of life* (Trans. P. Greenberg & R. Ripin). John Day.
Coates, S.W. (2004). John Bowlby and Margaret S. Mahler: Their lives and theories. *Journal of the American Psychoanalytic Association*, 52(2), 571–601. doi:10.1177/00030651040520020601
Cohn, J.F., & Tronick, E.Z. (1987). Mother–infant face-to-face interaction: The sequencing of dyadic states at 3, 6, and 9 months. *Developmental Psychology*, 23(1), 68–77. doi:10.1037/0012–1649.23.1.68
Cohn, J.F., & Tronick, E.Z. (1988). Mother–infant face-to-face interaction: Influence is bidirectional and unrelated to periodic cycles in either partner's behavior. *Developmental Psychology*, 24(3), 386–392. doi:10.1037/0012–1649.24.3.386
Collins, H., Evans, R., & Gorman, M. (2007). Trading zones and interactional expertise. *Studies in History and Philosophy of Science Part A*, 38(4), 657–666. doi:10.1016/j.shpsa.2007.09.003
Condon, W.S. (1982). Cultural microrhythms. In M. Davis (Ed.), *Interaction rhythms: Periodicity in communicative behavior* (pp. 53–77). Human Sciences Press.
Davis, M. (1981). Movement characteristics of hospitalized psychiatric patients. *American Journal of Dance Therapy*, 4(1), 52–71. doi:10.1007/BF02579526
Davis, M. (Ed.). (1982). *Interaction rhythms: Periodicity in communicative behavior.* Human Sciences Press.
Davis, M. (1992). Flowing into the mainstream isn't free. *American Journal of Dance Therapy*, 14(1), Spring/Summer.
Davis, M. (1997). Guide to movement analysis methods: Part 1 Movement Signature Analysis (MSA), Part 2 Movement Psychodiagnostic Inventory (MPI), Part 3 Nonverbal Interaction and States Analysis (NISA). Unpublished manuscript.
Davis, M. (2001). Film projectors as microscopes. Ray Birdwhistell and the microanalysis of interaction (1955–1975) [Conference presentation]. Origins of Visual Anthropology.
Davis, M., & Dulicai, D. (1992). Hitler's movement signature. *TDR: The Drama Review*, 36(2), 152–172. https://www.jstor.org/stable/1146204
Davis, M., Dulicai, D., Hadiks, D., & Berger, M.R. (1992, August). Body language of world leaders [Conference presentation]. Annual Convention of the American Psychological Association, Washington, DC [Unpublished conference paper]. Martha Davis Papers (Collection 0373-SCPA), Michelle Smith Performing Arts Library, University of Maryland.
Davis, M., & Hadiks, D. (1990). Nonverbal behavior and client state changes during psychotherapy. *Journal of Clinical Psychology*, 46(3), 340–351.

Eisold, K. (1994). The intolerance of diversity in psychoanalytic institutes. *The International Journal of Psychoanalysis*, 75(4), 785–800.

Eissler, K.R. (1953). The effect of the structure of the ego on psychoanalytic technique. *Journal of the American Psychoanalytic Association*, 1, 104–143.

Fantz, R. (1963). Pattern vision in newborn infants. *Science*, 140(3564), 296–297.

Fogelman, E. (1988). Intergenerational group therapy: Child survivors of the Holocaust and offspring of survivors. *Psychoanalytic Review*, 75(4), 619–640.

Fogelman, E. (2017). The evolution of a second-generation Holocaust survivor identity. Available at: https://evafogelman.com/publications/the-evolution-of-a-second-generation-holocaust-survivor-identity/

Fogelman, E., & Savran, B. (1979). Therapeutic groups for children of Holocaust survivors. *International Journal of Group Psychotherapy*, 29(2), 211–235.

Fogelman, E., & Savran, B. (1980). Brief group therapy with offspring of Holocaust survivors: Leaders' reactions. *American Journal of Orthopsychiatry*, 50(1), 96–108.

Fonagy, P. (2007). Embodied psychoanalysis? Or, on the confluence of psychodynamic theory and developmental science [Commentary]. In L. Mayes, P. Fonagy, & M. Target (Eds.), *Developmental science and psychoanalysis: Integration and innovation* (pp. 39–45). Karnac Books.

Freedman, N., & Bucci, W. (1981). On kinetic filtering in associative monologue. *Semiotica*, 34(3–4), 225–249.

Freud, S. (1961). The ego and the id. In J. Strachey (Ed. & Trans.), *The standard edition of the complete psychological works of Sigmund Freud* (Vol. 19, pp. 3–66). Hogarth Press & Institute of Psycho-Analysis. (Original work published 1923)

Freud, S. (2001). Formulations on the two principles of mental functioning. In J. Strachey (Ed. & Trans.), *The Standard Edition of the Complete Psychological Works of Sigmund Freud* (Vol. 12, pp. 213–226). Vintage. (Original work published 1911)

Galenson, E. (1971, 23 February). Discussion of Judith S. Kestenberg: Development of the young child expressed through bodily movement I. 565th Meeting Proceedings, New York Psychoanalytic Association and Society Meeting Notes, A. A. Brill Library, Archives and Special Collections.

Galison, P. (1996). Computer simulations and the trading zone. In P. Galison & D.J. Stump (Eds.), *The disunity of science: Boundaries, contexts, and power* (pp. 118–157). Stanford University Press.

Galison, P., & Stump, D.J. (Eds.). (1996). *The disunity of science: Boundaries, contexts, and power*. Stanford University Press.

Gergely, G. (2000). Constancy from cognitive developmental theory: Reapproaching Mahler: New perspectives on normal autism, symbiosis, splitting and libidinal object. *Journal of the American Psychoanalytic Association*, 48, 1197–1228. doi:10.1177/00030651000480040801

Gesell, A., & Amatruda, C.S. (1947). *Developmental diagnosis* (2nd ed.). Paul B. Hoeber.

Gilani, H.Z., Bucci, W., & Freedman, N. (1985). The structure and language of a silence. *Semiotica*, 56(1–2),99–113.

Gober, S. (2014). The development of a measure of Margaret Mahler's theory integrating the infant, the mother, and their dyadic relationship during the infant's first five months of life. Doctoral dissertation, Rutgers, State University of New Jersey. Rutgers University Community Repository (RUcore). https://rucore.libraries.rutgers.edu/rutgers-lib/42338/

Greenacre, P. (1966). Problems of training analysis. *The Psychoanalytic Quarterly*, 35 (4), 540–567.

Grob, G.N. (1991). *From asylum to community mental health policy in modern America*. Princeton University Press.

Hacking, I. (1996). The disunities of the sciences. In P. Galison & D.J. Stump (Eds.), *The disunity of science: Boundaries, contexts, and power* (pp. 37–74). Stanford University Press.

Hale, N.G. (1995). *The rise and crisis of psychoanalysis in the United States: Freud and the Americans, 1917–1985*. Oxford University Press.

Hartmann, H. (1958). *Ego psychology and the problem of adaptation*. International Universities Press.

Hartmann, H., Kris, E., & Loewenstein, R.M. (1949). Notes on the theory of aggression. *Psychoanalytic Study of the Child*, 3/4, 9–36.

Herzog, D. (2016a). The libido wars. In *Cold War Freud: Psychoanalysis in an age of catastrophes* (pp. 21–55). Cambridge University Press. doi:10.1017/9781139680455.002

Herzog, D. (2016b). Homophobia's durability and the reinvention of psychoanalysis. In *Cold War Freud: Psychoanalysis in an age of catastrophes* (pp. 56–86). Cambridge University Press. doi:10.1017/9781139680455.003

Jurist, E. (2022). Mentalizing from/to/with the body. In *Psychoanalysis and the mind-body problem* (pp. 186–203). Routledge. doi:10.4324/9781003090755-9

Kaye, K.L., & Bower, T.G.R. (1994). Learning and intermodal transfer of information in newborns. *Psychological Science*, 5, 286–288.

Kestenberg Amighi, J., Loman, S., Lewis, P., & Sossin, K.M. (Eds.). (1999). *The meaning of movement: Developmental and clinical perspectives of the Kestenberg Movement Profile*. Gordon & Breach.

Kestenberg, J.S. (1945). Early reactions to tensions. Presentation at the 283rd Meeting of the New York Psychoanalytic Society. Documents of Judith S. Kestenberg (1937–1999). New York Psychoanalytic Association and Society A. A. Brill Library, Archives and Special Collections. New York, USA.

Kestenberg, J.S. (1946). Early fears and early defenses. *The Nervous Child*, 4(1), 56–70.

Kestenberg, J.S. (1953). Notes on ego development. *International Journal of Psychoanalysis*, 34(2), 1–12.

Kestenberg, J.S. (1956a). Vicissitudes of female sexuality. *Journal of the American Psychoanalytic Association*, 4, 453–475.

Kestenberg, J.S. (1956b, 16 March). On the development of maternal feelings in early childhood: Observations and reflections [Presentation]. Meeting of the New York Psychoanalytic Society, Documents of Judith S. Kestenberg (1937–1999). New York Psychoanalytic Association and Society A. A. Brill Library, Archives and Special Collections, New York, USA.

Kestenberg, J.S. (1965a). The role of movement patterns in development. I. Rhythms of movement. *Psychoanalytic Quarterly*, 24(1), 1–36. doi:10.1080/21674086.1965.11926334

Kestenberg, J.S. (1965b). The role of movement patterns in development. II. Flow of tension and effort. *Psychoanalytic Quarterly*, 24(4), 517–563. doi:10.1080/21674086.1965.11926363

Kestenberg, J.S. (1967). The role of movement patterns in development. III. Control of shape. *Psychoanalytic Quarterly*, 26(3), 356–409. doi:10.1080/21674086.1967.11926431

Kestenberg, J.S. (1973). Comments on movement therapy as a psychotherapeutic tool. *Journal of the American Psychoanalytic Association*, 21(2), 347–350. doi:10.1177/000306517302100208

Kestenberg, J.S. (1974). Profiles [Unpublished archival document]. Laban/Bartenieff Institute of Movement Studies (LIMS) records (0339-SCPA), Student files, Certification projects. Michelle Smith Performing Arts Library, University of Maryland, United States.

Kestenberg, J.S. (1975a). Preface. In *Children and parents: Psychoanalytic studies in development* (pp. xv–xxvii). Jason Aronson.

Kestenberg, J.S. (1975b). Attunement and clashing in mother–child interaction. In *Children and parents: Psychoanalytic Studies in Development*. Jason Aronson.

Kestenberg, J.S. (1978). Transsensus-outgoingness and Winnicott's intermediate zone. In S. A. Grolnick & L.B. Barkin (Eds.), *Between reality and fantasy; Winnicott's concepts of transitional objects and phenomena* (pp. 61–75). Jason Aronson.

Kestenberg, J.S. (1980a). Pregnancy as a developmental phase. *Journal of Biological Experience: Studies in the Life of the Body*, 3, 58–66.

Kestenberg, J.S. (1980b). The three faces of femininity. *Psychoanalytic Review*, 67(3), 313–335.

Kestenberg, J.S. (1980c). Maternity and paternity in the developmental context. *Psychiatric Clinics of North America*, 3(1), 61–79.

Kestenberg, J.S. (1981). The Centre for Parents and Children. How do we do things in the Centre? *Child Development Research News*, 3(2).

Kestenberg, J.S. (1985). The role of movement patterns in diagnosis and prevention. In D.A. Shaskan & W.I. Roller (Eds.), *Paul Schilder: Mind explorer* (pp. 97–161). Human Sciences Press.

Kestenberg, J.S. (1987). Empathy for the fetus. In T. Verny (Ed.), *Pre- and perinatal psychology: An introduction* (pp. 138–150). Human Sciences Press.

Kestenberg, J.S. (1989). What are the ingredients of bonding postnatally? Paper presented at the International Congress on Pre and Perinatal Psychology and Medicine, Jerusalem.

Kestenberg, J.S. (1990a) What are the ingredients of bonding prenatally? *International Journal for Prenatal and Perinatal Studies*, 119–124.

Kestenberg, J.S. (1990b). Future directions of the KMP: Panel discussion: Goldman, E., LaBarre, F., Lewis, P., Merman, H., & Sossin, K. M. In S. Loman & P. Lewis (Eds.), *The Kestenberg Movement Profile: Its past, present applications, and future directions* (pp. 155–173). Retrieved from https://aura.antioch.edu/facbooks/25

Kestenberg, J.S. (1991). Dr Judith S. Kestenberg talks to Kristina Stanton. *Free Associations*, 2(2), 157–174.

Kestenberg, J.S. (1992). Kindheit und Wissenschaft. Eine biographische Skizze. In. *Psychoanalyse in Selbstdarstellungen* (Vol. 1, pp. 147–202). Ludger M. Hermanns. Edition Diskord.

Kestenberg, J.S., Berlowe, J., Buelte, A., Hershey, M., & Robbins, E. (1971). Development of the young child as expressed through bodily movement I. *Journal of the American Psychoanalytic Association*, 19(4), 746–764.

Kestenberg, J.S., & Borowitz, E. (1990). On narcissism and masochism in the fetus and the neonate. *Pre- and Perinatal Psychology Journal*, 5(1), 87. Retrieved from ProQuest Central.

Kestenberg, J.S., & Buelte, A (1977a). Prevention, infant therapy and the treatment of adults: 1. Towards understanding mutuality. *International Journal of Psychoanalytic Psychotherapy*, 6, 339–367.

Kestenberg, J.S., & Buelte, A. (1977b). Prevention, infant therapy and the treatment of adults: 2. Mutual holding and holding oneself up. *International Journal of Psychoanalytic Psychotherapy*, 6, 368–396.

Kestenberg, J.S., & Marcus, H. (1979). Hypothetical monosex and bisexuality: A psychoanalytic interpretation of sex difference as they reveal themselves in movement patterns of men and women. In N.M. Coleman & J. Ikenberry (Eds.), *Psychosexual imperatives* (pp. 146–181). Human Sciences Press.

Kestenberg, J.S., & Sossin, K.M. (1979). *The role of movement patterns in development* (Vols. 1–2). Dance Notation Bureau Press.

Kestenberg, J.S., & Weinstein, J. (1978). Transitional objects and body-image formation. In S.A. Grolnick & L.B. Barkin (Eds.), *Between reality and fantasy; Winnicott's concepts of transitional objects and phenomena* (pp. 75–97). Jason Aronson.

Kirsner, D. (2009). *Unfree associations: Inside psychoanalytic institutes.* Jason Aronson.

Knoblauch, S.H. (2017). The fluidity of emotions and clinical vulnerability: A field of rhythmic tensions. *Psychoanalytic Perspectives*, 14(3), 283–308. doi:10.1080/1551806X.2017.1342421

Knorr Cetina, K. (1999). *Epistemic cultures: How the sciences make knowledge.* Harvard University Press.

Kormos, J. (2023a). Dance becomes therapeutic in the mid to late 20th century. *Journal of the History of the Behavioral Sciences*, 59(3), 268–282.

Kormos, J. (2023b). A modernitás kinetikus projektje a humántudományok területén: Tánc- és tudománytörténet találkozása a mozgáskutatás területén [The kinetic project of modernity in the field of humanities: The encounter of dance and science history in the field of movement research]. In L. Fuchs, J. Fügedi, & P. Péter (Eds.), *Tánctudományi Tanulmányok 2022–2023* [Dance Studies 2022–2023] (pp. 121–153). Magyar Táncm⊠vészeti Egyetem, Magyar Tánctudományi Társaság.

Laban, R. (1950). *The mastery of movement on stage.* Macdonald & Evans.

Laban, R. (1954). *Principles of dance and movement notation.* Macdonald & Evans.

Laban, R. (2008). *Koreográfia* [Choreography] (Trans. J. Fugedi). L'Harmattan. (Original work published 1926)

Laemmli, W.E. (2016). The choreography of everyday life: Rudolf Laban and the making of modern movement. Doctoral dissertation, University of Pennsylvania. Retrieved from: https://repository.upenn.edu/entities/publication/8f9a810d-1d39-46f7-a40a-2f57f833f645

Lamb, W. (1965, 18 January, 6 April). Letters to Irmgard Bartenieff. In I. Bartenieff papers (0390-SCPA), Correspondence, 1929–1981. Michelle Smith Performing Arts Library, University of Maryland, United States.

Lausberg, H. (2014). Movement behaviour research through history and in current scientific disciplines. In H. Lausberg (Ed.), *Understanding body movement: A guide to empirical research on nonverbal behaviour – with an introduction to the NEUROGES* (pp. 1–13). Peter Lang.

Leeds-Hurwitz, W., & Kendon, A. (2021). The natural history of an interview and the microanalysis of behavior in social interaction: A critical moment in research practice. In J. McElvenny & A. Ploder (Eds.), *Holisms of communication: The early history of audio-visual sequence analysis* (pp. 145–200). Language Science Press. doi:10.5281/zenodo.5142288

Levy, F. (1988). *Dance/movement therapy: A healing art*. The American Alliance for Health, Physical Education, Recreation and Dance.
Mahler, M.S., Pine, F., & Bergman, A. (1975). *The psychological birth of the human infant: Symbiosis and individuation*. Basic Books.
Makari, G. (2008). *Revolution in mind: The creation of psychoanalysis*. Harper Collins.
Martin-Nielsen, J. (2010). This war for men's minds: The birth of a human science in Cold War America. *History of the Human Sciences*, 23(5), 131–155. doi:10.1177/0952695110378952
Mason, E.A. (Director & Producer), & Fogelman, E. (Writer & Producer). (1984). *Breaking the silence* [Documentary film]. Documentaries for Learning, Public Broadcasting Service.
McQuown, N.A. (Ed.). (1971). *The natural history of an interview* [Microfilm]. University of Chicago, Joseph Regenstein Library, Department of Photoduplication.
Meltzoff, A.N., & Moore, M.K. (1977). Imitation of facial and manual gestures by human neonates. *Science*, 198(4312), 75–78.
Meltzoff, A.N., & Moore, M.K. (1989). Imitation in newborn infants: Exploring the range of gestures imitated and the underlying mechanisms. *Developmental Psychology*, 25, 954–962.
Midgley, N. (2013). *Reading Anna Freud*. Routledge. doi:10.4324/9780203078876
Murray, H.A. (1943). Analysis of the personality of Adolph Hitler: With predictions of his future behavior and suggestions for dealing with him now and after Germany's surrender [OSS confidential report]. Office of Strategic Services. Donovan Nuremberg Trials Collection, Cornell University Law Library.
Peterson, D. (2017). The depth of fields: Managing focus in the epistemic subcultures of mind and brain science. *Social Studies of Science*, 47(1), 53–74. https://www.jstor.org/stable/26107046
Pickren, W. (2007). Tension and opportunity in post-World War II American psychology. *History of Psychology*, 10(3), 279–299. doi:10.1037/1093-4510.10.3.279
PiusXII. (1952, 14 September). The moral limits of medical research and treatment. Address to the First International Congress on the Histopathology of the Nervous System. Papal Encyclicals. Available at: https://www.papalencyclicals.net/pius12/p12psych.htm
Polat, B. (2021). Mental hygiene, psychoanalysis, and interwar psychology: The making of the maternal deprivation hypothesis. *Isis*, 112(2), 266–290. doi:10.1086/714599
Saslow, G., Matarazzo, J.D., & Guze, S.B. (1955). The stability of interaction chronograph patterns in psychiatric interviews. *Journal of Consulting Psychology*, 19(6), 417–430. doi:10.1037/h0047036
Scheflen, A.E. (1965). *Stream and structure of communicational behavior. Context analysis of a psychotherapy session*. Mental Health Research Foundation.
Scheflen, A.E. (1970). Communicational arrangements which further specify meaning. *Family Process*, 9, 457–472.
Sheets-Johnstone, M. (2011). *The primacy of movement* (Expanded 2nd ed.). John Benjamins.
Siegel, E.V. (1973). Movement therapy as a psychotherapeutic tool. *Journal of the American Psychoanalytic Association*, 21(2), 327–349. doi:10.1177/000306517302100210
Solnit, A. (1971, 23 February). Discussion of Judith S. Kestenberg: Development of the young child expressed through bodily movement I. 565th Meeting Proceedings,

New York Psychoanalytic Association and Society Meeting Notes, A. A. Brill Library, Archives and Special Collections.

Solnit, A. (1973). Commentary on movement therapy as a psychotherapeutic tool. *Journal of the American Psychoanalytic Association*, 21(2), 344–346. doi:10.1177/000306517302100207

Spitz, R.A. (1950). Relevancy of direct infant observation. *The Psychoanalytic Study of the Child*, 5(1), 66–73. doi:10.1080/00797308.1950.11822885

Stein, A. (2009). Feminism, therapeutic culture, and the Holocaust in the United States: The second-generation phenomenon. *Jewish Social Studies*, 16(1), 27–53. doi:10.2979/jss.2009.16.1.27

Stern, D. (1971). A microanalysis of mother–infant interaction. *Journal of the American Academy of Child Psychiatry*, 10, 501–517. doi:10.1016/S0002-7138(09)61752-0

Stern, D. (1982). Some interactive functions of rhythm changes between mother and infant. In M. Davis (Ed.), *Interaction rhythms: Periodicity in communicative behavior* (pp. 101–118). Human Sciences Press.

Stern, D.N. (1998a). *The interpersonal world of the infant: A view from psychoanalysis and developmental psychology.* Karnac Books. (Original work published in 1985)

Stern, D.N. (1998b). The sense of a subjective self: II. Affect attunement. In D.N. Stern, *The interpersonal world of the infant* (pp. 138–161). Karnac Books. (Original work published 1985)

Stern, D.N. (2010). *Forms of vitality: Exploring dynamic experience in psychology, the arts, psychotherapy, and development.* Oxford University Press.

Thompson, C. (1958). A study of the emotional climate of psychoanalytic institutes. *Psychiatry*, 21(1), 45–51. doi:10.1080/00332747.1958.11023113

Trevarthen, C. (1979). Communication and cooperation in early infancy: A description of primary intersubjectivity. In M. Bullowa (Ed.), *Before speech: The beginnings of human communication* (pp. 321–347). Cambridge University Press.

Tronick, E. (1989). Emotions and emotional communication in infants. *American Psychologist*, 44(2), 112–119. doi:10.1037/0003-066X.44.2.112

Tronick, E., & Cohn, J. (1989). Infant–mother face-to-face interaction: Age and gender differences in coordination and the occurrence of miscoordination. *Child Development*, 60, 85–92. doi:10.2307/1131074

Wallerstein, R.S. (2002). The growth and transformation of American ego psychology. *Journal of the American Psychoanalytic Association*, 50(1), 135–168. doi:10.1177/00030651020500011401

Watson, J.S. (1972). Smiling, cooing, and "the game." *Merrill-Palmer Quarterly*, 18, 323–339.

Weinstein, D. (2013). *The pathological family: Postwar America and the rise of family therapy.* Cornell University Press.

Wolff, P. (1959). Observations of newborn infants. *Psychosomatic Medicine*, 21, 110–118.

Yadlin-Gadot, S. (2022). Lacan on mind and body. In J. Mills (Ed.), *Psychoanalysis and the mind–body problem* (pp. 119–136). Routledge. doi:10.4324/9781003090755–6

Zwerling, I. (1989). The creative arts therapies as real therapies. *American Journal of Dance Therapy*, 11, 19–26. doi:10.1007/BF00844263

Chapter 5

Echoes and Afterlives

Afterlives of Body Concepts

Kestenberg's body–mind concepts and movement analysis method have been applied most widely in the clinical practice of dance/movement therapy and creative arts therapies (Loman, 1998; Loman, 2016; Loman et al., 2021; Johnson, 2018; Gass et al., 2013; Gonzalez-Dolginko, 2021) and more rarely in psychoanalytic and parent–child psychotherapy (La Barre, 2001, 2018; Birklein, 2018; Sossin & Birklein, 2006) and in psychology research, in areas such as developmental psychopathology, and infant mental health (Araki, 2017; Bromberg, 2015; Koch, 2007; Koch et al., 2001; Fuchs & Koch, 2014; Feniger-Schaal & Lotan, 2017; Shaw et al., 2010; Sossin & Shaw, 2011). Today, the Kestenberg Movement Profile (KMP) forms an integral part of the academic curriculum of dance/movement therapy under the jurisdiction of the American Dance Therapy Association. It is also included in accredited courses leading to the Swiss higher diploma in dance/movement therapy. It appears as an optional component in programmes accredited by the European Dance Therapy Association. The following section provides an illustrative overview of current studies employing the KMP.

Most recently, Gonzalez-Dolginko (2021) developed an adaptation of the KMP applicable to art therapy. Gonzalez-Dolginko retained the developmental and psychodynamic roots of the KMP and extended it with a more pronounced object-relations perspective. In 2015, to advance operationalisation and coding criteria in the KMP and to support its use beyond specialist movement and dance contexts, Loman, Johnson-French, and Serasis conducted the KMP video project. It compiled video material for all movement patterns listed in the KMP, with added voice-over explanations, providing a visual and didactic reference for the system.[1]

Araki's study (2017), conducted in the Mind, Movement, Interaction and Development Research Group at Pace University, investigated relationships between maternal movement patterns coded with the KMP. Both constellations of patterns and sequential patterns (e.g., *Direct* followed by *Strong Effort*, or *Acceleration* followed by *Direct Effort*) were examined in relation to

DOI: 10.4324/9781003559955-6

personality dimensions such as extraversion, neuroticism, and agreeableness. Findings suggested that particular movement qualities and sequences may be associated with distinct interaction styles and potential defensive functions. The study provided a basis for further investigations of maternal personality and relational qualities through the lens of sequential movement processes (Sossin, 2018). Feniger-Schaal and Lotan (2017) examined associations between movement patterns and attachment styles in adults. Study participants engaged in the mirror game (a nonverbal interaction in which partners mirror each other's movements), which was then analysed using the KMP's *Shaping in Directions* and *Shaping in Planes* categories. Feniger-Schaal and Lotan (2017) identified significant links between shaping patterns in the vertical, horizontal, and sagittal planes and the dimensions of attachment anxiety and avoidance. They suggested that the persistence and elaboration of early-acquired movement patterns into adulthood may relate to the complexity of attachment orientations, and that analysing movement interactions can offer a nonverbal window on to attachment-related tendencies. Bromberg (2015) applied KMP-based analysis to the micro-sequencing of facial movements in mother–infant interactions. In addition to focusing on overall movement frequencies, specific facial movement sequences were examined in relation to maternal depressive tendencies. This sequential approach highlighted the KMP's sensitivity to capturing nuanced nonverbal processes and to exploring how maternal depressive tendencies may be reflected in the unfolding of mother–infant interactions (cf. Sossin, 2018).

An experimental study drawing on KMP concepts investigated the impact of *Light* versus *Strong* movement qualities on affect and memory (Koch et al., 2014). A Movement-Based Affect Scale (MBAS) was used based on the KMP. The results indicated that distinct movement qualities were associated with different affective states. These findings were interpreted as supporting the significance of dynamic body feedback in cognitive and affective processes and highlighting the role of movement qualities in shaping such feedback. A quasi-experimental pilot study involving a child diagnosed with Down syndrome employed the KMP, along with standardised behavioural measures and naturalistic observation, to assess nonverbal social skills, developmental movement, and relational patterns. The authors suggested that an embodied, movement-focused intervention based on the KMP could highlight the child's "strengths in visual memory, imitation, receptive language, and nonverbal communication" (Gass et al., 2013, p. 13). Additionally, they argued that the KMP could be used to address misattunements in child–caregiver interactions.

Shaw et al. (2010) examined mother–child dyads, focusing on how observed movement patterns and emotional availability within the caregiver–infant dyad related to maternal personality traits and child temperament. Movements in free play were notated using the KMP. Significant associations were reported between distinct movement patterns, maternal personality dimensions (such as neuroticism, extraversion, and conscientiousness), and child temperament, suggesting that movement behaviour could serve as a channel through which aspects of parental personality and child disposition are expressed. In related work, Sossin and Shaw (2011) identified movement patterns associated with heightened emotion, such as *Widening* and *Lengthening* in *Bipolar Shape-Flow* and *Unipolar Lengthening Up*, that occur during sequences of mind-to-mindedness and joint attention. These patterns were later discussed as potential indices of *Tension-Flow* and *Shape-Flow* configurations associated with pre-mentalising events, where communication conveys empathy and understanding without a complete sharing of feeling (cf. Sossin, 2018).

Sossin (2007, 2015, 2018), Frances La Barre (2001, 2018), and Birklein (2018) highlighted the applicability of Kestenberg's embodied framework to the interpretation of nonverbal phenomena in the analytic space. Sossin (2015) proposed integrating the KMP with mentalisation-based therapy for individuals with high-functioning autism spectrum disorder (ASD). He argued that the KMP provides therapists with insights into intra- and intersubjective regulation patterns, sense of self, and self–other representations. Sossin (2015) added that Kestenberg's concepts of *Shape-Flow* adjustment and *Tension-Flow* attunement may facilitate the development of shared affective states and a sense of being recognised. He proposed that therapeutic interventions for individuals with ASD should focus on self-regulation patterns manifested in the alignment or discord between *Tension-Flow* and *Shape-Flow*, as well as between *Efforts* and *Shaping*, within the individual's movement repertoire.

La Barre (2018) emphasised that the KMP equips analysts with embodied attention and a vocabulary for understanding "the flow of movement in kinetic text" (p. 245). She highlighted that the analyst's kinaesthetic attunement to a patient's *Tension-Flow* and corresponding adjustments in *Shape-Flow* thereby support the development of a therapeutic alliance and holding environment (La Barre, 2018). She also noted that psychoanalytic dialogue is co-created not only through words but also through nonverbal behaviour, kinaesthetic text, and bodily attention. By tracking and responding to patterns of *Tension-Flow*, via vocal intonation or slight shifts in gesture and posture, feeling states rooted in early experiences can be evoked in the therapeutic space. Birklein (2018, pp. 247–251) illustrated the use of the KMP in analytic therapy with a client who had experienced childhood trauma and sexual abuse. She described the client's movement as marked by a loss of *Tension-Flow* plasticity and absence of temporality, conveying a state of psychic withdrawal. Birklein initially adopted a *Neutral Flow* and *Low Intensity*, constricted posture and subsequently introduced expanding and *Bulging* movement patterns to regulate the client's tension and foster a sense of safety. The client slowly responded with new *Tension-Flow* and *Shape-Flow* patterns, deeper breathing, lifting her head, and establishing eye contact (Birklein, 2018, p. 250). Birklein concluded that the KMP allowed the embodied dimension of the therapeutic process to emerge, thus deepening clinical understanding and illuminating the relational dynamics of the analytic relationship. Birklein further noted that Kestenberg's work offers a clearly articulated movement language already linked to psychoanalytic developmental theory, providing a foundation for enriching psychoanalysis with greater embodied depth. Additionally, she (Birklein, personal communication, 11 November 2022) emphasised that the next, urgent steps for the future of the KMP are to deliberately foreground cultural and gender diversity so that the framework more accurately reflects and responds to a broader range of human experience.

Afterlives of Transgenerational Trauma Concepts

Kestenberg's concept of transposition and her Holocaust studies have been reflected upon by various contemporary trauma researchers (Eickhoff, 2006; Eisold, 2012; Kangisser Cohen et al., 2017; Brenner, 2020; Bakó & Zana, 2021; Békés & Starrs, 2021; Naszkowska, 2023). Eickhoff (2006) cited Kestenberg's formulations on the unconscious, embodied aspect of trauma transmission. Eisold (2012) also drew on Kestenberg's concept of transposition in her study of historical trauma and prejudice among first-generation Chinese Americans.

In 2017, an anthology entitled *Children in the Holocaust and Its Aftermath* compiled interdisciplinary studies on testimonies from the Kestenberg Holocaust Child Survivor Archive (originally known as the Jerome Riker International Study of Organised Persecution of Children at the Hebrew University, Israel). "The archive consists of more than 1,500 testimonies from child survivors across the world, war children from Germany and Poland, and caretakers, and additional post-liberation depositions collected by the Central Jewish Historical Commission in Poland" (Kangisser Cohen et al., 2017, p. 5). The volume introduced readers to the complexities of studying the testimonies of child survivors of the Nazi Holocaust from historical, psychological, and ethical perspectives, considering both wartime and postwar contexts. Several chapters analyse non-Jewish childhoods under Nazism. Person (2017) compared Polish, Jewish, and non-Jewish testimonies, and Brüning (2017) explored how perpetrators' children negotiated their parents' crimes. Quindeau, Einert, and Teuber (2017) analysed new interviews with those who grew up in the Third Reich. Turning to reconstruction after the Nazi Holocaust, Cohen (2017) traced the reconstitution of Jewish families. Mihăilescu (2017) assessed how family structure informs memory and personality. Bass-Wichelhaus (2017) considered resilience, and Isserman (2017) examined survivors' attitudes towards perpetrators. Horváth and Zana (2017) showed how Hungarian specificities and the postwar context conditioned coping and identity, thereby initiating a comparative frame. Methodologically, Saban, Sossin, and Yasik (2017) combined qualitative and quantitative analyses to demonstrate that parental adjustment predicts children's later psychological functioning. Young (2017) examined how public memory inflects individual testimony.

Another recent volume, edited by Ira Brenner (2020), gathered leading scholars and clinicians to examine the effects of the Nazi Holocaust from multiple angles. Contributors from four continents wove together research, clinical work, and personal accounts to explore themes of resilience, memory, testimony, ageing, and mourning. Central throughlines of the volume are how trauma reverberates across generations, for both victims and perpetrators, including comparative contexts, and the politicisation and misuse of Holocaust memory. Therapeutic chapters address the distinct needs of survivors and their second and third generations, drawing on psychoanalysis alongside other treatment approaches. Bekerman-Greenberg (2020) expanded Holocaust studies into the third generation and reported on her psychoanalytically oriented group work with grandchildren of survivors. Her case studies underscored Kestenberg's notion of *transposition* and the unique combination of ego-strength and weakness among survivors (p. 125). Also drawing on Kestenberg's *transposition*, Gampel (2020) introduced the notions of "radioactive identification" and "radioactive transmission" to describe how large-scale political violence leaves enduring, clinically palpable effects. Gampel explained this concept, centring on the idea that events distant in time and place still exert psychic effects. These impacts can be received passively and transmitted onwards, so that residues of socio-political violence can persist as lingering traces of dread contributing to distress or illness across generations. Gampel's formulations emphasised the layered, embodied forms of inheritance, described as crypt-like deposits in the body, "vampiric" identifications, and displacements into past worlds (pp. 105–106). Eickhoff (2020) exemplified Kestenberg's pioneering influence on psychoanalytic approaches to Holocaust-related transmission in his case study of a patient who was a child of Nazi persecutors and developed a dissociative identity disorder. Kestenberg Amighi (2020) extended core questions of her parents' studies to two cases of mass violence – the Rwandan genocide of the Tutsi people and the oppression and mass murder of Palestinians in Gaza. Drawing on the conceptual tools of the studies on the Nazi Holocaust conducted by her parents, Kestenberg Amighi argued that genocide always leaves in survivors a persistent "tension beyond diagnosis" (J. Kestenberg, cited in Valent, 1998). She clarified that conventional notions of post-traumatic stress are inadequate for understanding children who grow up during mass violence, because, in these cases, the effects of trauma are rarely 'post'. The trauma persists beyond the end of armed conflict, continuing within survivors' psyches and within their postwar environments. Kestenberg Amighi (2020) illuminated that ongoing denial, silencing, lack of reparations, incomplete reconciliation, and the absence of supportive contexts for survivor communities to develop their own narratives shape the long-term consequences of genocide.

Devastated by the ongoing genocide of Palestinians in Gaza and the West Bank, I found myself lamenting many of Kestenberg's concepts. For me, perhaps the most important aspect of her legacy is the unwavering ethical commitment to children. Her studies on the effects of the Nazi Holocaust showed the specific vulnerabilities of children living under persecution. She was vocal that the impacts of trauma and dehumanisation do not end with persecution; they reach into bodies, family histories, and generations not yet born. Her *International Study of the Organised Persecution of Children* widened its scope to include trauma narratives of non-Jewish children and children of Nazi persecutors, expanding the category of survivor to all those who were children during the German Nazi regime. These studies showed us that genocidal projects not only victimise their chosen 'other' but also injure their own children through positing a world-view in which one's survival is contingent upon killing others. It is difficult not to hear the echo of Kestenberg's warnings today, when "Jewish safety" is politically mobilised to justify the genocide against the Palestinians. Here, the language of protection becomes entangled with practices of mass destruction, only creating further divisions, endangering both Palestinian and Jewish life. The mass atrocities, gender-based violence, and ongoing humanitarian catastrophes in Sudan and the eastern region of the Democratic Republic of Congo further echo Kestenbergian notions that death-driven ideologies and violence only imperil our collective survival. Kestenberg's work also exemplified the care and sensitivity one needs to support survivors to process the various intricate ways such horrific trauma affects them. Instead of focusing solely on pathology, she also highlighted survivors' creative attempts at working-through. She also insisted that telling one's story can be healing. I believe her oeuvre embodies our task of creating and protecting spaces where survivors of persecution today can begin to reclaim their narratives.

Contemporary Echoes

There are palpable echoes between contemporary concepts in infant mental health and Kestenberg's embodied developmental concepts. The following section traces these echoes and consonances.

Kestenberg's notion of kinaesthetic attunement through *Tension-* and *Shape-Flow* and its significance in the development of early self-and-other schemas seem to be resonant with current concepts of marked affect mirroring (Fonagy et al., 2002; Fonagy, Bateman et al., 2012; Gergely, 2004, 2007; Gergely & Unoka, 2008; Gergely & Watson, 1996, 1999), synrhythmia (Malloch & Trevarthen, 2009), vitality affects, and interaffectivity (Stern, 1971, 1998). The psychoanalytically informed, embodied child guidance interventions at Kestenberg's Center for Parents and Children align with the approach of current mentalisation-based treatments in analytic therapy and parent–child psychotherapy (Knoblauch, 1997, 2007, 2017; Bucci, 1997). Several contemporary researchers in child development commented on the relevance and richness of Kestenberg's developmental framework in understanding body–mind processes. Jonathan Delafield-Butt[2] praised the KMP as a highly detailed and sensitive methodology that provides a structure for approaching the affective and embodied mind. Beatrice Beebe[3] commented that the *Movement Profile* offers an invaluable approach to understanding nonverbal communication.

The backbone of Kestenberg's developmental movement studies was the understanding that somatic and movement experiences of the early years are not only forerunners but organisers of psychic development (Kestenberg et al., 1971; Kormos, 2021). In consonance, Luyten et al. (2012) stated that "there can be little doubt that the first experiences of reflective thinking are somatic in nature" (p. 404). Delafield-Butt and Trevarthen (2015) posited that the primary conscious perceptions of the self emerge from experiences of muscle action as the body stretches during contact or shrinks away in detachment. Kestenberg captured this phenomenon in her *Shape-Flow* category (Kestenberg et al., 1971; Kestenberg, 1967). Furthermore, Delafield-Butt and Trevarthen (2015, p. 1) located the "origins of narrative within the innate sensorimotor intelligence of a highly mobile human body and traced its development from initial manifestations in movement. They contended that aspects of intelligent planning, coupled with self-awareness, are observable in the gestures and movement expressions of the mid-gestation fetus. After birth, these individual intentions are sequentially structured into projects with increasingly ambitious objectives and social significance". They further explained that shared cultural rituals depend on foundational corporeal practices and psychomotor structures. These serve as "generative processes of thought-in-action," organising nonverbal actions into complex, expressive, and exploratory sequences of sense-making that lead to the establishment of conventional meanings with narrative power. In a similar vein to Kestenberg, Delafield-Butt and Trevarthen (2015) recognised the importance of embodied experiences and the organisation and function of motor action in the process of meaning-making.

The developmental and clinical concept of mentalisation, pioneered by Fonagy, Watson, Gergely, and Target (Gergely & Watson, 1996, 1999; Fonagy et al., 2002; Fonagy, Bateman et al., 2012; Fonagy & Allison, 2012; Mayes et al., 2007), has attracted considerable interest across fields spanning psychoanalysis, neuroscience, child development, genetics, and existential philosophy and phenomenology. Fonagy, Allison et al. (2012) defined mentalisation as a complex, imaginative, and predominantly preconscious mental state that is essential for affect regulation and enables the interpretation of others' intentions, feelings, and mental states (p. 11). From a developmental perspective, Jurist (2002, p. 190) argued that children become able to mentalise when their caregivers actively engage in mentalising about them. This account integrates psychoanalytic and attachment theories by situating the child's developing sense of mind within reflective caregiving (cf. Fonagy et al., 2002). Fonagy and Target (2007) and Mayes et al. (2007) used the concept of "embodied cognition" to challenge attachment theory's reliance on disembodied information-processing models, emphasising that mentalising grows from sensorimotor and affective exchanges (Jurist, 2022, p. 190). Shai and Belsky (2011, p. 175) described parental embodied mentalising as the process by which the parent implicitly infers and anticipates the infant's mental state from the infant's kinaesthetic expression and synchronises their own somatic patterns accordingly. Gergely and Watson (1996) emphasised that the healthy development of a sense of self requires the caregiver to contingently mirror the infant's emotional cues. They viewed contingent mirroring as a process that goes beyond mere timing, spatial alignment, and emotional resonance. It also requires markedness – that is, the exaggeration or slight distortion of the infant's emotional signals by the caregiver. Apparent cues that accompany the caregiver's affective response signal a pedagogical situation that prompts the infant to search for the intended referent. The 'markedness' of mirroring, characterised by subtle biological cues that signal that the displayed affect is not the caregiver's own, enables the infant to recognise that the expressed emotion does not reflect the caregiver's emotional state (Gergely & Watson, 1996, p. 1197). The infant must then identify the referent of this marked emotional display, often relying on external cues such as the caregiver's gaze direction. As the caregiver produces these marked affect mirroring displays while looking at and orienting towards the infant, the infant's attention is drawn to their own face and body. This contingent feedback supports the infant's developing understanding of both others' emotions and intentions and their own (Fonagy, Bateman et al., 2012, p. 24). Marked mirroring therefore enables the infant to attribute the displayed emotional experience to themselves, rather than to the caregiver (Fonagy et al., 2002; Gergely, 2004). Through this process, infants internalise representations of their experiences, thus developing a representational system for understanding internal states akin to a social "biofeedback mechanism" (Gergely & Watson, 1996).

Trevarthen and Aitken (2001) argued that primary intersubjectivity may be an early innate capacity of the human infant, expressed at the perceptual level through the recognition of movements, prosodic features, gestures, and rhythmic qualities. Beebe and Lachmann (1988, p. 305) further clarified that structures of interaction are created through patterns of mutual influence between the infant and caregivers, which the infant comes to expect. These patterns can be cognitively recalled even though they lack semantic meaning. They are encoded at a nonverbal level and can be affectively experienced, yet are difficult to elaborate symbolically. Stern (1971, 1998, 2010) examined the process of attunement between infant and caregiver, which he defined as a continuous process of interactive patterning of matching and mismatching across various perceptual and motion-based modalities. Tronick and Cohn (1989) emphasised the importance of matching and mismatching somatic interactions between infants and caregivers. They argued that mismatching is especially necessary for the growth of the relationship when it is accompanied by responsive attempts at repair in the attunement. Malloch and Trevarthen (2009) coined the term "synrhythmia" to denote the subtle processes of rhythmic and movement-based harmonisation between infant and caregiver, which provide the basis for intersubjectivity and play a significant role in mentalisation.

Mentalisation-based treatment models highlight increased vulnerability to psychopathology among individuals exposed to stressful psychosocial situations during early attachment, particularly when affect mirroring is inadequate (Fonagy et al., 2012; Gergely & Watson, 1996). Similarly, Kestenberg aimed to train parents in kinaesthetic attunement at the Center for Parents and Children to prevent attachment issues, childhood trauma, and subsequent psychopathology. Contemporary mentalisation-based treatment approaches aim to reconfigure body-image distortions, resulting in hyper-embodied states (when the individual experiences their somatic and internal states as immediate and 'too real') or in disembodied disconnection from somatic and affective states (Skårderud & Fonagy, 2012, p. 475). Mechanisms to enable patients to mind their own bodies are at the centre of these approaches. Within models of embodied mentalisation, the therapist, analogous to a securely attached mother, might engage in marked mirroring, demonstrating attunement and kinaesthetic empathy while maintaining a clear distinction between self and other. This process may include the explicit display of affective coping strategies through exaggerated, slowed, and schematic movements that differ from the therapist's typical movement repertoire (Fonagy et al., 2002; Fonagy, Bateman et al., 2012; Gergely, 2004, 2007; Gergely & Unoka, 2008; Gergely & Watson, 1996).

Kestenberg's movement-analytic system offers a detailed vocabulary for specifying the bodily parameters of precisely these processes of attunement and markedness within mentalisation-based models. Within this framework, kinaesthetic attunement, shaped by modulations of intensity, temporal, and gravity factors in *Tension-Flow Attributes* and the dimensions of *Bipolar* and *Unipolar Shape-Flow* (Kestenberg, 1965a, 1965b, 1967, 1985), can be conceptualised as the motor mechanisms underlying marked mirroring, affect attunement, and synrhythmicity. Consistent with Fonagy, Bateman et al. (2012) and contemporary mentalisation-based treatments, Kestenberg (1965a) argued that different forms of partial, selective, and complete attunement (varying across *Tension-Flow* and *Shape-Flow*) have distinct implications for the development of relationality and intersubjective affect-regulation.

The basic tenet of Kestenberg's work was that the systematic analysis of movement behaviour allows for a deeper understanding of intra- and intersubjective processes; the cataloguing of movement patterns furthers knowledge of the nature, function, and organisation of bodily movement, thereby enabling clinicians to develop sophisticated interventions to address body–mind processes. In consonance with this, Knoblauch (1997, 2005, 2007, 2017, 2018) emphasised the need to expand the understanding of embodied experience in analytic therapy to include the body's ability to express emotional states and its role in guiding the analyst's attention. He argued that attention to subsymbolic embodied registrations enables therapists to engage with distinct self-states during the analytic process. Furthermore, alternating between symbolic and subsymbolic levels of experience may facilitate the construction of meaning regarding the affective states of both the analyst and the patient (Knoblauch, 2005).

Stern's (1971, 2010) vitality affects, Bucci's (1997) subsymbolic layers of experience, Fonagy et al. (2002) and Knoblauch's (2005, 2017) fluid emotional activity and embodied registrations of rhythmic patterning all denote somatically based processes that, owing to their affective density and transmodally fluid organisational structures, cannot be symbolically represented and yet play a vital role in the development of self-and-other schemas. Kiersky and Beebe (1994, p. 390) defined interaction structures as shaped by the "dimensions of affective stimulation, temporal patterns, spatial relationships, and related proprioceptive arousal." Volume, tone, rhythm, tempo, and visual cues – in other words, process contours – contribute to structuring these patterns into a recognisable shape. Schore (2003) asserted that the therapist's awareness and understanding of changes in their own embodied states could be crucial for evaluating the differences between constructive and potentially destructive countertransferential influences on the therapeutic process. Bucci (1997) distinguished between symbolic and subsymbolic processes. She explained that "the categorical function, by which the continuous gradients of perceptual experience are chunked into discrete prototypical images, is the core of the symbolising process" (p. 142). By contrast, subsymbolic processing is continuous rather than discrete and can proceed in parallel across multiple pathways. The recognition of another's feeling state is grounded in subtle shifts in posture or facial expression (Bucci, 1997, p. 197). Kestenberg's psychodynamic vocabulary of movement explicitly addressed these concerns about the multilayered and intertwined nature of psychological and somatic processes; her notion of *Tension-Flow* was intended to capture the precise vitality features of changing affective states.

Jurist (2022) proposed the method of mentalised affectivity, a psychoanalytic approach to emotion that integrates body and mind by regulating feeling through autobiographical memory, focusing on how emotions have been lived in one's personal, familial, and cultural history. Rather than prioritising cognitive appraisal, this model brings cognition and affect together via the re-experiencing of emotion. Jurist (2022, p. 194) organised this work into three interlocking processes: identifying emotions (naming them and situating them in personal meaning and history); processing emotions (modulating intensity and duration, tolerating and differentiating complex blends, and comparing them with how one wishes to feel); and expressing emotions (communicating feelings outwardly to others and inwardly to oneself). As a contribution to body–mind perspectives in psychoanalysis, mentalised affectivity highlights how felt bodily states, memory, and meaning co-constitute one another. Jurist's (2022) considerations of the subprocess involved in emotional expression resonate with Kestenberg's notions of degree of intensity and degree and rate of change in relation to *Tension-Flow Attributes*, which she considered somatic, qualitative features of emotional expression. Applying variations of Kestenberg's *Tension-Flow Attributes* could contribute to a more varied somatic perspective on Jurist's (2022) approach of mentalised affectivity. Levit (2018) argued for the use of body-oriented methods, such as somatic experiencing, encouraging a more sustained attention to moment-to-moment bodily states in psychoanalytic therapy. Echoing Kestenberg, he stressed the need for a rapprochement between psychoanalysis and body-oriented therapies. In his view, careful tracking of bodily sensations supports regulation of emotions and access to their symbolic elaboration. As demonstrated in earlier chapters, creating a closer proximal relationship between analytic and embodied therapies was also a central focus of Kestenberg's work.

Kestenberg's concepts of kinaesthetic attunement and *Tension-* and *Shape-Flow* dynamics align with embodied notions in current discourse of the psy-sciences. These echoes suggest that Kestenberg's work on the somatic mechanisms underlying early developmental processes could be considered as conceptual antecedent to contemporary concepts in infant mental health and embodied mentalisation. Tracing these continuities not only enriches the historical record but also deepens our current understanding of the varied pathways through which affect and cognition are embodied.

Notes

1 I encourage readers to visit the KMP Video Project's website, see https://kestenbergmovementprofile.org/kmp-training-videos. And consult the demonstration videos available on the YouTube channel of the KMP Video Project, see https://www.youtube.com/@kmpvideoproject4908.

2 Lecturer in Developmental Psychology and Director of the Autism Innovation Laboratory at the University of Strathclyde. Read the critics' reviews here: https://www.routledge.com/The-Meaning-of-Movement-Embodied-Developmental-Clinical-and-Cultural-Perspectives-of-the-Kestenberg-Movement-Profile/KestenbergAmighi-Loman-Sossin/p/book/9781138484634

3 Clinical Professor of Medical Psychology, Columbia University Medical Center. Read the critics' reviews here: https://www.routledge.com/The-Meaning-of-Movement-statothers'Embodied-Developmental-Clinical-and-Cultural-Perspectives-of-the-Kestenberg-Movement-Profile/KestenbergAmighi-Loman-Sossin/p/book/9781138484634

References

Araki, M. (2017). Maternal movement patterns in relation to personality features and emotional availability. Doctoral dissertation, Pace University, New York, NY.

Bakó, T., & Zana, K. (2021). *A transzgenerációs atmoszféra: kollektív társadalmi traumák átörökítésének mélylélektani modellje* [Transgenerational atmosphere: Psychoanalytic model of collective trauma transmission]. In K. Bárdos, M. Heller, and

K. Vörös (Eds.), *A holokauszt nemzedékei. Traumatizált generációk az interperszonális, szociális és kulturális térben* [Generations of the Holocaust. Traumatised generations in the interpersonal, social and cultural space]. Konferenciakötet [Conference publication]. Animula.

Bass-Wichelhaus, H. (2017). Resilience in child survivors: History and application of coding of the international study of organized persecution of children. In S.K. Cohen, E. Fogelman, & D. Ofer (Eds.), *Children in the Holocaust and its aftermath: Historical and psychological studies of the Kestenberg Archive* (1st ed., pp. 170–184). Berghahn Books. doi:10.2307/j.ctvw04hks.12

Beebe, B., & Lachmann, F.M. (1988). The contribution of mother–infant mutual influence to the origins of self- and object representations. *Psychoanalytic Psychology*, 5(4), 305–337. doi:10.1037/0736–9735.5.4.305

Bekerman-Greenberg, R. (2020). Third generation. In I. Brenner (Ed.), *The handbook of psychoanalytic Holocaust studies: International perspectives* (pp. 119–126). Routledge. doi:10.4324/9780429292965–15

Békés, V., & Starrs, J.C. (2021). A transzgenerációs és történelmi traumaátadás egyéni és családi mechanizmusai: sérülékenység és reziliencia tényezők [The mechanisms of transgenerational trauma transmission: Factors of vulnerability and resilience]. In K. Bárdos, M. Heller, & K. Vörös (Eds.), *A holokauszt nemzedékei. Traumatizált generációk az interperszonális, szociális és kulturális térben* [Generations of the Holocaust. Traumatised generations in the interpersonal, social and cultural space]. Konferenciakötet [Conference publication]. Animula.

Birklein, S. (2018). Contours of vitality in movement. In J. Kestenberg Amighi, S. Loman, & K.M. Sossin (Eds.), *The meaning of movement: Embodied developmental, clinical, and cultural perspectives of the Kestenberg Movement Profile* (2nd ed., pp. 247–251). Routledge. doi:10.4324/9781351038706

Brenner, I. (Ed.). (2020). *The handbook of psychoanalytic Holocaust studies: International perspectives*. Routledge. doi:10.4324/9780429292965

Bromberg, Y. (2015). Sequential shape flow facial patterns among 12-month-olds correspondent to maternal dependency and self-criticism: A microanalytic application of the Kestenberg Movement Profile. Dissertations and theses, Pace University, New York, NY. Retrieved from https://search.proquest.com/docview/1749873092?accountid=13044

Brüning, C.I. (2017). Insights into the German interviews of the Kestenberg Archive: Children of perpetrators and how they dealt with their parents' actions. In S. Kangisser Cohen, E. Fogelman, & D. Ofer (Eds.), *Children in the Holocaust and its aftermath: Historical and psychological studies of the Kestenberg Archive* (1st paperback ed., pp. 224–246). Berghahn Books. doi:10.1515/9781785334399–011

Bucci, W. (1997). *Psychoanalysis and cognitive science: A multiple code theory*. Guilford.

Cohen, B.B. (2017). Starting over: Reconstituted families after the Holocaust. In S. Kangisser Cohen, E. Fogelman, & D. Ofer (Eds.), *Children in the Holocaust and its aftermath: Historical and psychological studies of the Kestenberg Archive* (1st ed., pp. 62–80). Berghahn Books. doi:10.2307/j.ctvw04hks.7

Delafield-Butt, J.T., & Trevarthen, C. (2015). The ontogenesis of narrative: From moving to meaning. *Frontiers in Psychology*, 6. doi:10.3389/fpsyg.2015.01157

Eickhoff, F. (2006). Nachträglichkeit from the perspective of the phylogenetic factor in Freud's Moses and monotheism. *The Scandinavian Psychoanalytic Review*, 29(1), 53–59. doi:10.1080/01062301.2006.10592780

Eickhoff, F.W. (2020). Transmitted unatoned guilt. In I. Brenner (Ed.), *The handbook of psychoanalytic Holocaust studies: International perspectives* (pp. 143–152). Routledge. doi:10.4324/9780429292965

Eisold, B. (2012). The implications of family expectations, historical trauma, and prejudice in psychoanalytic psychotherapy with naturalized and first-generation Chinese Americans. *Contemporary Psychoanalysis,* 48(2), 238–266. doi:10.1080/00107530.2012.10746500

Feniger-Schaal, R., & Lotan, N. (2017). The embodiment of attachment: Directional and shaping movements in adults' mirror game. *Journal of Infant, Child, and Adolescent Psychotherapy,* 14, 294–310. doi:10.1080/15289168.2015.1066630

Fonagy, P., & Allison, E., (2012). What is mentalization? The concept and its foundations in developmental research. In N. Midgley & I. Vrouva (Eds.), *Minding the child: Mentalization-based interventions with children, young people and their families* (pp. 11–34). Routledge.

Fonagy, P., Bateman, A.W., & Luyten, P. (2012). Introduction and overview. In *Handbook of mentalizing in mental health practice* (pp. 3–43). American Psychiatric Association.

Fonagy, P., Gergely, G., Jurist, E.L., & Target, M. (2002). *Affect regulation, mentalization, and the development of the self.* Other Press.

Fonagy, P., & Target, M. (2007). The rooting of the mind in the body: New links between attachment theory and psychoanalytic thought. *Journal of the American Psychoanalytic Association*, 55, 411–456.

Fuchs, T., & Koch, S.C. (2014). Embodied affectivity: On moving and being moved. *Frontiers in Psychology,* 5. doi:10.3389/fpsyg.2014.00508

Gampel, Y. (2020). Trans-generational fallout. In I. Brenner (Ed.), *The handbook of psychoanalytic Holocaust studies: International perspectives* (pp. 103–110). Routledge. doi:10.4324/9780429292965-13

Gass, K.R., Kennedy, J.R., Hastie, S., & McCardell Wentworth, H. (2013). Somatic assessment of nonverbal social skills in children with Down syndrome: Using the Kestenberg Movement Profile as a tool for treatment planning. *Body, Movement and Dance in Psychotherapy: An International Journal for Theory, Research and Practice.* doi:10.1080/17432979.2012.744354

Gergely, G. (2004). The role of contingency detection in early affect-regulative interactions and in the development of different types of infant attachment. *Social Behavior,* 13, 468–478.

Gergely, G. (2007). The social construction of the subjective self: The role of affect-mirroring, markedness, and ostensive communication in self-development. In L. Mayes, P. Fonagy, & M. Target (Eds.), *Developmental science and psychoanalysis: Integration and innovation* (pp. 45–88). Karnac.

Gergely, G., & Unoka, Z. (2008). Attachment, affect-regulation and mentalization: The developmental origins of the representational affective self. In C. Sharp, P. Fonagy, & I. Goodyer (Eds.), *Social cognition and developmental psychopathology* (pp. 305–342). Oxford University Press.

Gergely, G., & Watson, J. (1996). The social biofeedback model of parental affect-mirroring. *International Journal of Psychoanalysis,* 77, 1181–1212.

Gergely, G., & Watson, J.S. (1999). Early socio-emotional development: Contingency perception and the social-biofeedback model. In P. Rochat (ed.) *Early social cognition: Understanding others in the first months of life* (pp. 101–136). Lawrence Earlbaum.

Gonzalez-Dolginko, B. (2021). *Applying developmental art theory in art therapy treatment and interventions: Illustrative examples through the life cycle.* Routledge.

Horváth, R., & Zana, K. (2017). Both valuable and difficult: A meeting point between historical and psychological interviews. In S. Kangisser Cohen, E. Fogelman, & D. Ofer (Eds.), *Children in the Holocaust and its aftermath: Historical and psychological studies of the Kestenberg Archive* (1st ed., pp. 81–96). Berghahn Books. doi:10.2307/j.ctvw04hks.8

Isserman, N. (2017). Symbolic revenge in Holocaust child survivors. In S. Kangisser Cohen, Fogelman, E., & Ofer, D. (Eds.), *Children in the Holocaust and its aftermath: Historical and psychological studies of the Kestenberg Archive* (1st paperback ed., pp. 150–170). Berghahn Books. doi:10.1515/9781785334399–011

Johnson, M. (2018). A KMP approach to treating adults with developmental disabilities in group therapy. In J. Kestenberg Amighi, S. Loman, & M.K. Sossin (Eds.), *The meaning of movement, embodied developmental, clinical and cultural perspectives of the Kestenberg Movement Profile* (2nd ed., pp. 251–255). Routledge.

Jurist, E. (2022). Mentalizing from/to/with the body. In *Psychoanalysis and the mind–body problem* (pp. 186–203). Routledge. doi:10.4324/9781003090755-doi:9

Kangisser Cohen, S., Fogelman, E., & Ofer, D. (Eds.). (2017). *Children in the Holocaust and its aftermath: Historical and psychological studies of the Kestenberg Archive* (1st paperback ed.). Berghahn Books.

Kestenberg Amighi, J. (2020). Holocaust, Rwanda, and Palestine. In I. Brenner (Ed.), *The handbook of psychoanalytic Holocaust studies: International perspectives* (pp. 219–230). Routledge. doi:10.4324/9780429292965–25

Kestenberg, J.S. (1965a). The role of movement patterns in development. I. Rhythms of movement. *Psychoanalytic Quarterly*, 24(1), 1–36. doi:10.1080/21674086.1965.11926334

Kestenberg, J.S. (1965b). The role of movement patterns in development. II. Flow of tension and effort. *Psychoanalytic Quarterly*, 24(4), 517–563. doi:10.1080/21674086.1965.11926363

Kestenberg, J.S. (1967). The role of movement patterns in development. III. Control of shape. *Psychoanalytic Quarterly*, 26(3), 356–409. doi:10.1080/21674086.1967.11926431

Kestenberg, J.S. (1985). The role of movement patterns in diagnosis and prevention. In D.A. Shaskan & W.I. Roller (Eds.), *Paul Schilder: Mind explorer* (pp. 97–161). Human Sciences Press.

Kestenberg, J.S., & Berlowe, J., Buelte, A., Hershey, M., & Robbins, E. (1971). Development of the young child as expressed through bodily movement I. *Journal of the American Psychoanalytic Association*, 19(4), 746–764.

Kiersky, S., & Beebe, B. (1994). The reconstruction of early nonverbal relatedness in the treatment of difficult patients: A special form of empathy. *Psychoanalytic Dialogues*, 4 (4), 389–408.

Knoblauch, S.H. (1997). Beyond the word in psychoanalysis: The unspoken dialogue. *Psychoanalytic Dialogues: The International Journal of Relational Perspectives*, 7(4), 491–516. doi:10.1080/10481889709539199

Knoblauch, S.H. (2005). Body rhythms and the unconscious: Toward an expanding of clinical attention. *Psychoanalytic Dialogues*, 15(6), 807–827. doi:10.2513/s10481885pd1506_2

Knoblauch, S.H. (2007). The perversion of language in the analyst's activity: Navigating the rhythms of embodiment and symbolization. *International Forum of Psychoanalysis,* 16(1), 38–42. doi:10.1080/08037060601020393

Knoblauch, S.H. (2017). The fluidity of emotions and clinical vulnerability: A field of rhythmic tensions. *Psychoanalytic Perspectives,* 14(3), 283–308.doi:10.1080/1551806X.2017.1342421

Knoblauch, S.H. (2018). Attention and narration to micro-moment registrations of embodied dialogue in the clinical interaction: How are we doing? *Psychoanalytic Inquiry,* 38(7), 502–510. doi:10.1080/07351690.2018.1504577

Koch, S.C. (2007). Defenses in movement: Video-analysis of conflict patterns in group communication. *Body, Movement and Dance in Psychotherapy,* 2(1), 29–45. doi:10.1080/17432970601025386

Koch, S.C. (2014). Rhythm is it: Effects of dynamic body feedback on affect and attitudes. *Frontiers in Psychology,* 5, 537. doi:10.3389/fpsyg.2014.00537

Koch, S.C., Fuchs, T., & Summa, M. (2014). Body memory and kinesthetic body feedback: The impact of light versus strong movement qualities on affect and cognition. *Memory Studies,* 7(3), 272–284.

Koch, S.C., Cruz, R.F., & Goodill, S. . (2001). The Kestenberg Movement Profile: Performance of novice raters. *American Journal of Dance Therapy,* 23(2), Fall/Winter.

Kormos, J. (2021). Kinaesthetic attunement, clashing and mismatches of early interactions and their influence in later development – theoretical introduction to the Kestenberg Movement Profile. *Imágó Budapest: Pszichoanalízis Társadalom Kultúra,* 10(1), 42–54.

La Barre, F. (2001). *On moving and being moved: Nonverbal behavior in clinical practice.* Routledge.

La Barre, F. (2018). The kinetic text: Using the KMP in psychoanalysis. In J. Kestenberg Amighi, S. Loman, & M.K. Sossin (Eds.), *The meaning of movement, embodied developmental, clinical and cultural perspectives of the Kestenberg Movement Profile* (2nd ed., pp. 243–246). Routledge.

Levit, D. (2018). Somatic experiencing: In the realms of trauma and dissociation – what we can do, when what we do is really not good enough. *Psychoanalytic Dialogues,* 28(5), 586–601.

Loman, S. (1998). Employing a developmental model of movement patterns in dance/movement therapy with young children and their families. *American Journal of Dance Therapy,* 20(2), 101–115. doi:10.1023/A:1022100511657

Loman, S. (2016). Judith S. Kestenberg's dance/movement therapy legacy: Approaches with pregnancy, young children, and caregivers. *American Journal of Dance Therapy,* 38(2), 225–244.

Loman, S., White, H., & Johnson French, M. (2021). Kestenberg Movement Profile (KMP) approaches to working with young children and caregivers in dance/movement therapy. *Journal of Infant, Child, and Adolescent Psychotherapy,* 20(1), 36–50. doi:10.1080/15289168.2021.1875703

Luyten, P., Fonagy, P., Lemma, A., & Target, M. (2012). Depression. In A.W. Bateman & P. Fonagy (Eds.), *Handbook of mentalizing in mental health practice* (pp. 385–418). American Psychiatric Publishing.

Malloch, S., & Trevarthen, C. (Eds.). (2009). *Communicative musicality: Exploring the basis of human companionship.* Oxford University Press.

Mayes, L., Fonagy, P., & Target, M. (Eds.). (2007). *Developmental science and psychoanalysis: Integration and innovation*. Karnac Books.

Mihăilescu, D. (2017). Shadows of memory and intergenerational legacies in child survivors' testimonies from the Kestenberg Archive. In S. Kangisser Cohen, E. Fogelman, & D. Ofer (Eds.), *Children in the Holocaust and its aftermath: Historical and psychological studies of the Kestenberg Archive* (1st ed., pp. 122–149). Berghahn Books. doi:10.2307/j.ctvw04hks.10

Naszkowska, K. (2023). Give me permission to remember: Judith S. Kestenberg and the memory of the Holocaust. In L. Henik & L. Aron (Eds.), *Contemporary psychoanalysis and Jewish thought: Answering a question with more questions* (pp. 197–217). Routledge.

Person, K. (2017). They were Jews, but they were very kind people: Polish language testimonies in the Kestenberg Child Survivor Archive. In S. Kangisser Cohen, E. Fogelman, & D. Ofer (Eds.), *Children in the Holocaust and its aftermath: Historical and psychological studies of the Kestenberg Archive* (1st paperback ed., pp. 187–199). Berghahn Books. doi:10.1515/9781785334399–011

Quindeau, I., Einert, K., & Teuber, N. (2017). War children in Nazi Germany and World War II. In S. Kangisser Cohen, E. Fogelman, & D. Ofer (Eds.), *Children in the Holocaust and its aftermath: Historical and psychological studies of the Kestenberg Archive* (1st ed., pp. 200–223). Berghahn Books. doi:10.2307/j.ctvw04hks.14

Saban, G.S., Sossin, K.M., & Yasik, A. (2017). Age, circumstance, and outcome in child survivors of the Holocaust: Considerations of the literature and a report of a study using narrative content analysis. In S. Kangisser Cohen, E. Fogelman, & D. Ofer (Eds.), *Children in the Holocaust and its aftermath: Historical and psychological studies of the Kestenberg Archive* (1st ed., pp. 15–40). Berghahn Books. doi:10.2307/j.ctvw04hks.5

Schore, A.N. (2003). *Affect regulation and the repair of the self.* Norton.

Shai, D., & Belsky, J. (2011). When words just won't do: Introducing parental embodied mentalizing. *Child Development Perspectives*, 5(3), 173–180.

Shaw, J., Sossin, K.M., & Salbod, S. (2010). Shape-Flow in embodied parent–child affect regulation: Heightened emotional expression in dyadic interaction. Paper presented at the World Association for Infant Mental Health, 12th World Congress: Infancy in Times of Transition. 1 July 2010. Leipzig, Germany.

Skårderud, F., & Fonagy, P. (2012). Eating disorders. In A.W. Bateman & P. Fonagy (Eds.), *Handbook of mentalizing in mental health practice* (pp. 347–383). American Psychiatric Publishing.

Sossin, K.M. (2007). The history and future of the Kestenberg Movement Profile. In S. Koch & S. Bender (Eds.), *Movement analysis – Bewegungsanalyse* (pp. 103–119). Logos.

Sossin, K.M. (2015). A movement-informed mentalization lens applied to psychodynamic psychotherapy of children and adolescents with high functioning autism spectrum disorder. *Journal of Infant, Child, and Adolescent Psychotherapy*, 14(3), 294–310. doi:10.1080/15289168.2015.1066630

Sossin, K.M. (2018). Musings on theoretical and research contributions of the KMP within the context of nonverbal studies. In J. Kestenberg Amighi, S. Loman, & M. K. Sossin (Eds.), *The meaning of movement, embodied developmental, clinical and cultural perspectives of the Kestenberg Movement Profile* (2nd ed., Kindle edition, pp. 287–316). Routledge.

Sossin, K.M., & Birklein, S.C. (2006). Nonverbal indices of stress in parent–child dyads: Implications for individual and interpersonal affect regulation and intergenerational transmission. In S. Koch & I. Bräuninger (Eds.), *Advances in dance/movement therapy: Theoretical perspectives and empirical findings* (pp. 128–141). Logos.

Sossin, K.M., & Shaw, J. (2011). Tension and shape-flow in marked moments: Nonverbal qualities embodied in parent–child affect regulation. *Infant Mental Health Journal*, 31 (Suppl. 3), 239.

Stern, D. (1971). A microanalysis of mother–infant interaction. *Journal of the American Academy of Child Psychiatry*, 10, 501–517. doi:10.1016/S0002-7138(09)61752-0

Stern, D.N. (1998). *The interpersonal world of the infant: A view from psychoanalysis and developmental psychology.* Karnac Books. (Original work published in 1985)

Stern, D.N. (2010). *Forms of vitality: Exploring dynamic experience in psychology, the arts, psychotherapy, and development*. Oxford University Press.

Trevarthen, C., & Aitken, K.J. (2001). Infant intersubjectivity: Research, theory, and clinical applications. *Journal of Child Psychology and Psychiatry*, 42(1), 3–48. doi:10.1111/1469-7610.00701

Tronick, E., & Cohn, J. (1989). Infant–mother face-to-face interaction: Age and gender differences in coordination and the occurrence of miscoordination. *Child Development*, 60, 85–92. doi:10.2307/1131074

Valent, P. (1998). *Children surviving persecution: An international study of trauma and healing*. Transaction.

Young, S. (2017). Performative memory-making and the future of the Kestenberg Archive. In S. Kangisser Cohen, E. Fogelman, & D. Ofer (Eds.), *Children in the Holocaust and its aftermath: Historical and psychological studies of the Kestenberg Archive* (1st ed., pp. 99–121). Berghahn Books. doi:10.2307/j.ctvw04hks.9

Chapter 6

Patterns of a Life

> I think she was what we call in movement studies a spreader. She did so many different things. I suppose when you spread your attention like that, you find integration.
>
> (Kestenberg Amighi, personal communication, 13 November 2021)

Judith S. Kestenberg belonged to the group of early-twentieth-century Jewish women who pursued university education during the interwar period and defied traditional gender expectations by seeking a professional identity in traditionally male-dominated fields (Freidenreich, 2002; Naszkowska, 2023). Her life illustrates the distinct challenges and opportunities encountered by Eastern European Jewish women in the shifting sociocultural context of the early twentieth century, including expanding professional opportunities for women, loss of home and family resulting from the rise of German Fascism, forced migration, the struggle to find belonging within new professional and cultural contexts, language barriers, and financial hardship.

The growing involvement of women in intellectual and artistic spheres during this era entailed moving beyond the private family domain and into public life, often while remaining subject to traditional gender expectations. This shift produced an intermediary social status, positioning many women as inside-outsiders, a role they had to actively navigate. Many served as intermediaries between groups, disciplines, and movements, bridging private and public domains and contributing significantly to the evolution of cultural, social, and artistic norms (Borgos, 2018, 2019; Gambrell, 1997). The lives of many early women psychoanalysts exemplify this process, as psychoanalysis was more accessible to middle-class women in early-twentieth-century Central Europe than any other scientific discipline (Borgos, 2019; Appignanesi & Forrester, 2000; Zaretsky, 2005). Kestenberg's career also demonstrated the potential of the inside-outsider position. She pursued underexplored, neglected topics, thereby introducing new perspectives to the male-dominated fields of American psychiatry and psychoanalysis (Borgos, 2018, 2019). Her work expanded the conceptual space of psychoanalysis with an embodied dimension. Through her psychosomatic vocabulary, concepts of bodily attunement,

DOI: 10.4324/9781003559955-7

and method of muscle-tension inscription, she was able to discuss child development in unique detail. Her career also poignantly shows the mediation between private and public domains, women's roles, motherhood, and academic aspirations. Through her contributions to child guidance, she aimed to enhance the status of parenting by providing specialised support and training for parents. She introduced the concept of a maternal developmental phase and argued that parenthood constitutes a distinct stage of development.

Kestenberg pursued a unique integration of artistic and scientific methods. In doing so, she contributed to the transfer of European modern dance ideals – particularly the legacy of Rudolf von Laban – into American clinical discourse. Although Kestenberg encountered Laban's work only after arriving in the United States, she was receptive to émigré networks, as her first movement teacher was the German Laban-trained dancer Irmgard Bartenieff. Kestenberg's theory and movement assessment remained closely tied to Laban's ideas of the moving body, especially the vibratory potential of gesture and its cultural and therapeutic significance, thus contributing to the migration and uptake of European intellectual traditions in the United States.

Kestenberg, like many early-twentieth-century educated women, primarily identified herself through her profession rather than gender identity (Naszkowska, 2022; Borgos, 2018, 2019). She was an independently minded person who was always proud to be herself and follow her own ideas (Kestenberg, 1991, 1992, p. 172; Naszkowska, 2023). In her daughter's view: "She always pursued and did what she wanted to do" (Kestenberg Amighi, personal communication, 13 November 2021). Across her oeuvre, themes of embodiment, prevention, and community development come to the fore. In the first epoch of her professional career, immersed in the psychodynamic study of movement, she established a community centre for families. Later, during a period devoted to the psychoanalytic study of the Nazi Holocaust, she founded the Child Survivors Association to connect survivors worldwide. Throughout her life, she was a dedicated advocate for vulnerable groups – especially children – and was committed to amplifying the voices of neglected groups of Holocaust survivors.

Kestenberg's body of work reveals a life in which personal experience and professional commitments were deeply intertwined. Her pursuits in psychiatry, psychoanalysis, infant observation, and trauma studies were mutually co-constructed by her own journey. According to Naszkowska's (2023, p. 200) studies of Jewish women in the psychoanalytic movement, Judith's case was somewhat atypical. Her family was observant and Orthodox, unlike most other Jewish women psychoanalysts in her cohort, whose families were generally non-observant. Another difference in Judith's upbringing was her mother's strong intellectual interests and commitment to supporting her daughter's university education (Naszkowska, 2023). This stands in contrast to the backgrounds of many early women psychoanalysts, whose mothers often discouraged their training. More often, their fathers were role models for them to pursue further education.

Both parents served as role models for Kestenberg. She attributed her analytic interests to both her mother's curiosity and psychological giftedness and to her father's innovative and indulgent temperament (Kestenberg, 1992, p. 156). Her father's democratic socialist convictions shaped her politics throughout her life (Kestenberg, 1975), a legacy her daughter recalled: "She advocated for civil rights and instilled in me a commitment to socialist values, which she also lived by in her daily life. She encouraged our housekeeper and nanny to pursue further education and offered to cover their expenses" (Kestenberg Amighi, personal communication, 13 November 2021). Although Kestenberg's parents supported her pursuit of higher education, they disapproved of her choice of medicine, considering it inappropriate for a woman to examine male corpses during medical training (Naszkowska, 2023, p. 201). She nevertheless stepped out of the parental prescription and pursued psychiatry. Kestenberg (1992) recalled that her mother's love of children shaped her career as a child development researcher, and her father's philanthropic spirit inspired her strong dedication to community development.

Family legacies took on various meanings for Kestenberg. Paternal figures remained important to her throughout her life, perhaps owing to her father's sporadic absences during her childhood. Educated in an Orthodox Jewish household, she described having a close relationship with God (Kestenberg, 1992). She recalled a condensed representation of her father, Freud, and God merged in a single parental imago. As she wrote: "for me, Freud has God's features. He knows so many things that no one else knows. [...] I learned a lot from the patriarchs. I can criticise Freud or develop new ideas that would interest him" (Kestenberg, 1992, p. 163). This fused image may explain her unwavering lifelong commitment to Freudian drive-theory, which she consistently maintained, even at the expense, at times, of aligning her work with dominant paradigms in psychoanalysis.

Kestenberg's early life was also marked by important somatic memories. The daily experience of lying in a scoliosis corset with her mother by her side may have sparked her interest in somatic sensations and the intimacy of early interactions between mother and child. From a young age, she felt drawn to dance; her imagination swirled with choreographic visions. In gymnastics, she delighted in the rush of leaping and soaring through the air (Kestenberg, 1992). These early experiences may have seeded her later interest in the psychic significance of somatic and kinaesthetic sensations.

Kestenberg's vocational choices were also shaped by loss and responsibility. The economic struggles her family endured in the 1920s pushed her towards a profession that promised security and the means to support her family. She indicated that her interest in neurology and psychiatry was shaped by her wish to heal her family members, and it was perhaps also a way to understand parts of herself that others (reportedly Max Schur and Heinz Hartmann) had interpreted as "neurotic" (Kestenberg, 1992, p. 165). Kestenberg stated that being a young child during the First World War was one of the most important aspects of her life, an experience through which she acquired a deep understanding of individual and societal hardship. She cherished fond memories of visiting with her mother a war orphanage that her father had established. Following the tragic loss of her parents in the Nazi Holocaust, she coped by throwing herself into work and began her infant observation studies. The decision to study child development was perhaps both an attempt to return to her parents' legacy and a way to process their inexplicable loss; a professional focus perhaps born out of the need to work through her personal trauma; a thread that wove through her life-work.

Kestenberg arrived in the United States in 1937. The economic depression of the 1930s, heightened concerns about foreign political influence, and the impending threat of the war contributed to widespread ethnic prejudice in American society. Anti-Semitism was on the rise, peaking in 1946 and persisting into the postwar period. Jewish émigrés encountered prejudices in the United States that closely resembled those they had previously faced in Europe (Aron & Starr, 2013, pp. 111–112). Forced to settle in New York by the outbreak of the Second World War, Kestenberg reportedly lacked fluency in English and struggled to express herself in her new professional environment (Kestenberg, 1992). As a foreigner in a discriminatory, tension-filled social environment that fractured her sense of identity and belonging, she sought a medium that could bridge these divisions; this was bodily movement. Her studies on the Nazi Holocaust could also be seen as further attempts to integrate the multiple losses she experienced, including the loss of her parents, her homes in Vienna and Poland, and significant aspects of her Polish-Jewish identity. Sossin expressed that the primary objective of Kestenberg's work was prevention, including both developmental trauma and trauma resulting from social-political atrocities (Sossin, personal communication, 1 November 2022). Throughout her career, she spoke out against oppressive authorities – parental and governmental – shining a light on their psychological and social consequences.

Looking at the life and work of Kestenberg, we can see a confluence of family inheritances, somatic sensibilities shaped by childhood constraints (scoliosis corset) and dance experience (gymnastics classes), the pragmatic demands of migration, and reparative attempts born of loss. These threads led to a career that, as Laemmli (2016, pp. 132–138) also argued, treated bodily movement as both evidence of and instrument for personal and social development, and as a way to reckon with the traumas of the twentieth century.

Examining Kestenberg's intellectual legacy has contributed to the current understanding of the history of the psy-sciences in the mid- to late twentieth century. Her oeuvre exemplified the centrality of infant observation and developmental assessment to efforts to legitimise psychoanalytic developmental concepts within the changing landscape of mid-century American psy-sciences. Her career also reflected the shift towards community-based settings and prophylactic approaches in the 1960s (Grob, 1991; Hale, 1995; Midgley,

2013; Polat, 2021). Her focus on bodily movement in the service of individual and societal well-being reflected Cold War discourses in the psy-sciences, in which the psychological analysis, paralinguistic interpretation, and the diagrammatic and therapeutic regulation of movement behaviour came to occupy a central place in the pursuit of the Western democratic project (Martin-Nielsen, 2010; Weinstein, 2013; Laemmli, 2016). Her formulations on sex-specific identity, parental attitudes, and parenthood as a developmental phase also exemplified the strong gender-stereotyped and heteronormative tendencies of American psychoanalysis, born out of internal debates on the centrality of the libido and external demands by religious critiques and emerging sexology research in the Cold War period (Herzog, 2016a, 2016b). The selective reception of her work exposed the power dynamics underpinning the circulation of ideas in mid- to late-twentieth-century American psychoanalysis and psy-sciences. In particular, the contrasting receptions of Kestenberg's and Stern's attunement concepts reveal how evidence hierarchies and scientific representational norms governed perceptions of knowledge.

Applying Bergmann's (1993, 1997) view of pioneers across categories of extenders, modifiers, and heretics, Kestenberg was a modifier. Her propositions generated controversy because they were perceived as threatening the theoretical continuity of psychoanalysis and unsettling the institutional and epistemic alliances of the time. Importantly, Bergmann (1993, 1997) argued that taking modifiers seriously requires an acknowledgement that development is neither linear nor neatly demarcated. Such recognition in American psychoanalysis between the 1950s and 1970s would perhaps have allowed the integration of Kestenberg's somatic concepts and movement vocabulary. Since the 1980s, generative collaborations between artistic and scientific approaches have become increasingly prominent in the psy-sciences, evidenced by the growing relevance of creative arts therapies and the emergence of arts-based research (Levy, 1988; Karkou & Sanderson, 2006, pp. 13–21). In parallel, an emphasis on embodiment sparked renewed interest in somatic processes in psychoanalysis (Shai & Fonagy, 2014; Lombardi, 2008, 2018, 2019, 2020; Lemma, 2014, 2020; Levit, 2018). These developments present a timely opportunity to integrate Judith S. Kestenberg's work into the historical narrative of American psychological sciences. I have sought to advance this integration by establishing a dedicated archival collection of Kestenberg's materials at the Manuscript Division of the Library of Congress, where her extensive body of work is now accessible to the public.

References

Appignanesi, L., & Forrester, J. (2000). *Freud's women*. Penguin Books.

Aron, L., & Starr, K. (2013). Psychoanalysis as Holocaust survivor. In *A psychotherapy for the people: Toward a progressive psychoanalysis* (pp. 111–127). Routledge.

Bergmann, M.S. (1993). Reflections on the history of psychoanalysis. *Journal of the American Psychoanalytic Association*, 41(4), 929–955. doi:10.1177/000306519304100402

Bergmann, M.S. (1997). The historical roots of psychoanalytic orthodoxy. *International Journal of Psychoanalysis*, 78, 69–86.

Borgos, A. (2018). *Holnaplányok: Nők a pszichoanalízis budapesti iskolájában* [Girls of tomorrow: Women in the Budapest school of psychoanalysis]. Noran Libro Kiadó.

Borgos, A. (2019). Nőtörténeti dokumentumok a pszichoanalízis-történetben [Documents of women's history in the history of psychoanalysis]. In C. Pléh, *A pszichológiatörténet-írás módszerei és a magyar pszichológiatörténet* [Methodologies of the history of psychology and the history of Hungarian psychology] (pp. 76–90). Gondolat.

Freidenreich, H.P. (2002). *Female, Jewish and educated*. Indiana University Press.

Gambrell, A. (1997). *Women intellectuals, modernism, and difference: Transatlantic culture, 1919–1945*. Cambridge University Press.

Grob, G.N. (1991). *From asylum to community mental health policy in modern America*. Princeton University Press.

Hale, N.G. (1995). *The rise and crisis of psychoanalysis in the United States: Freud and the Americans, 1917–1985*. Oxford University Press.

Herzog, D. (2016a). The libido wars. In *Cold War Freud: Psychoanalysis in an age of catastrophes* (pp. 21–55). Cambridge University Press. doi:10.1017/9781139680455.002

Herzog, D. (2016b). Homophobia's durability and the reinvention of psychoanalysis. In *Cold War Freud: Psychoanalysis in an age of catastrophes* (pp. 56–86). Cambridge University Press. doi:10.1017/9781139680455.003

Karkou, V., & Sanderson, P. (2006). Professional development of arts therapies. In V. Karkou & P. Sanderson (Eds.), *Arts therapies: A research-based map of the field* (pp. 8–29). Elsevier Science.

Kestenberg, J.S. (1975). Preface. In *Children and parents: Psychoanalytic studies in development* (pp. xv–xxvii). Jason Aronson.

Kestenberg, J.S. (1991). Dr. Judith S. Kestenberg talks to Kristina Stanton. *Free Associations*, 2(2), 157–174.

Kestenberg, J.S. (1992). Kindheit und Wissenschaft. Eine biographische Skizze. In L. M. Hermanns (Ed.) *Psychoanalyse in Selbstdarstellungen* (Vol. 1, pp. 147–202). Edition Diskord.

Laemmli, W.E. (2016). The choreography of everyday life: Rudolf Laban and the making of modern movement. Doctoral dissertation, University of Pennsylvania. Retrieved from: https://repository.upenn.edu/entities/publication/8f9a810d-1d39-46f7-a40a-2f57f833f645

Lemma, A. (2014). *Minding the body: The body in psychoanalysis and beyond*. Routledge.

Lemma, A. (2020). The aesthetic link: The patient's use of the analyst's body and the body of the consulting room. *Psychoanalytic Perspectives*, 17, 57–73. doi:10.1080/1551806X.2020.1769453

Levit, D. (2018). Somatic experiencing: In the realms of trauma and dissociation – what we can do, when what we do is really not good enough. *Psychoanalytic Dialogues*, 28(5), 586–601.

Levy, F. (1988). *Dance/movement therapy: A healing art*. The American Alliance for Health, Physical Education, Recreation and Dance.

Lombardi, R. (2008). The body in the analytic session: Focusing on the body–mind link. *International Journal of Psychoanalysis*, 89(1), 89–109. doi:10.1111/j.1745-8315.2007.00008.x

Lombardi, R. (2018). Beyond the psychosexual: The body–mind relationship discussion of somatic experiencing. *Psychoanalytic Dialogues*, 28(5), 629–639. doi:10.1080/10481885.2018.1483977

Lombardi, R. (2019). Mysteries, abysses, and impasses in body–mind dissociation. *International Journal of Psychoanalysis*, 100(6), 1371–1389. doi:10.1080/00207578.2019.1696647

Lombardi, R. (2020). Coronavirus, social distancing, and the body in psychoanalysis. *Journal of the American Psychoanalytic Association*, 68(3), 455–462. doi:10.1177/0003065120937024

Martin-Nielsen, J. (2010). This war for men's minds: The birth of a human science in Cold War America. *History of the Human Sciences*, 23(5), 131–155. doi:10.1177/0952695110378952

Midgley, N. (2013). *Reading Anna Freud*. Routledge. doi:10.4324/9780203078876

Naszkowska, K. (2022). Psychoanalyst, Jew, woman, wife, mother, emigrant: The émigré foremothers of psychoanalysis in the United States. *European Judaism*, 55 (1), 112–137. doi:10.3167/ej.2022.550109

Naszkowska, K. (2023). Give me permission to remember: Judith S. Kestenberg and the memory of the Holocaust. In L. Henik & L. Aron (Eds.), *Contemporary psychoanalysis and Jewish thought: Answering a question with more questions* (pp. 197–217). Routledge.

Polat, B. (2021). Mental hygiene, psychoanalysis, and interwar psychology: The making of the maternal deprivation hypothesis. *Isis*, 112(2), 266–290. doi:10.1086/714599

Shai, D., & Fonagy, P. (2014). Beyond words: Parental embodied mentalizing and the parent–infant dance. In M. Mikulincer & P.R. Shaver (Eds.), *Mechanisms of social connection: From brain to group* (pp. 185–203). American Psychological Association. doi:10.1037/14250-011

Weinstein, D. (2013). *The pathological family: Postwar America and the rise of family therapy*. Cornell University Press.

Zaretsky, E. (2005). *Secrets of the soul: A social and cultural history of psychoanalysis*. Vintage Books.

Index

Note: Kestenberg's terminology and publications are in *italics.*

For Product Safety Concerns and Information please contact our EU representative GPSR@taylorandfrancis.com Taylor & Francis Verlag GmbH, Kaufingerstraße 24, 80331 München, Germany